Liver Regeneration Techniques In Hepatic Surgery

Luca Aldrighetti • Elio Jovine
Francesca Ratti • Matteo Serenari
Editors

Liver Regeneration Techniques In Hepatic Surgery

Springer

Editors
Luca Aldrighetti
Dept. of Hepato-biliary Surgery
San Raffaele Hospital
Milano, Italy

Francesca Ratti
Dept. of Hepato-biliary Surgery
IRCCS Ospedale San Raffaele
Milan, Italy

Elio Jovine
Department of General Surgery
IRCCS Azienda Ospedaliero-Universitaria
Di Bologna
Bologna, Bologna, Italy

Matteo Serenari
Hepato-Biliary Surgery and Transplant Unit
IRCCS Azienda Ospedaliero-Universitaria
Di Bologna
Bologna, Italy

ISBN 978-3-032-10996-5 ISBN 978-3-032-10997-2 (eBook)
https://doi.org/10.1007/978-3-032-10997-2

This Springer imprint is published by the registered company Springer Nature Switzerland AG
The registered company address is: Gewerbestrasse 11, 6330 Cham, Switzerland

The book is dedicated to the memory of Luca Aldrighetti

"Always remember where you come from"
L. Aldrighetti

Foreword

Postoperative liver failure due to an insufficient remnant liver represents the single most important cause of poor outcome following complex liver surgery. This book, edited by four Italian experts in liver surgery, covers in a systematic and comprehensive way all relevant aspects of liver regeneration. The chapters are beautifully written by international authorities in liver pathophysiology, radiology, hepatology, and surgery, linking established and innovative techniques with enhanced liver regeneration and function.

While the exclusive ability of the liver to regenerate remains enigmatic in many aspects with the involvement of not only well-known, but also "to discover," molecular pathways, this book offers an essential resource for all physicians looking to stay ahead of the curve in liver surgery and provide the best possible care to their patients.

This collaborative endeavor will undoubtedly become a "must-have" source of information in the complex field of liver regeneration.

Professor of Surgery
and Transplantation
University of Zurich
and Swiss Medical Network
Zurich, Switzerland

Pierre-A. Clavien

Preface

Modern vogue of liver surgery focuses on advanced technologies and complex prediction and navigation systems: in this scenario, a book whose roots extend back to mythology may seem unfashionable.

Belonging to the new generation of liver surgeons, we strongly believe that the topic of hepatic regeneration can resist trends and maintain its mysterious charm.

Indeed, the modern reinterpretation of the myth of Prometheus finds an ideal ground for discussion in the heterogeneity of methods currently available to induce liver hypertrophy and in the multidisciplinary of figures involved (i.e., surgeons, radiologists, hepatologists, pathologist, basic researchers).

Our ancient interest in the prevention of liver failure—the most life-threatening complication of hepatic surgery—has led us to outline a table of contents ranging from the biological bases of liver regeneration, to the methods of hypertrophy induction before surgery with their strengths and weaknesses, to the analyses on the disease-specific aspects, up to the synergic combination of new technologies and liver regeneration... in a travel from the origins toward the future. As surgeon-scientists we support and underline the importance of clinical and translational research as decision-making tools in the bedside management of patients.

We thank our mentors, Luca Aldrighetti and Elio Jovine, for supporting the idea of this exciting journey, for nurturing in us the love for this topic, and for having made this approach to science our standard. Thanks also to the authors who contributed to this text, not only for drafting the chapters and trusting in this idea but also for carrying forward research on the topic of liver regeneration, contributing to the improvement of clinical practice and to the always lively discussion.

We recognize the dynamism of the topic "Liver regeneration techniques in liver surgery" as one of the most fascinating aspects of this issue, but we hope that this text can provide a milestone for defining the current state of the art and hopefully pave the way for new ideas.

Milan, Italy — Francesca Ratti
Bologna, Italy — Matteo Serenari

Contents

Part I

Liver Regeneration and Liver Failure

Mechanisms of Liver Regeneration

1

Alexander Kofler, Lukas Pölsler, Rupert Oberhuber, and Florian Primavesi

1.1 Cellular and Molecular Basis of Liver Regeneration

The liver is responsible for several critical biological functions in the human body, including the regulation of metabolism, the detoxification of endogenous and exogenous compounds, and the synthesis of a diverse array of proteins with essential extrahepatic functions. Liver disease causes more than two million deaths each year, making up about 4% of all global fatalities. Conditions such as cirrhosis, viral hepatitis, and liver cancer are among the leading causes of these deaths [1].

Throughout their lives, adult humans frequently experience episodes of liver damage, particularly under normal physiological conditions. The liver's ability to regenerate plays a crucial role in maintaining the vital functions necessary for the survival of the human body following different types of injury. Research has shown that effective liver repair relies not only on the proliferation of individual hepatocytes but also on complex crosstalk between various cell types. Ensuring a stable liver function is fundamental to overall physiological balance. Various regenerative mechanisms have evolved to uphold optimal liver performance at all times. Liver size can fluctuate under different physiological conditions, expanding, for example, during pregnancy and shrinking in cases of cachexia or extreme weight loss. While the precise signaling pathways governing these changes remain incompletely

A. Kofler · L. Pölsler · R. Oberhuber
Department of Visceral, Transplant and Thoracic Surgery, Medical University of Innsbruck, Innsbruck, Austria

F. Primavesi (✉)
Department of Visceral, Transplant and Thoracic Surgery, Medical University of Innsbruck, Innsbruck, Austria

Department of Surgery, Ordensklinikum Linz, Linz, Austria
e-mail: florian.primavesi@i-med.ac.at; florian.primavesi@leberchirurgie.at

L. Aldrighetti et al. (eds.), *Liver Regeneration Techniques In Hepatic Surgery*, https://doi.org/10.1007/978-3-032-10997-2_1

understood, it is evident that a regulatory system operates to preserve liver size in proportion to the body's overall size and functional demands. This system employs multiple strategies to ensure that the liver remains adequately scaled to meet the body's needs. This section gives an overview of the liver's remarkable regenerative capacity in response to various forms of damage, including toxin- or drug-induced injury, infections, trauma, and surgical resection [2–4].

1.1.1 Hepatocytes: Proliferation and Cell Cycle Regulation

Hepatocytes are the predominant cell type in the liver, making up approximately 80% of its mass and carrying out the majority of its essential functions. Hepatocyte proliferation is the process by which hepatocytes multiply to maintain liver homeostasis and regenerate the liver after injury. The liver is unique in its ability to regenerate apparently without relying on a dedicated stem cell population. Instead, mature hepatocytes themselves re-enter the cell cycle and divide to restore liver mass. Even after surgical removal of up to 70–80% of its mass, the remnant liver tissue expands to restore both its size and function, ensuring continued physiological balance [5]. Besides cell division, also hypertrophy of hepatocytes plays a major role in the early phase of liver regeneration [6].

Hepatocytes are of central importance in the adaptability of the hepatic epithelial cell populations, not only by re-entering the cell cycle to replenish their own population but also by transforming into biliary epithelial cells (BECs) when liver damage occurs. This plasticity allows hepatocytes to contribute to bile duct formation when needed. BECs, in turn, initiate a ductular reaction that serves as a backup biliary system and can step in to replace hepatocytes that have lost their ability to replicate. However, whether a distinct population of hepatic stem cells is responsible for liver regeneration during normal conditions or injury remains an open question [7–10].

1.1.1.1 The Role of Quiescent Hepatocytes and Cell Division

A healthy liver is characterized by mitotically quiescent hepatocytes with a particularly low proliferation rate (about 0.005% per day) until an aggression occurs. In this case, in order to maintain a homeostatic role, the remaining hepatocytes initiate proliferation to re-establish the functional mass of the liver. A necessary condition for cell growth and division is an increased protein synthesis and amino acid availability [9, 11].

While hepatocytes exhibit differences in proliferative capacity depending on their location within the liver lobule, a crucial question remains about the specific roles of these zonally distinct hepatocyte populations in maintaining liver homeostasis and driving regeneration [12]. Clonal studies on hepatocyte expansion have demonstrated that hepatocytes across all three lobular zones (periportal, central, and midzonal) participate in liver homeostasis, with midzonal hepatocytes exhibiting significantly higher proliferative activity compared to those in the other zones. Hepatocyte renewal occurs across all liver zones in a pattern that follows a Poisson distribution, suggesting that cell turnover happens randomly and independently rather than being confined to specific regions or triggered by uniform signals [13].

In the starting or priming phase, quiescent hepatocytes receive mitogenic signals from cytokines and growth factors and switch from the G_0-state, where cells are known to be outside the proliferative cycle, to the G_1-state. While hepatocytes in G_0 phase carry out essential liver functions, those transitioning into G_1 re-enter the cell cycle in preparation for division. This process permits mature hepatocytes to divide self-sufficiently without relying on stem cells [11].

1.1.1.2 Cell Cycle Checkpoints and Regulatory Mechanisms

Liver regeneration is a tightly controlled process that relies on accurate regulation of the cell cycle, safeguarding hepatocyte proliferation occurs proficiently without leading to excessive growth or tumor formation. This regulation is achieved through cell cycle checkpoints and signaling pathways. It is widely recognized that cyclins and cyclin-dependent kinases (CKDs) are essential regulators in driving progression through the various cell cycle phases [14].

The entry into the cell cycle and the step toward hepatocyte DNA replication are stimulated by hepatocyte growth factor (HGF) and epidermal growth factor (EGF). These factors activate cyclin D/CDK4/6, which endorses cell cycle entry [14]. In the G_0/G_1 transition phase, cyclin D/CDK4/6 complexes are formed and stabilized by Cip/Kip proteins (in the liver $p21^{Cip1/Waf1}$, $p27^{Kip1}$, $p57^{Kip2}$) alongside Ink proteins ($p15^{Ink4b}$, $p16^{Ink4a}$, $p18^{Ink4c}$, $p19^{Ink4d}$), which switch from stalling to supporting cell division [15]. The G_1 checkpoint (or DNA damage checkpoint) checks whether a cell has enough nutrients and no DNA damage [16]. When cyclin D/CDK4/6 is activated in early G_1, phosphorylation of the tumor suppressor protein retinoblastoma (Rb) occurs, releasing transcription factors (e.g., E2F), which turn on genes needed for S-phase and DNA synthesis. As the cycle moves forward to late G_1, cyclin E binds to CDK2, which further phosphorylates Rb, removes Cip/Kip inhibitors (e.g., the highly expressed p27 during quiescence) and fully activates E2F, pushing the cycle into S-phase. Before the cell fully commits to DNA replication, the G_1/S checkpoint (or restriction point) makes sure there are no major DNA errors. From this point on, no more external growth factors are needed [17–19].

In the S phase, cyclin A/CDK2 ensures a smooth DNA replication. Here, the S-phase checkpoint (DNA replication checkpoint) checks for stalled DNA replication forks or DNA damage before moving on to the G_2 phase [20].

In G_2, hepatocytes prepare for mitosis by increasing protein synthesis and organelle duplication. Crucial at this stage is the G_2/M checkpoint, which ensures that cells do not enter mitosis with damaged or unreplicated DNA. This occurs primarily by ATM (ataxia-telangiectasia mutated) and ATR (ataxia-telangiectasia and rad3-related), two closely related protein kinases that play a central role in the damage response that detect DNA damage and activate the serine/threonine kinase CHK1, preventing premature activation of the cyclin B/CDK1 complex. Once the DNA integrity check is complete, cyclin B/CDK1 is fully activated, allowing hepatocytes to proceed to mitosis. The metaphase checkpoint ensures that chromosomes are lined up correctly before separation, preventing genetic mistakes [21].

These checkpoints and regulatory mechanisms ensure precise cell cycle progression, enabling effective liver regeneration while preventing unchecked cell division that could compromise tissue integrity. However, when cells experience excessive stress or DNA damage during this regenerative process, an additional safeguard mechanism can be activated: cellular senescence is a state of permanent cell cycle arrest that is triggered by various cellular stresses, serving as a key mechanism to maintain tissue integrity. In the context of liver regeneration, senescence acts as a protective mechanism when DNA damage peaks alongside increased DNA synthesis. However, if the balance shifts from hepatocyte proliferation to excessive senescence, the liver's regenerative capacity can be impaired. Additionally, senescence may serve as a regulatory mechanism to prevent overgrowth once liver function and tissue integrity have been restored [22].

1.1.2 Liver Progenitor Cells and Stem Cells

Stem cells are distinct by their capability to self-renew and differentiate into multiple cell types. In the liver, the stem cell is a progenitor that gives rise to both hepatocytes and BECs, the two primary epithelial cell types of the liver [23].

In embryonic development, the fetal liver bud is made up of hepatoblasts, cells that express alpha-fetoprotein (AFP), along with markers for both hepatocytes and bile duct cells. These hepatoblasts are thought to function as fetal liver stem cells, with the ability to generate both hepatocytes and the biliary system, playing a key role in liver development and regeneration [24]. Nevertheless, their ability to proliferate and to change their phenotype throughout development may make them more appropriately defined as liver progenitor cells (LPCs).

The role of stem/progenitor cells in the adult liver is more complex and remains a subject of discussion. In adult tissues, stem cells typically serve two key functions: maintaining homeostasis under normal physiological conditions and facilitating tissue repair and regeneration in response to injury [24]. In many tissues, mature cells have a relatively concise lifespan and require continuous replacement from stem cell compartments to sustain the tissue integrity. The liver operates differently with a slow exchange of mature hepatocytes with a lifespan of 200–300 days, raising the question of whether stem cells are necessary for normal liver maintenance [23, 24].

The prevailing view in the field is that under normal physiological conditions liver homeostasis is maintained primarily through the proliferation of mature hepatocytes across the liver parenchyma. The liver's high regenerative capacity has led to the debate about whether stem cells contribute to liver regeneration. In studies on partial hepatectomy, the surgical removal of specific liver lobes does not damage the remaining liver tissue, and regeneration occurs primarily through hypertrophy and proliferation of existing mature hepatocytes. Also, genetic lineage-tracing studies in rodents show that hepatocyte-driven regeneration is the dominant mechanism [3].

However, some evidence suggests a backup regenerative LPC-pathway when hepatocyte proliferation is impaired, providing bipotent potential to regenerate both hepatocytes and BECs. Hepatocytes and BEC appear to act as facultative stem cells

(FSCs) for each other contributing to liver maintenance and regeneration, depending on the circumstances. Processes like normal liver turnover and injury repair may involve both mature hepatocytes and FSCs [23, 25].

This topic, while supported by many experimental findings, remains an area of active investigation.

1.1.3 Non-parenchymal Cells and Their Contributions in Liver Regeneration

Hepatocytes are the main type of parenchymal cells in the liver. In addition to these, the liver contains a diverse population of non-parenchymal cells, which are involved in liver regeneration. BECs are differentiated epithelial cells involved in bile excretion and maintaining liver homeostasis. Beyond their primary function, BECs exhibit remarkable plasticity, a trait often associated with stem cells. When hepatocyte damage surpasses the capacity for self-replication, BECs can become activated and contribute to liver regeneration through cellular reprogramming [2, 26].

Of note are also Kupffer cells (KCs), which are known as resident macrophages, hepatic stellate cells (HSCs), and liver sinusoidal endothelial cells (LSECs) (Fig. 1.1). KCs act as the liver's immune sentinels, clearing pathogens, debris, and dysfunctional cells. HSCs are located in the space of Disse and play a crucial role in

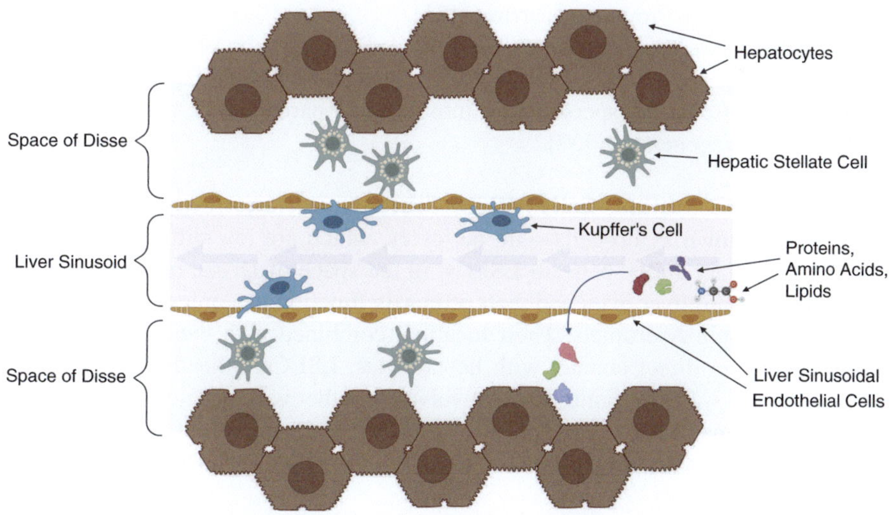

Fig. 1.1 Illustration of the hepatic sinusoidal interface highlighting the space of Disse between liver sinusoidal endothelial cells and hepatocytes. Hepatic stellate cells are located within the space of Disse, where they remain quiescent under normal conditions but become activated during injury to regulate extracellular matrix remodeling and fibrogenesis. They extend into the space, enabling the exchange of metabolites, nutrients, and signaling molecules. Kupffer cells, the liver-resident macrophages situated within the sinusoidal lumen, interact closely with endothelial cells and influence the microenvironment of the space of Disse. The figure emphasizes the space of Disse as a dynamic niche coordinating metabolic exchange, immune responses, and regenerative signaling. (Created in BioRender. Primavesi, F. (2025) https://BioRender.com/27c5n93)

extracellular matrix production and remodeling. LSECs form the lining of the sinusoids, allowing the exchange of metabolites, proteins, and drugs between the bloodstream and liver cells. They also regulate filtration, ensuring that essential substances reach hepatocytes and HSCs in the space of Disse. These non-parenchymal cells support liver function by maintaining homeostasis, immune defense, and structural integrity [27].

1.1.3.1 Kupffer Cells and Inflammatory Responses

Traditionally referred to as Kupffer cells (KCs), resident macrophages constitute 15% of liver's mass and are also involved in maintaining liver homeostasis and immune defense. These macrophages originate from fetal precursors and do clear pathogens, remove damaged cells, and process metabolites [27, 28].

Liver injury and liver disease lead to depletion of KCs, which in turn causes an influx of monocyte-derived macrophages, impairing liver regeneration [29, 30]. These infiltrating macrophages cluster around necrotic areas [31]. During liver damage, monocyte-derived macrophages become the dominant macrophage population, adopting proinflammatory functions [30, 32]. Over time, a shift toward curative macrophages occurs, which endorse liver regeneration by secreting anti-inflammatory cytokines and remodeling fibrosis [33, 34]. Furthermore, studies indicate that monocyte-derived macrophages can integrate into the perisinusoidal space, mimicking KCs in phenotype and function. This supports the idea that the macrophage pool in the liver changes over time, influenced by cycles of damage and regeneration, termed "immune scarring" [35].

KCs have also effects on the activation and differentiation of BECs to hepatocytes during liver regeneration as they are activated before BEC expansion [36]. Additionally, KCs help disperse BECs into the liver parenchyma, facilitating their contribution to regeneration [37].

1.1.3.2 Hepatic Stellate Cells (HSCs): Fibrosis vs. Regeneration

HSCs—also known as Ito-cells—are pericytes, which are low-differentiated cells along the capillary walls, beneath LSECs, in the space of Disse. In the liver, they constitute 3–5% of liver mass and their primarily function in a quiescent state is the storage of vitamin A droplets. Their location, combined with their dendritic processes, enables a direct contact with hepatocytes, LSECs, other HSCs and KCs. HSCs (collagen I, III, IV, laminin) are involved together with hepatocytes (collagen I, fibronectin) and LSECs (collagen I, IV) in the production of ECM components [27, 38]. In case of liver injury, HSCs receive promigratory and proliferation signals by dying hepatocytes [39].

KCs and infiltrating macrophages release transforming growth factor beta (TGF-β) and platelet-derived growth factor (PDGF) besides other proinflammatory cytokines. PDGF is the most potent mitogen for HSCs and TGF-β is the most potent stimulus for HSCs to produce collagen I. Once activated, HSCs produce molecules enhancing angiogenesis, inflammation, and fibrogenesis. They acquire their contractile function by adopting a myofibroblast-like phenotype and produce a substantial amount of ECM components culminating in scar tissue (central event in hepatic fibrosis where collagen IV is replaced by scar-forming collagen I) [38, 40]. On the other hand, activated HSCs produce matrix metalloproteinases (MMPs), which break down structural ECM components such as collagens, also clearing damaged ECM and allowing for replacement during tissue remodeling. More, activated HSCs produce also tissue inhibitors of metalloproteases (TIMPs), which protects collagen cells from apoptosis inhibiting the MMPs function. During fibrosis, an imbalance occurs where TIMPs outweigh MMPs, resulting in excessive ECM accumulation. In contrast, during regeneration, MMP activity rises, breaking down ECM, supporting hepatocyte migration, and promoting fibrosis resolution [38, 41]. Additionally, HSCs can replenish the liver mass by differentiating into hepatocytes and BECs under certain circumstances [2, 42].

1.1.3.3 Liver Sinusoidal Endothelial Cells (LSECs) and Angiogenesis

LSECs are the major endothelial cell type in the liver and compose 2–3% of the liver mass. They are specialized endothelial cells exceptional to the liver, characterized by lacking a basement membrane and the existence of transcellular pores (fenestrae), representing a distinct subset within the liver's vascular system. This permeable barrier enables direct contact with hepatocytes and the bloodstream, permitting involvement in vascular tone regulation (nitric oxide) and consequently assuring quiescence of HSCs [43, 44].

Throughout acute and chronic liver injury, hepatic cell types undergo functional and phenotypic alterations. LSECs lose their characteristic fenestrae and develop a basement membrane (so-called capillarization), which provides features resembling conventional capillary endothelium. This structural alteration impairs oxygenation of hepatocytes, contributing to cell death through apoptosis and necrosis. This also triggers the release of damage-associated molecular patterns (DAMPs). These DAMPs, together with factors released by LSECs, activate HSCs, leading to ECM overproduction and fibrosis formation. Simultaneously, LSECs acquire vasoconstrictive, pro-inflammatory, and pro-thrombotic properties, further worsening liver damage and vascular dysfunction [43, 45, 46].

In the early stages of liver regeneration, angiogenesis in LSECs plays a key role in initiating hepatocyte proliferation. As hepatocytes divide and expand the liver mass, the demand for an increased blood supply rises. Hepatocyte growth is mediated by angiocrine factors, including Wnt and HGF, which are released by LSECs. In response, LSECs proliferate and migrate, forming new sinusoidal networks through VEGF-dependent angiogenesis mainly from hepatocytes and HSCs, ensuring the growing liver is adequately vascularized, driving both LSEC proliferation and vascular remodeling, which are essential for restoring liver structure and function [47].

1.1.4 Key Signaling Pathways in Liver Regeneration

As discussed previously, the liver possesses unique and remarkable capacities for regeneration, and these processes rely on the coordinated response of various liver cell types, including hepatocytes, BECs, KCs, HSCs, and LSECs. However, successful liver regeneration is not driven by a single mechanism but is the result of multiple interconnected pathways involving growth factors, cytokines, and other signaling networks, of which the most important are outlined (Fig. 1.2).

1.1.4.1 Growth Factor Signaling

- *Hepatocyte Growth Factor (HGF)*

Liver regeneration depends profoundly on HGF, a powerful stimulator of hepatocyte proliferation and survival. This involves a complex interplay between various liver cells and proteases. HGF is not active by default but is produced in an inactive form (pro-HGF). The primary source of pro-HGF are HSCs, with LSECs contributing to secretion. Once secreted into the ECM, pro-HGF is bound there until it is required to drive regeneration. At this point, the ECM must be degraded to release pro-HGF, a task largely carried out by MMPs, which are produced by both HSCs and LSECs. Once pro-HGF is liberated, proteolytic activation is necessary before it can bind to its MET receptor on hepatocytes and stimulate their growth. This activation is driven by proteases, with urokinase-type plasminogen activator (uPA) playing a key role. HSCs, LSECs, and KCs all produce uPA, which converts plasminogen into plasmin. Plasmin, in turn, cleaves pro-HGF into its active form. Another activator is HGF activator (HGFA), secreted by HSCs and LSECs, which can also directly cleave and activate pro-HGF. Finally, LSECs (and to a lesser extent, HSCs) produce tissue plasminogen activator (tPA), which further boosts plasmin formation, amplifying pro-HGF activation. Together, these cells and enzymes orchestrate the HGF release and activation when and where it is needed, allowing the liver to initiate and sustain its regenerative response after injury [3, 48–50]. HGF is considered a complete mitogen, which means that it is sufficient to induce hepatocyte re-entry in the cell cycle and division [51].

- *Epidermal Growth Factor (EGF)*

As a key regulator of hepatocyte proliferation, cell survival, and tissue repair, EGF is crucial for liver regeneration following injury or tissue loss. EGF activation often works alongside other pathways, such as the already mentioned HGF-MET pathway, with evidence suggesting MET signaling can enhance EGF activity to further support hepatocyte proliferation and regeneration. EGF acts by binding and activating the EGF-receptor (EGFR). Besides by EGF, EGFR is activated by several ligands, including transforming growth factor-α (TGF-α), and others. EGFR and its ligands are upregulated during liver injury and regeneration, and their partially overlapping roles create a reliable system, ensuring EGFR activation even if individual ligands are reduced or absent [5, 52–54]. EGFR-ligand

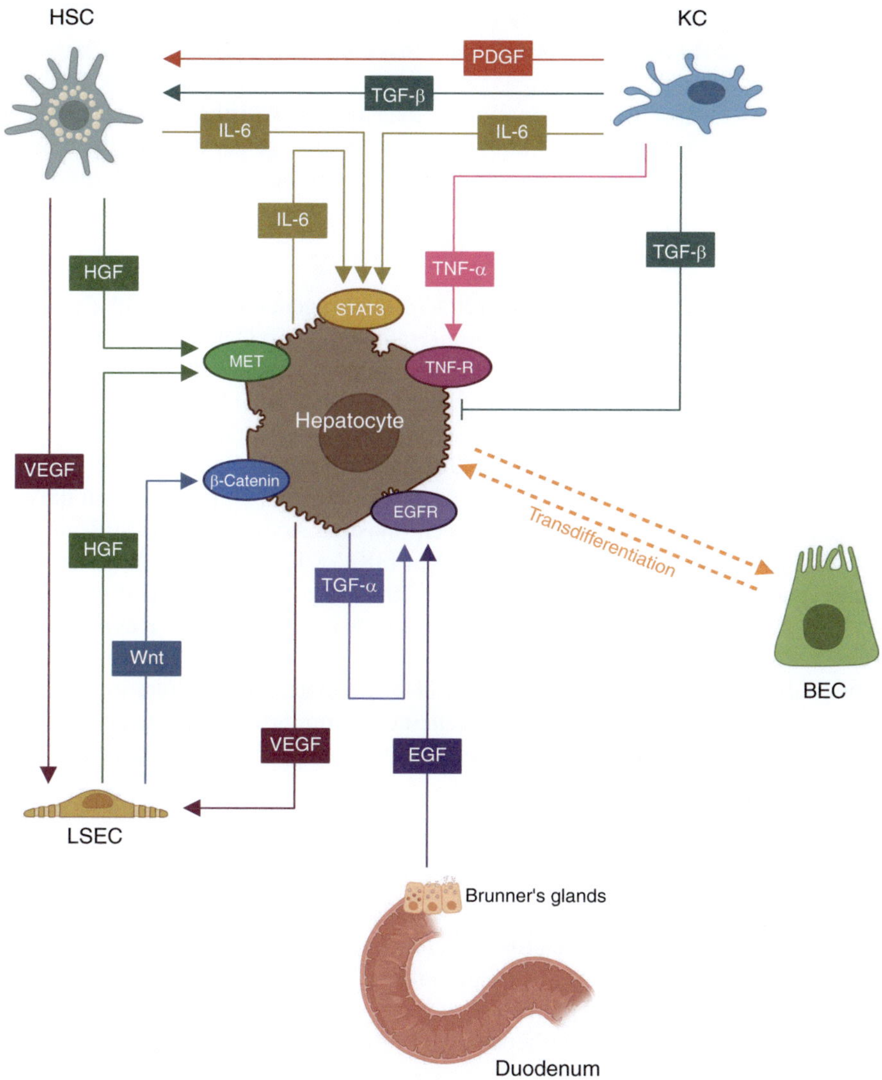

Fig. 1.2 Schematic representation of the dynamic interactions between hepatocytes, Kupffer cells (KCs), liver sinusoidal endothelial cells (LSECs), hepatic stellate cells (HSCs), and biliary epithelial cells (BECs) during liver regeneration. Key signaling pathways are illustrated, highlighting the coordinated balance between inflammation, proliferation, and tissue remodeling. Abbreviations: EGF epidermal growth factor, EGFR epidermal growth factor receptor, HGF hepatocyte growth factor, IL-6 interleukin 6, MET hepatocyte growth factor receptor, PDGF platelet-derived growth factor, STAT3 signal transducer and activator of transcription 3, TGF-α transforming growth factor-alpha, TGF-β transforming growth factor-beta, TNF-α tumor necrosis factor-alpha, TNF-R tumor necrosis factor receptor, VEGF vascular endothelial growth factor, Wnt Wnt signaling pathway. (Created in BioRender. Primavesi, F. (2025) https://BioRender.com/hyyh4n0)

binding initiates downstream signaling pathways (RAS/RAF/MEK/ERK cascade, PI3K/AKT, and the STAT signaling route) that control cell proliferation, survival, and tissue repair.

The importance of EGFR signaling in liver repair Is further demonstrated by genetic studies, where rodents lacking EGFR or certain ligands specifically in hepatocytes show defective liver regeneration and impaired hepatocyte proliferation.

- *Transforming Growth Factor-Alpha (TGF-α)*

TGF-α is a fundamental growth factor in liver regeneration, principally acting across EGFR to promote hepatocyte proliferation and survival. TGF-α is produced by hepatocytes, functioning in autocrine and paracrine means during normal liver homeostasis as well as in response to injury. Under normal conditions, TGF-α is expressed at low levels in hepatocytes. However, its expression is rapidly upregulated following liver injury or during regenerative processes [55, 56]. The increase in TGF-α levels is crucial in promoting the transition from G_1 phase to S in the cell cycle, allowing for DNA synthesis and cell division. Activation of EGFR initiates essential pathways (RAS/RAF/MEK/ERK, PI3K/AKT, STAT), which collectively stimulate hepatocyte proliferation and augment tissue repair. TGF-α is thought to act as an autocrine mitogen, stimulating hepatocyte proliferation. Overexpression of TGF-α leads to sustained hepatocyte DNA synthesis and tumor formation. TGF-α is not only a mitogen for hepatocytes but also stimulates the proliferation of endothelial and stromal cells during liver regeneration, supporting angiogenesis and tissue remodeling and ensuring a proper reconstruction of liver architecture after injury [56].

- *Transforming Growth Factor-Beta (TGF-β)*

TGF-β is a pivotal regulator in liver regeneration, mainly acting negatively on hepatocyte proliferation. While growth factors like HGF, EGF, and TGF-α stimulate hepatocyte proliferation, TGF-β strongly inhibits this process, even at low concentrations. It suppresses epithelial cell growth, promotes differentiation, and induces apoptosis, helping to terminate hepatocyte proliferation and restore tissue balance after the initial regenerative phase.

Its expression increases in necrotic areas after liver injury and is associated with impaired regeneration and hepatocyte senescence. Macrophage-derived TGF-β1 is a key source, as mice lacking TGF-β1 in myeloid cells show improved liver regeneration. Blocking TGF-β signaling), even with delayed treatment, enhances liver regeneration [57, 58].

1.1.4.2 Cytokine Networks

- *Tumor Necrosis Factor-Alpha (TNF-α)*

TNF-α plays a dual role in liver regeneration, acting as both a pro-proliferative and pro-apoptotic cytokine. Primarily produced by KCs and other immune and stromal cells, TNF-α signaling is crucial for hepatocyte proliferation following liver injury. Binding to one of its two receptors, TNF-R1 and TNF-R2, TNF-α triggers distinct signaling pathways. TNF-R1 activation can induce both pro-survival and apoptotic pathways. However, apoptosis is usually prevented by anti-apoptotic molecules like TRAF2 and NF-κB. TNF-R2 primarily activates pro-inflammatory pathways. During liver regeneration, TNF-α stimulates hepatocyte priming, making them responsive to mitogenic signals from HGF and EGF. Despite its potential to induce apoptosis, TNF-α-driven NF-κB activation is essential for hepatocyte survival and proliferation, ensuring successful tissue repair after injury [59, 60].

- *Interleukin 6 (IL-6)*

IL-6 is a multifunctional cytokine with diverse roles throughout the body. In the liver, it serves as a key inducer of the acute phase response and infection defense, while also being crucial for hepatocyte homeostasis, metabolic regulation, and acting as a potent hepatocyte mitogen. IL-6 is essential for liver regeneration following injury; however, its role is complex and context-dependent [61]. After liver injury, particularly hepatectomy, TNF-α levels rise as early as 2 h post-surgery, followed by a marked increase in IL-6 levels. KCs, stimulated by gut-derived factors, secrete IL-6 in a TNF-α-dependent manner. Additionally, IL-6 is produced by hepatocytes, further contributing to its rapid surge in the blood. This IL-6 signaling is vital for initiating hepatocyte proliferation and tissue repair as it binds to its receptor on hepatocytes, which activates the STAT3 signaling pathway. However, IL-6 alone may not always be sufficient to promote robust regeneration, particularly after severe liver injury. Furthermore, persistent or excessive activation of IL-6/STAT3 signaling has been linked to impaired regeneration in partial hepatectomy models and is associated with liver pathology, including the development of liver tumors. This highlights the biphasic nature of IL-6 signaling, with both regenerative and potentially detrimental effects depending on the circumstances and extent of activation [3–5, 61].

1.1.4.3 Essential Signaling Networks in Liver Regeneration

- *Wnt/β-catenin*

The Wnt/β-catenin signaling pathway is fundamental to liver homeostasis. It underpins key processes such as embryonic liver development, bile duct formation, postnatal hepatic growth, and hepatocyte differentiation. Beyond its physiological role, dysregulated β-catenin activity is closely linked to the emergence and advancement of liver disorders, including nonalcoholic steatohepatitis, liver fibrosis, and hepatocellular carcinoma. Importantly, Wnt/β-catenin signaling is also recognized as a central regulator of liver regeneration, orchestrating tissue repair and hepatocyte proliferation following hepatic resection or toxic liver injury, restoring hepatic structure and function after damage [62, 63].

After liver resection, increased shear stress within the hepatic sinusoids stimulates LSECs to release Wnt ligands. These ligands activate β-catenin signaling in adjacent hepatocytes within minutes and remain active for up to 24 h. A similar activation pattern is observed during drug-induced liver injury, where elevated Wnt ligand levels drive sustained β-catenin signaling, lasting up to 12 h. Once β-catenin signaling occurs, transcription factors induce the expression of proliferation-associated target genes, including cyclin D, which is critical for hepatocyte cell cycle progression. By promoting hepatocyte entry into the cell cycle and enhancing their proliferative capacity, Wnt/β-catenin signaling ensures effective liver repair and restoration of tissue mass [64].

- *Notch*

The Notch signaling pathway is unique because it enables cells to communicate with their direct neighbors by cell–cell ligand–receptor interaction to convey the signal into transcriptional responses [65]. During embryogenesis, Notch is essential for bile duct formation, and in the adult liver, it is crucial for ductal repair following injury. Beyond its function in biliary cells, Notch activation in hepatocytes can induce hepatocyte reprogramming into biliary-like cells, even under homeostatic conditions. This cellular plasticity not only supports bile duct regeneration but is also implicated in the development of intrahepatic cholangiocarcinoma. Notch signaling is further Involved In progenitor cell-mediated repair mechanisms, particularly in response to severe or chronic liver injury. Under these circumstances, the goal of liver repair is to restore the hepatic lobule and biliary architecture, yet persistent activation of Notch can shift this regenerative response toward a maladaptive repair program. This is characterized by an excessive ductular reaction, fibrogenesis, and architectural distortion, which can ultimately drive the progression to liver fibrosis and cancer. Thus, while Notch is indispensable for bile duct formation and tissue repair, its dysregulation in chronic liver disease can promote pathological remodeling and tumorigenesis [65–67].

- *Hippo/YAP*

The highly conserved Hippo/YAP signaling pathway is a central regulator of liver size, regeneration, and cellular plasticity. It controls organ growth and hepatocyte proliferation under homeostatic and regenerative conditions [68]. Under normal conditions, the Hippo pathway is active, suppressing Yes-associated protein (YAP) by promoting its phosphorylation, which leads to its sequestration in the cytoplasm or degradation. After liver injury or resection, Hippo signaling is downregulated, allowing YAP to translocate into the nucleus, where it interacts with transcription factors. Following liver injury, YAP activation promotes hepatocyte proliferation and tissue repair, but dysregulated or excessive YAP activity can disrupt hepatocyte identity. In such cases, hepatocytes may undergo trans-differentiation into cholangiocyte-like cells, a process associated with impaired liver regeneration. This highlights the dual role of YAP in both promoting regeneration and, when overactivated, driving hepatocyte dedifferentiation and limiting the regenerative capacity of the liver. Tight regulation of Hippo/YAP signaling is critical as excessive YAP activation can contribute to liver overgrowth, fibrosis, and tumor development [69, 70].

1.2 Microenvironmental and Metabolic Factors

1.2.1 Vascular Contributions and Angiogenesis

1.2.1.1 Sinusoidal Remodeling and Liver Perfusion

The liver sinusoidal endothelial cells (LSECs) are fundamental to hepatic development and the formation of its unique microvascular and functional architecture. The terminal branches of the portal vein and hepatic artery converge into hepatic sinusoids, which drain into the central vein. LSECs are exposed to nutrient-rich blood from the gut but also to potential toxins and waste products. This dual exposure contributes to the recruitment of inflammatory cells and triggering systemic inflammatory responses to harmful stimuli [71]. Liver regeneration depends not only on hepatocytes but also significantly on the activity of LSECs. These cells demonstrate adaptive responses to hepatic needs, facilitating neoangiogenesis, immune regulation, and the modulation of bone marrow activity [72, 73].

Surgical interventions often compromise hepatic blood flow, leading to microvascular damage and ischemia–reperfusion injury (IRI). While hepatocytes are primarily affected by warm ischemia, cold ischemia has a more profound impact on LSECs, with additional injury frequently occurring during reperfusion [74]. Following partial hepatectomy, LSECs initiate a regenerative response involving three distinct phases. Initially, hepatocytes are primed by signals from various cells, including non-parenchymal types. This is followed by an angiogenic phase, driven by hepatocyte proliferation, and finally, a termination phase marks the conclusion of regeneration [5, 75, 76]. Although LSEC proliferation is typically observed around 72 h post-resection, intracellular signaling begins immediately after surgical intervention. The altered hemodynamics following hepatectomy increase portal blood flow through the reduced liver volume, raising sinusoidal pressure and activating mechanosensitive pathways that convert mechanical stimuli into biological responses [56, 75, 77, 78]. Another proposed mechanism for regeneration involves the increased delivery of endothelial growth factors via the portal vein, promoting hepatic hypertrophy [5, 79–82].

1.2.1.2 Role of Vascular Endothelial Growth Factor

Hepatocyte regeneration begins immediately after liver resection, peaking within 24–48 h. The concurrent proliferation of hepatocytes and LSECs often results in transient ischemia, prompting hepatocytes to secrete vascular endothelial growth factor (VEGF) to improve oxygen delivery and reduce ischemia-induced damage [83]. In addition to local angiogenic effects, VEGF activates signaling pathways in the bone marrow, supporting the recruitment of new LSECs [84]. Hepatocytes expressing VEGF are typically located near blood vessels, and VEGF directly facilitates LSEC differentiation. Mature LSECs then release chemokines, such as CXCL12, which interact with receptors like CXCR7 on bone marrow-derived progenitor cells, attracting those cells and promoting their maturation into functional endothelial cells [85–87].

1.2.2 Extracellular Matrix and Fibrosis Regulation

1.2.2.1 ECM Composition and Its Role in Tissue Remodeling

The extracellular matrix (ECM), once viewed as a passive structural scaffold, is now recognized as a dynamic participant in liver regeneration. Composed of various proteins and macromolecules, the ECM influences critical processes such as receptor signaling, cell proliferation, angiogenesis, inflammation, and apoptosis [88–90]. Structural alterations in the ECM affect liver microarchitecture and the elasticity of hepatocyte clusters. Furthermore, ECM-regulated protein factors like vitronectin and olfactomedin 4 play pivotal roles in activating regenerative pathways [90]. The ECM also recruits inflammatory cells, which contribute to chronic liver disease. This persistent inflammation alters ECM structure, increasing stiffness and diminishing its regulatory capacity, ultimately impairing regenerative potential [91].

1.2.2.2 Interaction Between Fibrosis and Regeneration

Chronic liver injury profoundly alters ECM composition. In fibrotic tissue, both the quantity and structure of the ECM components change, with some proteins increasing up to sixfold compared to healthy liver samples [92]. This leads to scar formation and disrupts hepatic microarchitecture, severely affecting liver function [93]. Multiple pro-fibrogenic cell types such as hepatic stellate cells (HSCs), portal fibroblasts, and vascular smooth muscle cells are involved [94]. In healthy livers, HSCs reside in the space of Disse, but upon inflammatory activation, however, they differentiate into myofibroblast-like cells with pro-inflammatory and fibrogenic properties. Once activated, HSCs migrate and primarily become the principal source of type I collagen. The interplay among ECM, Kupffer cells, and HSCs is central to fibrotic progression [93, 95–98].

1.2.3 Oxygen Supply and Hypoxia-Driven Regeneration

1.2.3.1 Hypoxia-Inducible Factors in Liver Repair

Hypoxia contributes significantly to liver disease progression and regulation of hepatic homeostasis. Hypoxia-inducible factors (HIFs) are transcriptional regulators activated in response to low oxygen levels across various cell types, including hepatocytes [99]. HIFs are complexes out of alpha and beta subunits, with three known alpha isoforms (HIF-1α, HIF-2α, and HIF-3α) binding to HIF-1β [100]. Under hypoxic conditions, hydroxylation of HIFs is inhibited, allowing their stabilization and binding to HIF-1β. This complex then translocates to the nucleus and binds to hypoxia response elements (HREs), activating genes that support regeneration and angiogenesis, such as VEGF [101–103].

1.2.3.2 Impact of Ischemia and Reperfusion Injury

Ischemia–reperfusion injury (IRI) is a major cause of hepatic damage during liver surgery, significantly influencing regenerative outcomes. The liver's regenerative response involves both parenchymal (e.g., hepatocytes) and non-parenchymal cells (e.g., Kupffer cells, LSECs, and HSCs), with macrophages playing a pivotal role. Experimental studies have demonstrated that depleting macrophages impairs liver regeneration, underlining their essential contribution [104–106]. During IRI, endogenous danger-associated molecular patterns (DAMPs) are released from damaged cells, activating Kupffer cells and initiating regenerative pathways. These DAMPs also stimulate toll-like receptors, leading to local inflammation and recruitment of pro-inflammatory cells [107, 108]. Other immune cells also respond to IRI: dendritic cells adopt a reparative phenotype, secreting IL-13, which modulates macrophage activity through IL-10. Natural killer T cells (NKT), which constitute up to 30% of liver lymphocytes, remain inactive in liver sinusoids until triggered by IRI. Upon activation, NKT release chemokines (e.g., IL-4) and interferons, promoting immune recruitment and monocyte transition from inflammatory to pro-regenerative states [109–111].

During liver IRI, neutrophils infiltrate the tissue intensely, and their dysregulated activity leads to excessive production of proteinases and reactive oxygen species (ROS), thereby aggravating tissue damage [112, 113]. However, neutrophils also exhibit a dual role by contributing to tissue repair. They release lytic enzymes and ROS that help eliminate damaged cells and necrotic debris [114] and accumulate at injury sites where they function as phagocytes, supporting tissue remodeling [115]. For instance, during the later stages of acetaminophen (APAP)-induced liver injury, neutrophils are recruited to clear cellular debris, thus promoting the regenerative process [116].

The overall impact of neutrophils is highly context-dependent, as the resolution of their activity at the appropriate time is critical for proper healing. When reparative Ly6C^{hi} monocytes and macrophages are depleted, such as through CCR2 blockade, apoptotic neutrophils producing ROS accumulate, aggravating liver injury and impairing regeneration [117]. Similarly, neutrophil depletion during the recovery phase of carbon tetrachloride (CCl_4)-induced liver injury delays resolution of inflammation by disrupting the macrophage phenotype switch from pro-inflammatory to reparative [118] Notably, neutrophil-derived ROS can promote macrophage transition to a reparative phenotype, facilitating liver recovery after APAP-induced damage [119]. Additionally, neutrophils secrete lipocalin, which recruits pro-inflammatory macrophages to sites of injury, aiding in the clearance of debris and apoptotic cells, otherwise observed in myocardial IRI and associated with improved tissue repair [120].

In models of focal sterile heat injury in the liver, neutrophils not only migrate into the damaged vasculature but also create tunnels, likely via MMP-9 and VEGF secretion. This stimulates microvascular growth and regeneration [115, 121]. Despite these pro-reparative roles, the detailed mechanisms governing neutrophil–macrophage interactions during liver IRI remain incompletely understood [122].

1.2.4 Nutritional and Metabolic Regulation of Regeneration

1.2.4.1 Energy Demand and Mitochondrial Function

Liver regeneration places significant metabolic stress on individual cells, making sufficient energy supply essential for effective tissue recovery. Mitochondria, as the primary source of cellular energy, undergo dynamic changes throughout the cell cycle and their energetic status is particularly vulnerable during intensified periods of liver damage and regeneration [123, 124].

During the late G_1 phase, mitochondrial networks shift into a hyperfused, high-performance state in preparation for the S-phase, ensuring sufficient ATP production. This hyperfused configuration correlates with increased energy availability, whereas under nutrient-deprived conditions, mitochondria more commonly adopt a fragmented or reticular configuration. The marked increase in ATP demand during the G_1–S transition underscores the critical role of mitochondria in supporting hepatocyte proliferation during regeneration [125–127].

1.2.4.2 Role of Amino Acids, Lipids, and Glucose Metabolism

Amino acids are organic compounds containing both amine and carboxylic acid functional groups. They are fundamental building blocks of protein synthesis and play critical roles in lipid metabolism, glutathione production, redox regulation, and cell proliferation [128–130]. Several amino acids have been shown to significantly influence liver regeneration:

- Alanine

Alanine facilitates the transport of ammonia from peripheral tissues to the liver and contributes to glucose and urea production [131]. Under conditions of nutritional deficiency, it downregulates pyruvate kinase activity and suppresses gluconeogenesis [132]. Alanine is closely associated with the enzyme alanine transaminase (ALT), a key hepatic enzyme that exists in concentrations up to 3000 times higher in the liver than in bloodstream [133, 134]. When hepatocytes are damaged, ALT is released into circulation [135]. Alanine supplementation has shown hepatoprotective effects, including reduced liver necrosis and lower serum ALT levels following injury [136, 137].

- Glutamate

Glutamate modulates immune responses, particularly by dampening T-cell-mediated inflammation, and facilitates the transport of reductase enzymes across mitochondrial membranes. It also acts as a free radical scavenger, contributing to cellular homeostasis, and serves as a precursor for the synthesis of glutamine, GABA, and other amino acids [138, 139]. Evidence also supports its role in restoring hepatic architecture in metabolic-associated steatotic liver disease (MASLD) [140, 141].

- Aspartate

This nonessential amino acid is involved in the synthesis of purines, pyrimidines, asparagine, and arginine, as well as inositol and β-alanine. Through the production of oxaloacetate and aspartate, it also contributes to the reduction of oxidative stress. Studies indicate it can prevent hepatic steatosis and fibrogenesis. In the context of liver regeneration, it reduces inflammation by inhibiting TLR4 and downstream other pro-inflammatory signaling pathways [128, 142–144].

- Glycine

Glycine exerts cytoprotective effects during hypoxia, particularly in hepatocytes and renal tubular cells. It also activates chloride channels in Kupffer cells inhibiting their activation, reducing the release of pro-inflammatory mediators and fibrosis progression [145–149]. Additionally, glycine helps modulate vitamin A and E levels and downregulates TNF-α expression [150, 151]. In alcohol-induced liver damage (ALD), glycine has demonstrated regenerative benefits [152].

- Histidine

Histidine regulates hepatic copper accumulation and is used therapeutically in Wilson's disease to enhance copper excretion via urine. In animal models, a histidine-rich diet led to reductions in ALT and cholesterol levels, along with a decrease in pro-inflammatory cytokine expression [153, 154].

- Serine

In the context of ALD, serine has shown beneficial effects by reducing hepatic lipid accumulation. It also modulates hepatocyte function at the transcriptional level by regulating genes involved sphingosine synthesis and suppressing stress-related cellular pathways [155, 156].

1.2.4.3 Gut–Liver Axis and Microbiome Influence

Bile acids (BAs) are liver-specific molecules essential not only for lipid, vitamin, and cholesterol absorption but also for intrahepatic signaling. Approximately 90% of BAs are reabsorbed in the small intestine and returned to the liver via the portal vein through enterohepatic circulation. Following different types of liver injury (metabolic, ischemic, or surgical), BA accumulation increases. This is often linked to downregulation of Cyp7a1, a key enzyme in BA synthesis, suggesting impaired feedback regulation in damaged liver tissue [157–159].

Disruption of the enterohepatic circulation has been shown to inhibit liver regeneration, as BAs support hepatocyte proliferation [160–163]. Farnesoid X receptors (FXR), mainly expressed in the liver and small intestine, regulate BA levels by suppressing Cyp7a1. After major liver resections, elevated BA levels in peripheral blood indicate the liver remnant's impaired handling capacity [164, 165]. Fibroblast growth factors 15 and 19 may help protect against BA overload by modulation of FXR signaling [166, 167].

The gut–liver axis plays a crucial role in maintaining intestinal and hepatic homeostasis. Alterations in the gut microbiome composition can influence both healthy liver function and the progression of liver diseases. In conditions like metabolic-dysfunction-associated steatohepatitis (MASH), harmful bacterial strains are more prevalent. These strains can produce toxic metabolites, such as ethanol, and reduce the level of beneficial short-chain acids (SCFAs), contributing to hepatocellular injury. This dysbiosis, coupled with increased gut permeability, commonly referred to as a "leaky gut," promotes the development of MASH. Gut microbiota also impacts liver repair through multiple mechanisms: enhancing intestinal barrier integrity via tight junctions, boosting antioxidant defenses, and modulating oxidative stress. Additionally, microbiota-derived SCFAs influence hepatocyte regeneration and circadian rhythm regulation, further highlighting their role in liver regeneration [168–171].

1.2.5 Immune System and Inflammatory Modulation

1.2.5.1 Balance Between Regenerative and Pro-Fibrotic Responses

The immune system plays a dual role in liver regeneration, contributing to both tissue restoration and fibrotic progression. In the acute phase following liver injury, innate immune cells are the primary drivers of tissue repair. Kupffer cells and neutrophils rapidly release pro-regenerative cytokines such as IL-6 and TNF-α, which act to prime hepatocytes for cell cycle re-entry [172]. These cytokines activate key transcription factors, STAT3 via IL-6 and NF-κB via TNF-α, that drive hepatocyte proliferation. Adaptive immune cells also participate; for instance, certain T cell subsets, including αβ T cells, secrete regenerative signals like lymphotoxin that further support liver regrowth. This orchestrated inflammatory response serves to clear necrotic tissue and create a microenvironment for regeneration. The essential role of IL-6 and TNF-α is underscored by experimental models showing that their individual inhibition significantly impairs normal liver regeneration [173–175].

This regenerative process must be carefully regulated, as prolonged or dysregulated inflammation can shift immune activity toward fibrosis. TGF-β, predominantly secreted by activated macrophages and T cells (especially Th2 and regulatory subsets), is a potent inducer of HSC activation and collagen deposition, driving fibrosis. If resolution of inflammation fails, sustained TGF-β and Th2 cytokines such as IL-4 and IL-13 lead to excessive extracellular matrix accumulation and scar formation rather than functional tissue repair [173]. Macrophages are central in this immunological balance. Initially, they adopt a pro-inflammatory phenotype to support regeneration via IL-6 and TNF-α production. Over time, however, they must transition into a pro-resolutive state, characterized by the secretion of anti-inflammatory cytokines like IL-10 and MMPs, which help resolve inflammation and remodel fibrotic tissue. A successful regenerative outcome therefore hinges on a well-timed shift from immune activation to resolution. Too little immune stimulation can hinder regeneration, while prolonged or excessive activation may promote pathological fibrosis [176]. In summary, liver regeneration is tightly regulated by immune signals, those same mediators that stimulate hepatocyte proliferation must eventually be downregulated to prevent fibrotic complications.

1.2.5.2 Impact of Systemic Inflammation and Chronic Liver Diseases

In chronic inflammation, immune activation and tissue remodeling occur simultaneously. This persistent inflammatory state can be triggered by various underlying factors, including viral or autoimmune hepatitis, as well as toxic insults from alcohol or metabolic disorders. Regardless of the cause, chronic inflammation results in structural remodeling of both hepatocytes and non-parenchymal liver components, ultimately promoting fibrosis. Multiple growth factors, cytokines, and chemokines are involved in both the fibrogenic response and the chronic inflammatory process [177, 178].

In contrast, liver regeneration after acute injury depends on a precisely coordinated balance between pro-regenerative and pro-fibrotic signals. A key regulatory mechanism in this balance involves LSECs and their expression of CXCL12, interacting with CXCR4 and CXCR7. Following acute liver injury, upregulation of CXCR7 leads to the release of regenerative mediators such as Wnt2 and HGF, via activation of the transcription factor Id1, thereby promoting tissue repair [179]. However, in chronic hepatitis, sustained activation of fibroblast growth factor receptor 1 (FGFR1) skews the receptor balance in favor of CXCR4 signaling, which supports a fibrotic phenotype. An additional layer of regulation involves the phenotypic plasticity of hepatic macrophages. Their transition from a pro-inflammatory to a restorative phenotype is essential for effective regeneration. Restorative macrophages express higher levels of fibrinolytic enzymes such as matrix metalloproteinases MMP9 and MMP12, which contribute to extracellular matrix degradation and the resolution of fibrosis, ultimately facilitating liver tissue regeneration [180].

1.3 Regeneration After Human Partial Hepatectomy

1.3.1 The Regeneration Timeline: From Bench to Bedside

1.3.1.1 Early Post-hepatectomy Events (Minutes to Hours)

Liver regeneration after partial hepatectomy (PHx) begins within minutes of resection (Fig. 1.3). The abrupt hemodynamic changes—notably increased portal vein inflow per unit liver mass—exert shear stress on sinusoidal endothelium, triggering release of nitric oxide (NO) and cytokines such as IL-6 from liver sinusoidal endothelial cells [181]. At the same time, tissue injury and gut barrier perturbation lead to translocation of pathogen- and damage-associated molecular patterns (PAMPs/DAMPs), like endotoxin (LPS), into the portal circulation. These signals activate Kupffer cells via Toll-like receptors (e.g., TLR4), causing an immediate burst of TNF-α and IL-6 in the liver within the first hours post-hepatectomy. This constitutes the "priming phase" of regeneration. IL-6 and TNF-α are crucial pro-regenerative cytokines: they induce transcriptional programs in hepatocytes (through STAT3 and NF-κB, respectively) that shift quiescent hepatocytes from G0 into G1 of the cell cycle [173, 182]. For example, NF-κB activation in hepatocytes upregulates genes

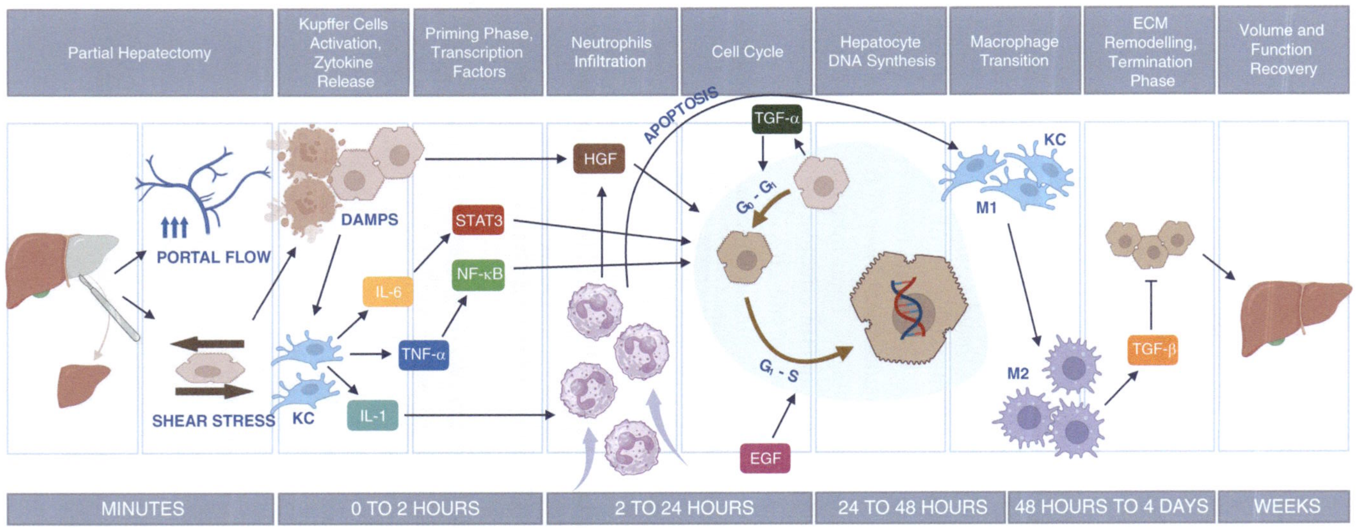

Fig. 1.3 Overview of the liver regeneration timeline in humans after liver surgery. Hepatic resection leads to an increase in portal flow and shear stress in the remnant liver within minutes. The resulting release of damage-associated molecular patterns (DAMPS) trigger activation of a Kupffer cell (KC)-related signaling cascade, including acute phase proteins such as interleukin-1 and 6 (IL-1/IL-6) and tumor necrosis factor-alpha (TNF-α). Within hours to days, this induces transcription programs, shifting quiescent hepatocytes from G0 into G1 of the cell cycle. Release of hepatocyte growth factor (HGF) within the liver further triggers proliferative signaling. Different immune cells infiltrate the damaged area to initially support clearance of cell debris and augment the inflammatory status, followed by macrophage transition, remodeling, and termination of the restorative process within days to weeks. Abbreviations: EGF epidermal growth factor, NF-kB nuclear factor kappa B, STAT3 signal transducer and activator of transcription 3, TGF-α/β transforming growth factor alpha/beta. (Created in BioRender. Primavesi (2025) https://BioRender.com/p3db398)

for IL-6 and growth factors, while IL-6/STAT3 signaling induces immediate early genes needed for cell cycle. Experiments in knockout mice have confirmed that without IL-6 or TNF-α signaling, the normal wave of hepatocyte proliferation is blunted. This early cytokine milieu also involves IL-1β and IL-18 from innate immune cells, which further promote hepatocyte priming.

1.3.1.2 Activation of Regenerative Pathways (Hours to First Days)

Following the priming phase, growth factor pathways are activated to drive DNA synthesis in the parenchyma. Hepatocyte growth factor (HGF) is one of the key mitogens in this stage. HGF is released from extracellular matrix stores and produced by stromal cells in response to the injury and cytokine signals; it binds the c-Met receptor on hepatocytes, triggering proliferative signaling. HGF levels rise quickly after resection (HGF mRNA peaks ~12 h post-PHx in rodents), and along with epidermal growth factor (EGF) and others, push hepatocytes through the G1/S transition [183]. By 12–18 h after surgery in rodent models, a first wave of hepatocytes enters DNA synthesis, peaking at ~24 h [181]. In humans, the timeline is slower: maximal hepatocyte DNA replication is observed around 2–3 days post-hepatectomy, and the full liver mass restoration unfolds over about 8–12 weeks. During this proliferative phase, IL-6/STAT3 and TNF-α/NF-κB pathways remain active to amplify regenerative signals. For instance, STAT3 activation leads to upregulation of cyclin D1, c-Myc, and other cell cycle drivers [173].

Concurrently, Kupffer cells and other non-parenchymal cells produce additional growth factors (HGF, EGF, Wnt ligands) to support the expanding hepatocyte population. The result is a wave of synchronized hepatocyte division that restores liver mass. Notably, each hepatocyte may undergo one or two rounds of replication; thus, in a 70% hepatectomy model, the liver can restore near-normal mass within 5–7 days in rodents, while this process takes several weeks in humans.

1.3.1.3 Immune Cell Infiltration and Cytokine Timeline

The regenerative process is closely entwined with an orchestrated immune cell infiltration. Neutrophils are among the first responders: they accumulate in the remnant liver within hours after resection. Clinical biopsy studies in patients have shown a significant increase in neutrophils in liver tissue as early as 2 h post-hepatectomy [184]. These neutrophils help clear surgical debris and release inflammatory mediators (like reactive oxygen species and proteases), but an excessive neutrophil influx can also cause collateral tissue damage. Kupffer cells, already activated in the first hour, continue to produce cytokines (TNF-α, IL-6, IL-1β) that sustain the regenerative signaling cascade [181]. Within about 24 h, monocytes from the bone marrow are recruited to the liver via chemokine signals. These monocytes infiltrate and differentiate into macrophages in the regenerating liver [173]. Early on, the newly arrived monocyte-derived macrophages adopt a pro-inflammatory profile (secreting IL-1β, TNF-α, etc., augmenting the regenerative stimulus). After the first 2–3 days, as necrotic material is cleared and hepatocyte proliferation slows, the immune response shifts: macrophages transition to an anti-inflammatory, pro-resolutive phenotype characterized by IL-10 secretion and release of matrix metalloproteinases (MMPs). This phenotypic switch is critical for remodeling the extracellular matrix and terminating the regenerative process before it becomes pathologic. Other immune cells also participate: for example, natural killer (NK) and NKT cells produce interferon-γ or IL-4 that can influence the balance of inflammatory vs. anti-inflammatory signals, and conventional T cells infiltrating later can secrete factors (like lymphotoxin-β and IL-22) that have been shown to support hepatocyte survival and growth [172, 176]. The net effect of this tightly timed immune involvement is to first create a pro-regenerative inflammatory milieu, and then to resolve inflammation and lay down new extracellular matrix as the liver architecture is restored.

1.3.1.4 Termination of Regeneration (Days to Weeks)

Liver regeneration is normally a self-limited process; once the liver-to-body size ratio is re-established, hepatocyte proliferation is shut down. Several mechanisms ensure this termination phase. One key player is TGF-β, a cytokine that potently inhibits hepatocyte proliferation. TGF-β is produced by Kupffer cells, monocyte-derived macrophages, and hepatic stellate cells in the later phase of regeneration. As local TGF-β levels rise, it causes hepatocytes to exit the cell cycle (e.g., by inducing cell cycle inhibitors) and promotes fibrous tissue remodeling of the provisional matrix laid down during regeneration [173]. Additionally, biomechanical signals and cell-contact inhibition come into play via pathways like Hippo/YAP—high cell density and restored architecture lead to Hippo pathway activation, which inactivates pro-growth transcriptional coactivator YAP, thereby halting further growth [181]. Apoptosis of excess cells is another facet of termination, with caspase-3 activity detectable as regeneration concludes. The result is that the liver ceases proliferating once sufficient mass is regained, avoiding over-shooting in size. In a healthy regeneration, the liver's architecture and function are fully normalized by the end of this process (approximately 1–2 weeks in rodents and 2–3 months in humans for complete structural recovery).

1.3.2 Clinical Laboratory and Imaging Indicators of Regeneration

Clinicians can monitor liver regeneration through a range of intraoperative and postoperative blood tests, imaging modalities, and hepatic functional tests. In the immediate postoperative period, a moderate elevation in liver enzymes (AST, ALT) is common due to the surgical injury, but a progressive decline in bilirubin and coagulopathy indicators is expected if regeneration is proceeding well. Laboratory trends such as a low (improving) total bilirubin by postoperative day 5 and a shortening prothrombin time indicate adequate functional recovery of the remnant liver; conversely, persistently rising bilirubin or INR after day 5 warns of impending liver failure [185]. Clinical research has noted the biochemical phenomenon of hypophosphatemia accompanying early liver regeneration—as hepatocytes rapidly uptake phosphate for nucleic acid synthesis, serum phosphate can drop—though severe or prolonged hypophosphatemia can also correlate with poorer outcomes in some cases [186]. Furthermore, other individual laboratory parameters such as lactate, CRP, and Antithrombin-III, or combinations such as the aspartate aminotransferase to platelet ratio (APRI) / albumin-bilirubin grade (ALBI) ratio (APRI-ALBI) and markers of oxidative stress activity have been proposed as early clinical predictors of patients at risk for post-hepatectomy liver failure [113, 187–190].

Beyond blood tests, imaging is invaluable to visualize and quantify regeneration. Volumetric CT or MRI of the liver is routinely used in the postoperative observational period, especially in case of delayed convalescence. On top of generating important information on perfusion and quality of the remaining liver, also volume dynamics can be effectively assessed. Within the first week after a major hepatectomy, the future liver remnant (FLR) volume increases markedly. For example, one study noted remnant volumes rising from ~800 mL immediately after surgery to ~1100 mL by postoperative day 5 in patients, correlating with substantial liver cell hyperplasia [191]. By 4–6 weeks post-hepatectomy, the liver volume often approaches 80–100% of its original size (at least in patients with healthy livers). However, volumetric recovery does not always equate to functional recovery. Hepatobiliary scintigraphy provides a dynamic assessment of liver function: using tracers like technetium-99 mebrofenin that are taken up and excreted by hepatocytes, one can measure the functional liver cell mass. Scintigraphy studies have shown that the majority of functional regeneration occurs in the first 5–7 days after resection, often preceding full anatomical regrowth. In patients without complications, the remnant liver's functional capacity (measured as percentage uptake per minute) nearly doubles in the first week. Interestingly, if the patient suffers postoperative complications (e.g., infection, persistent inflammation, or ischemia), functional gains are blunted even if the liver still increases in volume. Transient elastography (ultrasound-based stiffness measurement) can also track regeneration: the liver remnant becomes temporarily stiffer (higher kPa) in the first days—likely from congestion and extracellular matrix changes—then returns toward normal as regeneration completes. Imaging can also detect *qualitative* signs of regeneration, such as increased perfusion of the remnant and even visualization of enlarging regenerative nodules or bulky regenerating lobes on contrast scans.

A variety of hepatic functional assessment algorithms utilizing, for example, the maximal liver function capacity (LiMAx) test or indocyanine-green clearance have been proposed in the early perioperative regeneration phase during liver surgery [192–194]. Details on these will be covered in later chapters of the book.

1.3.3 Successful Regeneration vs. Post-hepatectomy Liver Failure

In an ideal scenario of appropriate regeneration, the patient remains clinically stable after surgery: the liver remnant rapidly hypertrophies and takes over necessary functions, preventing hepatic insufficiency. Clinically, this means bilirubin remains in a safe range (e.g., <2–3 mg/dL) and coagulation parameters normalize; the patient can often be discharged within a week or less. On imaging, the remnant liver shows progressive growth, and on functional tests, the clearance of bilirubin, lactate, and ammonia is adequate. By contrast, post-hepatectomy liver failure (PHLF) denotes an impaired regenerative outcome where the liver cannot maintain homeostasis. PHLF is typically defined by a sustained postoperative coagulopathy and hyperbilirubinemia [185, 195].

Patients with PHLF may develop jaundice, prolonged confusion (hepatic encephalopathy), ascites, and risk of multiorgan failure. The causes of PHLF are often multifactorial and relate to an insufficient functional liver mass or injury to the regenerative process [196]. Inadequate remnant size or quality is a primary risk factor—for example, a small-for-size remnant or a remnant with underlying cirrhosis/fibrosis has diminished regenerative capacity. Such livers cannot proliferate fast enough or provide necessary function, leading to failure. Ischemia and surgical complications also contribute. Excessive intraoperative blood loss and resultant shock can cause ischemia–reperfusion injury in the remnant liver, directly killing hepatocytes and impairing regeneration; indeed, requiring a large blood transfusion (>4–5 units) is associated with higher PHLF risk [185]. Similarly, if the liver suffers prolonged inflow occlusion (Pringle maneuver) or outflow obstruction, the resultant ischemic damage can tip the balance toward failure. Infection and sepsis are other key factors: sepsis activates a systemic inflammatory response that paradoxically can suppress the liver's regenerative cytokine signaling and induce further hepatocellular death. In patients with PHLF, sepsis is both a common consequence and aggravating cause—sepsis reduces perfusion to the regenerating liver and depletes functional Kupffer cells needed for regeneration. For example, an undrained intra-abdominal abscess or persistent bile leak (causing infected biloma) can incite sepsis that derails regeneration. Other factors like cholestasis, drug-induced injury, or postoperative portal vein thrombosis can likewise impair the regenerative process.

From bench to bedside, our understanding of liver regeneration underscores a critical principle: the speed and quality of regeneration determine clinical outcomes after hepatectomy. Surgeons now carefully assess future liver remnant volume and function preoperatively through predefined algorithms (using risk predictions, volumetry, and function tests) to ensure it will be sufficient [197]. Postoperatively, close monitoring of liver function tests guides early intervention—for instance, prolonged elevation of bilirubin might prompt imaging to check for complications or consideration of rescue therapies. While most patients with adequate preoperative planning regenerate successfully, PHLF remains a serious complication when the delicate balance of regeneration is upset. Ongoing research, integrating insights from the bench (molecular pathways like IL-6/STAT3, HGF/c-Met, etc.) with clinical practice (advanced imaging and perioperative care), continues to improve the safety of hepatic surgery by bolstering the liver's remarkable regenerative capacity.

References

1. Devarbhavi H, Asrani SK, Arab JP, Nartey YA, Pose E, Kamath PS. Global burden of liver disease: 2023 update. J Hepatol. 2023;79:516–37. https://doi.org/10.1016/j.jhep.2023.03.017.
2. Ma X, Huang T, Chen X, Li Q, Liao M, Fu L, et al. Molecular mechanisms in liver repair and regeneration: from physiology to therapeutics. Signal Transduct Target Ther. 2025;10:63. https://doi.org/10.1038/s41392-024-02104-8.
3. Michalopoulos GK, Bhushan B. Liver regeneration: biological and pathological mechanisms and implications. Nat Rev Gastroenterol Hepatol. 2021;18:40–55. https://doi.org/10.1038/s41575-020-0342-4.
4. Bhushan B, Apte U. Liver regeneration after acetaminophen hepatotoxicity: mechanisms and therapeutic opportunities. Am J Pathol. 2019;189:719–29. https://doi.org/10.1016/j.ajpath.2018.12.006.
5. Michalopoulos GK. Liver regeneration. J Cell Physiol. 2007;213:286–300. https://doi.org/10.1002/jcp.21172.
6. Miyaoka Y, Ebato K, Kato H, Arakawa S, Shimizu S, Miyajima A. Hypertrophy and unconventional cell division of hepatocytes underlie liver regeneration. Curr Biol. 2012;22:1166–75. https://doi.org/10.1016/j.cub.2012.05.016.
7. Esser H, Kilpatrick AM, Man TY, Aird R, Rodrigo-Torres D, Buch ML, et al. Primary cilia as a targetable node between biliary injury, senescence and regeneration in liver transplantation. J Hepatol. 2024;81:1005–22. https://doi.org/10.1016/j.jhep.2024.06.002.
8. Sun T, Pikiolek M, Orsini V, Bergling S, Holwerda S, Morelli L, et al. AXIN2(+) Pericentral hepatocytes have limited contributions to liver homeostasis and regeneration. Cell Stem Cell. 2020;26:97–107. e6. https://doi.org/10.1016/j.stem.2019.10.011.
9. Fabris G, Dumortier O, Pisani DF, Gautier N, Van Obberghen E. Amino acid-induced regulation of hepatocyte growth: possible role of Drosha. Cell Death Dis. 2019;10:566. https://doi.org/10.1038/s41419-019-1779-7.
10. Raven A, Lu WY, Man TY, Ferreira-Gonzalez S, O'Duibhir E, Dwyer BJ, et al. Cholangiocytes act as facultative liver stem cells during impaired hepatocyte regeneration. Nature. 2017;547:350–4. https://doi.org/10.1038/nature23015.
11. Mangnall D, Bird NC, Majeed AW. The molecular physiology of liver regeneration following partial hepatectomy. Liver Int. 2003;23:124–38. https://doi.org/10.1034/j.1600-0676.2003.00812.x.
12. He L, Pu W, Liu X, Zhang Z, Han M, Li Y, et al. Proliferation tracing reveals regional hepatocyte generation in liver homeostasis and repair. Science. 2021;371. https://doi.org/10.1126/science.abc4346.
13. Chen F, Jimenez RJ, Sharma K, Luu HY, Hsu BY, Ravindranathan A, et al. Broad distribution of hepatocyte proliferation in liver homeostasis and regeneration. Cell Stem Cell. 2020;26:27–33. e4. https://doi.org/10.1016/j.stem.2019.11.001.
14. Ramboer E, De Craene B, De Kock J, Vanhaecke T, Berx G, Rogiers V, et al. Strategies for immortalization of primary hepatocytes. J Hepatol. 2014;61:925–43. https://doi.org/10.1016/j.jhep.2014.05.046.
15. Ilyin GP, Glaise D, Gilot D, Baffet G, Guguen-Guillouzo C. Regulation and role of p21 and p27 cyclin-dependent kinase inhibitors during hepatocyte differentiation and growth. Am J Physiol Gastrointest Liver Physiol. 2003;285:G115–27. https://doi.org/10.1152/ajpgi.00309.2002.
16. Bisteau X, Caldez MJ, Kaldis P. The complex relationship between liver cancer and the cell cycle: a story of multiple regulations. Cancers (Basel). 2014;6:79–111. https://doi.org/10.3390/cancers6010079.
17. Pal D, Sur S, Mandal S, Das A, Roy A, Das S, et al. Prevention of liver carcinogenesis by amarogentin through modulation of G1/S cell cycle check point and induction of apoptosis. Carcinogenesis. 2012;33:2424–31. https://doi.org/10.1093/carcin/bgs276.

18. Toyoshima H, Hunter T. p27, a novel inhibitor of G1 cyclin-Cdk protein kinase activity, is related to p21. Cell. 1994;78:67–74. https://doi.org/10.1016/0092-8674(94)90573-8.
19. Polyak K, Lee MH, Erdjument-Bromage H, Koff A, Roberts JM, Tempst P, et al. Cloning of p27Kip1, a cyclin-dependent kinase inhibitor and a potential mediator of extracellular antimitogenic signals. Cell. 1994;78:59–66. https://doi.org/10.1016/0092-8674(94)90572-x.
20. Hanse EA, Nelsen CJ, Goggin MM, Anttila CK, Mullany LK, Berthet C, et al. Cdk2 plays a critical role in hepatocyte cell cycle progression and survival in the setting of cyclin D1 expression in vivo. Cell Cycle. 2009;8:2802–9. https://doi.org/10.4161/cc.8.17.9465.
21. Pellarin I, Dall'Acqua A, Favero A, Segatto I, Rossi V, Crestan N, et al. Cyclin-dependent protein kinases and cell cycle regulation in biology and disease. Signal Transduct Target Ther. 2025;10:11. https://doi.org/10.1038/s41392-024-02080-z.
22. Ferreira-Gonzalez S, Rodrigo-Torres D, Gadd VL, Forbes SJ. Cellular senescence in liver disease and regeneration. Semin Liver Dis. 2021;41:50–66. https://doi.org/10.1055/s-0040-1722262.
23. Miyajima A, Tanaka M, Itoh T. Stem/progenitor cells in liver development, homeostasis, regeneration, and reprogramming. Cell Stem Cell. 2014;14:561–74. https://doi.org/10.1016/j.stem.2014.04.010.
24. Duncan AW, Dorrell C, Grompe M. Stem cells and liver regeneration. Gastroenterology. 2009;137:466–81. https://doi.org/10.1053/j.gastro.2009.05.044.
25. Michalopoulos GK, Khan Z. Liver stem cells: experimental findings and implications for human liver disease. Gastroenterology. 2015;149:876–82. https://doi.org/10.1053/j.gastro.2015.08.004.
26. Kamimoto K, Kaneko K, Kok CY, Okada H, Miyajima A, Itoh T. Heterogeneity and stochastic growth regulation of biliary epithelial cells dictate dynamic epithelial tissue remodeling. Elife. 2016;5. https://doi.org/10.7554/eLife.15034.
27. Campana L, Esser H, Huch M, Forbes S. Liver regeneration and inflammation: from fundamental science to clinical applications. Nat Rev Mol Cell Biol. 2021;22:608–24. https://doi.org/10.1038/s41580-021-00373-7.
28. Bleriot C, Ginhoux F. Understanding the heterogeneity of resident liver macrophages. Front Immunol. 2019;10:2694. https://doi.org/10.3389/fimmu.2019.02694.
29. Stutchfield BM, Antoine DJ, Mackinnon AC, Gow DJ, Bain CC, Hawley CA, et al. CSF1 restores innate immunity after liver injury in mice and serum levels indicate outcomes of patients with acute liver failure. Gastroenterology. 2015;149:1896–909. e14. https://doi.org/10.1053/j.gastro.2015.08.053.
30. Holt MP, Cheng L, Ju C. Identification and characterization of infiltrating macrophages in acetaminophen-induced liver injury. J Leukoc Biol. 2008;84:1410–21. https://doi.org/10.1189/jlb.0308173.
31. Mossanen JC, Krenkel O, Ergen C, Govaere O, Liepelt A, Puengel T, et al. Chemokine (C-C motif) receptor 2-positive monocytes aggravate the early phase of acetaminophen-induced acute liver injury. Hepatology. 2016;64:1667–82. https://doi.org/10.1002/hep.28682.
32. Karlmark KR, Weiskirchen R, Zimmermann HW, Gassler N, Ginhoux F, Weber C, et al. Hepatic recruitment of the inflammatory Gr1+ monocyte subset upon liver injury promotes hepatic fibrosis. Hepatology. 2009;50:261–74. https://doi.org/10.1002/hep.22950.
33. Ryan PM, Bourdi M, Korrapati MC, Proctor WR, Vasquez RA, Yee SB, et al. Endogenous interleukin-4 regulates glutathione synthesis following acetaminophen-induced liver injury in mice. Chem Res Toxicol. 2012;25:83–93. https://doi.org/10.1021/tx2003992.
34. Bourdi M, Masubuchi Y, Reilly TP, Amouzadeh HR, Martin JL, George JW, et al. Protection against acetaminophen-induced liver injury and lethality by interleukin 10: role of inducible nitric oxide synthase. Hepatology. 2002;35:289–98. https://doi.org/10.1053/jhep.2002.30956.
35. Beattie L, Sawtell A, Mann J, Frame TCM, Teal B, de Labastida Rivera F, et al. Bone marrow-derived and resident liver macrophages display unique transcriptomic signatures but similar biological functions. J Hepatol. 2016;65:758–68. https://doi.org/10.1016/j.jhep.2016.05.037.

36. Viebahn CS, Benseler V, Holz LE, Elsegood CL, Vo M, Bertolino P, et al. Invading macrophages play a major role in the liver progenitor cell response to chronic liver injury. J Hepatol. 2010;53:500–7. https://doi.org/10.1016/j.jhep.2010.04.010.
37. Van Hul N, Lanthier N, Espanol Suner R, Abarca Quinones J, van Rooijen N, Leclercq I. Kupffer cells influence parenchymal invasion and phenotypic orientation, but not the proliferation, of liver progenitor cells in a murine model of liver injury. Am J Pathol. 2011;179:1839–50. https://doi.org/10.1016/j.ajpath.2011.06.042.
38. Puche JE, Saiman Y, Friedman SL. Hepatic stellate cells and liver fibrosis. Compr Physiol. 2013;3:1473–92. https://doi.org/10.1002/cphy.c120035.
39. Fazel Modares N, Polz R, Haghighi F, Lamertz L, Behnke K, Zhuang Y, et al. IL-6 trans-signaling controls liver regeneration after partial hepatectomy. Hepatology. 2019;70:2075–91. https://doi.org/10.1002/hep.30774.
40. Xiang DM, Sun W, Ning BF, Zhou TF, Li XF, Zhong W, et al. The HLF/IL-6/STAT3 feedforward circuit drives hepatic stellate cell activation to promote liver fibrosis. Gut. 2018;67:1704–15. https://doi.org/10.1136/gutjnl-2016-313392.
41. Tsuchida T, Friedman SL. Mechanisms of hepatic stellate cell activation. Nat Rev Gastroenterol Hepatol. 2017;14:397–411. https://doi.org/10.1038/nrgastro.2017.38.
42. Kordes C, Sawitza I, Gotze S, Haussinger D. Hepatic stellate cells support hematopoiesis and are liver-resident mesenchymal stem cells. Cell Physiol Biochem. 2013;31:290–304. https://doi.org/10.1159/000343368.
43. Gracia-Sancho J, Caparros E, Fernandez-Iglesias A, Frances R. Role of liver sinusoidal endothelial cells in liver diseases. Nat Rev Gastroenterol Hepatol. 2021;18:411–31. https://doi.org/10.1038/s41575-020-00411-3.
44. Furuta K, Guo Q, Hirsova P, Ibrahim SH. Emerging roles of liver sinusoidal endothelial cells in nonalcoholic steatohepatitis. Biology (Basel). 2020;9. https://doi.org/10.3390/biology9110395.
45. Ibrahim SH, Hirsova P, Gores GJ. Non-alcoholic steatohepatitis pathogenesis: sublethal hepatocyte injury as a driver of liver inflammation. Gut. 2018;67:963–72. https://doi.org/10.1136/gutjnl-2017-315691.
46. Deleve LD, Wang X, Guo Y. Sinusoidal endothelial cells prevent rat stellate cell activation and promote reversion to quiescence. Hepatology. 2008;48:920–30. https://doi.org/10.1002/hep.22351.
47. Ding BS, Nolan DJ, Butler JM, James D, Babazadeh AO, Rosenwaks Z, et al. Inductive angiocrine signals from sinusoidal endothelium are required for liver regeneration. Nature. 2010;468:310–5. https://doi.org/10.1038/nature09493.
48. Kim TH, Mars WM, Stolz DB, Michalopoulos GK. Expression and activation of pro-MMP-2 and pro-MMP-9 during rat liver regeneration. Hepatology. 2000;31:75–82. https://doi.org/10.1002/hep.510310114.
49. Mars WM, Liu ML, Kitson RP, Goldfarb RH, Gabauer MK, Michalopoulos GK. Immediate early detection of urokinase receptor after partial hepatectomy and its implications for initiation of liver regeneration. Hepatology. 1995;21:1695–701.
50. Naldini L, Vigna E, Bardelli A, Follenzi A, Galimi F, Comoglio PM. Biological activation of pro-HGF (hepatocyte growth factor) by urokinase is controlled by a stoichiometric reaction. J Biol Chem. 1995;270:603–11. https://doi.org/10.1074/jbc.270.2.603.
51. Zhang C, Sun C, Zhao Y, Ye B, Yu G. Signaling pathways of liver regeneration: biological mechanisms and implications. iScience. 2024;27:108683. https://doi.org/10.1016/j.isci.2023.108683.
52. Berasain C, Avila MA. The EGFR signalling system in the liver: from hepatoprotection to hepatocarcinogenesis. J Gastroenterol. 2014;49:9–23. https://doi.org/10.1007/s00535-013-0907-x.
53. Paranjpe S, Bowen WC, Tseng GC, Luo JH, Orr A, Michalopoulos GK. RNA interference against hepatic epidermal growth factor receptor has suppressive effects on liver regeneration in rats. Am J Pathol. 2010;176:2669–81. https://doi.org/10.2353/ajpath.2010.090605.

54. Paranjpe S, Bowen WC, Mars WM, Orr A, Haynes MM, DeFrances MC, et al. Combined systemic elimination of MET and epidermal growth factor receptor signaling completely abolishes liver regeneration and leads to liver decompensation. Hepatology. 2016;64:1711–24. https://doi.org/10.1002/hep.28721.
55. Kimura M, Moteki H, Ogihara M. Role of hepatocyte growth regulators in liver regeneration. Cells. 2023;12. https://doi.org/10.3390/cells12020208.
56. Michalopoulos GK, DeFrances MC. Liver regeneration. Science. 1997;276:60–6. https://doi.org/10.1126/science.276.5309.60.
57. Bird TG, Muller M, Boulter L, Vincent DF, Ridgway RA, Lopez-Guadamillas E, et al. TGFbeta inhibition restores a regenerative response in acute liver injury by suppressing paracrine senescence. Sci Transl Med. 2018;10. https://doi.org/10.1126/scitranslmed.aan1230.
58. Michalopoulos GK. Hepatostat: liver regeneration and normal liver tissue maintenance. Hepatology. 2017;65:1384–92. https://doi.org/10.1002/hep.28988.
59. Schwabe RF, Brenner DA. Mechanisms of liver injury. I. TNF-alpha-induced liver injury: role of IKK, JNK, and ROS pathways. Am J Physiol Gastrointest Liver Physiol. 2006;290:G583–9. https://doi.org/10.1152/ajpgi.00422.2005.
60. Wajant H, Pfizenmaier K, Scheurich P. Tumor necrosis factor signaling. Cell Death Differ. 2003;10:45–65. https://doi.org/10.1038/sj.cdd.4401189.
61. Schmidt-Arras D, Rose-John S. IL-6 pathway in the liver: from physiopathology to therapy. J Hepatol. 2016;64:1403–15. https://doi.org/10.1016/j.jhep.2016.02.004.
62. Nejak-Bowen K, Monga SP. Wnt-beta-catenin in hepatobiliary homeostasis, injury, and repair. Hepatology. 2023;78:1907–21. https://doi.org/10.1097/HEP.0000000000000495.
63. Perugorria MJ, Olaizola P, Labiano I, Esparza-Baquer A, Marzioni M, Marin JJG, et al. Wnt-beta-catenin signalling in liver development, health and disease. Nat Rev Gastroenterol Hepatol. 2019;16:121–36. https://doi.org/10.1038/s41575-018-0075-9.
64. Carson MD, Nejak-Bowen K. Wnt/beta-catenin signaling in liver pathobiology. Annu Rev Pathol. 2025;20:59–86. https://doi.org/10.1146/annurev-pathmechdis-111523-023535.
65. Geisler F, Strazzabosco M. Emerging roles of notch signaling in liver disease. Hepatology. 2015;61:382–92. https://doi.org/10.1002/hep.27268.
66. Merrell AJ, Peng T, Li J, Sun K, Li B, Katsuda T, et al. Dynamic transcriptional and epigenetic changes drive cellular plasticity in the liver. Hepatology. 2021;74:444–57. https://doi.org/10.1002/hep.31704.
67. Fiorotto R, Raizner A, Morell CM, Torsello B, Scirpo R, Fabris L, et al. Notch signaling regulates tubular morphogenesis during repair from biliary damage in mice. J Hepatol. 2013;59:124–30. https://doi.org/10.1016/j.jhep.2013.02.025.
68. Camargo FD, Gokhale S, Johnnidis JB, Fu D, Bell GW, Jaenisch R, et al. YAP1 increases organ size and expands undifferentiated progenitor cells. Curr Biol. 2007;17:2054–60. https://doi.org/10.1016/j.cub.2007.10.039.
69. Bou Saleh M, Louvet A, Ntandja-Wandji LC, Boleslawski E, Gnemmi V, Lassailly G, et al. Loss of hepatocyte identity following aberrant YAP activation: a key mechanism in alcoholic hepatitis. J Hepatol. 2021;75:912–23. https://doi.org/10.1016/j.jhep.2021.05.041.
70. Yimlamai D, Christodoulou C, Galli GG, Yanger K, Pepe-Mooney B, Gurung B, et al. Hippo pathway activity influences liver cell fate. Cell. 2014;157:1324–38. https://doi.org/10.1016/j.cell.2014.03.060.
71. Shetty S, Lalor PF, Adams DH. Liver sinusoidal endothelial cells - gatekeepers of hepatic immunity. Nat Rev Gastroenterol Hepatol. 2018;15:555–67. https://doi.org/10.1038/s41575-018-0020-y.
72. Marcu R, Choi YJ, Xue J, Fortin CL, Wang Y, Nagao RJ, et al. Human organ-specific endothelial cell heterogeneity. iScience. 2018;4:20–35. https://doi.org/10.1016/j.isci.2018.05.003.
73. De Rudder M, Dili A, Starkel P, Leclercq IA. Critical role of LSEC in post-hepatectomy liver regeneration and failure. Int J Mol Sci. 2021;22. https://doi.org/10.3390/ijms22158053.

74. de Vries RJ, Pendexter CA, Cronin SEJ, Marques B, Hafiz EOA, Muzikansky A, et al. Cell release during perfusion reflects cold ischemic injury in rat livers. Sci Rep. 2020;10:1102. https://doi.org/10.1038/s41598-020-57589-4.
75. Fausto N, Campbell JS, Riehle KJ. Liver regeneration. Hepatology. 2006;43:S45–53. https://doi.org/10.1002/hep.20969.
76. Sakamoto T, Liu Z, Murase N, Ezure T, Yokomuro S, Poli V, et al. Mitosis and apoptosis in the liver of interleukin-6-deficient mice after partial hepatectomy. Hepatology. 1999;29:403–11. https://doi.org/10.1002/hep.510290244.
77. Fausto N. Liver regeneration. J Hepatol. 2000;32:19–31. https://doi.org/10.1016/s0168-8278(00)80412-2.
78. Albinsson S, Hellstrand P. Integration of signal pathways for stretch-dependent growth and differentiation in vascular smooth muscle. Am J Physiol Cell Physiol. 2007;293:C772–82. https://doi.org/10.1152/ajpcell.00622.2006.
79. Shavandi A, Saeedi P, Gérard P, Jalalvandi E, Cannella D, Bekhit AE. The role of microbiota in tissue repair and regeneration. J Tissue Eng Regen Med. 2020;14:539–55. https://doi.org/10.1002/term.3009.
80. Jones DE, Tran-Patterson R, Cui DM, Davin D, Estell KP, Miller DM. Epidermal growth factor secreted from the salivary gland is necessary for liver regeneration. Am J Phys. 1995;268:G872–8. https://doi.org/10.1152/ajpgi.1995.268.5.G872.
81. Rubin RA, O'Keefe EJ, Earp HS. Alteration of epidermal growth factor-dependent phosphorylation during rat liver regeneration. Proc Natl Acad Sci USA. 1982;79:776–80. https://doi.org/10.1073/pnas.79.3.776.
82. Skov Olsen P, Boesby S, Kirkegaard P, Therkelsen K, Almdal T, Poulsen SS, et al. Influence of epidermal growth factor on liver regeneration after partial hepatectomy in rats. Hepatology. 1988;8:992–6. https://doi.org/10.1002/hep.1840080503.
83. Gadd VL, Aleksieva N, Forbes SJ. Epithelial plasticity during liver injury and regeneration. Cell Stem Cell. 2020;27:557–73. https://doi.org/10.1016/j.stem.2020.08.016.
84. DeLeve LD. Liver sinusoidal endothelial cells and liver regeneration. J Clin Invest. 2013;123:1861–6. https://doi.org/10.1172/JCI66025.
85. DeLeve LD, Wang X, Wang L. VEGF-sdf1 recruitment of CXCR7+ bone marrow progenitors of liver sinusoidal endothelial cells promotes rat liver regeneration. Am J Physiol Gastrointest Liver Physiol. 2016;310:G739–46. https://doi.org/10.1152/ajpgi.00056.2016.
86. Libermann TA, Baltimore D. Activation of interleukin-6 gene expression through the NF-kappa B transcription factor. Mol Cell Biol. 1990;10:2327–34. https://doi.org/10.1128/mcb.10.5.2327-2334.1990.
87. Fujiyoshi M, Ozaki M. Molecular mechanisms of liver regeneration and protection for treatment of liver dysfunction and diseases. J Hepatobiliary Pancreat Sci. 2011;18:13–22. https://doi.org/10.1007/s00534-010-0304-2.
88. De Franceschi N, Hamidi H, Alanko J, Sahgal P, Ivaska J. Integrin traffic - the update. J Cell Sci. 2015;128:839–52. https://doi.org/10.1242/jcs.161653.
89. Hynes RO. The extracellular matrix: not just pretty fibrils. Science. 2009;326:1216–9. https://doi.org/10.1126/science.1176009.
90. Klaas M, Kangur T, Viil J, Maemets-Allas K, Minajeva A, Vadi K, et al. The alterations in the extracellular matrix composition guide the repair of damaged liver tissue. Sci Rep. 2016;6:27398. https://doi.org/10.1038/srep27398.
91. McQuitty CE, Williams R, Chokshi S, Urbani L. Immunomodulatory role of the extracellular matrix within the liver disease microenvironment. Front Immunol. 2020;11:574276. https://doi.org/10.3389/fimmu.2020.574276.
92. Bataller R, Brenner DA. Liver fibrosis. J Clin Invest. 2005;115:209–18. https://doi.org/10.1172/JCI24282.
93. Arriazu E, Ruiz de Galarreta M, Cubero FJ, Varela-Rey M, Pérez de Obanos MP, Leung TM, et al. Extracellular matrix and liver disease. Antioxid Redox Signal. 2014;21:1078–97. https://doi.org/10.1089/ars.2013.5697.

94. Novo E, di Bonzo LV, Cannito S, Colombatto S, Parola M. Hepatic myofibroblasts: a heterogeneous population of multifunctional cells in liver fibrogenesis. Int J Biochem Cell Biol. 2009;41:2089–93. https://doi.org/10.1016/j.biocel.2009.03.010.
95. Mormone E, Lu Y, Ge X, Fiel MI, Nieto N. Fibromodulin, an oxidative stress-sensitive proteoglycan, regulates the fibrogenic response to liver injury in mice. Gastroenterology. 2012;142:612–21.e5. https://doi.org/10.1053/j.gastro.2011.11.029.
96. Nieto N. Ethanol and fish oil induce NFkappaB transactivation of the collagen alpha2(I) promoter through lipid peroxidation-driven activation of the PKC-PI3K-Akt pathway. Hepatology. 2007;45:1433–45. https://doi.org/10.1002/hep.21659.
97. Urtasun R, Lopategi A, George J, Leung TM, Lu Y, Wang X, et al. Osteopontin, an oxidant stress sensitive cytokine, up-regulates collagen-I via integrin α(V)β(3) engagement and PI3K/pAkt/NFκB signaling. Hepatology. 2012;55:594–608. https://doi.org/10.1002/hep.24701.
98. Nieto N. Oxidative-stress and IL-6 mediate the fibrogenic effects of [corrected] Kupffer cells on stellate cells. Hepatology. 2006;44:1487–501. https://doi.org/10.1002/hep.21427.
99. Jungermann K, Kietzmann T. Oxygen: modulator of metabolic zonation and disease of the liver. Hepatology. 2000;31:255–60. https://doi.org/10.1002/hep.510310201.
100. Kietzmann T, Cornesse Y, Brechtel K, Modaressi S, Jungermann K. Perivenous expression of the mRNA of the three hypoxia-inducible factor alpha-subunits, HIF1alpha, HIF2alpha and HIF3alpha, in rat liver. Biochem J. 2001;354:531–7. https://doi.org/10.1042/0264-6021:3540531.
101. Dimova EY, Kietzmann T. Hypoxia-inducible factors: post-translational crosstalk of signaling pathways. Methods Mol Biol. 2010;647:215–36. https://doi.org/10.1007/978-1-60761-738-9_13.
102. Kim WY, Safran M, Buckley MR, Ebert BL, Glickman J, Bosenberg M, et al. Failure to prolyl hydroxylate hypoxia-inducible factor alpha phenocopies VHL inactivation in vivo. EMBO J. 2006;25:4650–62. https://doi.org/10.1038/sj.emboj.7601300.
103. Nath B, Szabo G. Hypoxia and hypoxia inducible factors: diverse roles in liver diseases. Hepatology. 2012;55:622–33. https://doi.org/10.1002/hep.25497.
104. Hirao H, Nakamura K, Kupiec-Weglinski JW. Liver ischaemia-reperfusion injury: a new understanding of the role of innate immunity. Nat Rev Gastroenterol Hepatol. 2022;19:239–56. https://doi.org/10.1038/s41575-021-00549-8.
105. Krenkel O, Tacke F. Liver macrophages in tissue homeostasis and disease. Nat Rev Immunol. 2017;17:306–21. https://doi.org/10.1038/nri.2017.11.
106. Ito Y, Hosono K, Amano H. Responses of hepatic sinusoidal cells to liver ischemia-reperfusion injury. Front Cell Dev Biol. 2023;11:1171317. https://doi.org/10.3389/fcell.2023.1171317.
107. Jaeschke H. Molecular mechanisms of hepatic ischemia-reperfusion injury and preconditioning. Am J Physiol Gastrointest Liver Physiol. 2003;284:G15–26. https://doi.org/10.1152/ajpgi.00342.2002.
108. Shan Z, Ju C. Hepatic macrophages in liver injury. Front Immunol. 2020;11:322. https://doi.org/10.3389/fimmu.2020.00322.
109. Crosby CM, Kronenberg M. Tissue-specific functions of invariant natural killer T cells. Nat Rev Immunol. 2018;18:559–74. https://doi.org/10.1038/s41577-018-0034-2.
110. Van Kaer L. NKT cells: T lymphocytes with innate effector functions. Curr Opin Immunol. 2007;19:354–64. https://doi.org/10.1016/j.coi.2007.03.001.
111. Liew PX, Lee WY, Kubes P. iNKT cells orchestrate a switch from inflammation to resolution of sterile liver injury. Immunity. 2017;47:752–65.e5. https://doi.org/10.1016/j.immuni.2017.09.016.
112. Jaeschke H, Farhood A, Smith CW. Neutrophils contribute to ischemia/reperfusion injury in rat liver in vivo. FASEB J. 1990;4:3355–9.
113. Primavesi F, Senoner T, Schindler S, Nikolajevic A, Di Fazio P, Csukovich G, et al. The interplay between perioperative oxidative stress and hepatic dysfunction after human liver resection: a prospective observational pilot study. Antioxidants (Basel). 2024;13. https://doi.org/10.3390/antiox13050590.

114. Bratton DL, Henson PM. Neutrophil clearance: when the party is over, clean-up begins. Trends Immunol. 2011;32:350–7. https://doi.org/10.1016/j.it.2011.04.009.
115. Wang J, Hossain M, Thanabalasuriar A, Gunzer M, Meininger C, Kubes P. Visualizing the function and fate of neutrophils in sterile injury and repair. Science. 2017;358:111–6. https://doi.org/10.1126/science.aam9690.
116. Williams CD, Bajt ML, Sharpe MR, McGill MR, Farhood A, Jaeschke H. Neutrophil activation during acetaminophen hepatotoxicity and repair in mice and humans. Toxicol Appl Pharmacol. 2014;275:122–33. https://doi.org/10.1016/j.taap.2014.01.004.
117. Graubardt N, Vugman M, Mouhadeb O, Caliari G, Pasmanik-Chor M, Reuveni D, et al. Ly6Chi monocytes and their macrophage descendants regulate neutrophil function and clearance in acetaminophen-induced liver injury. Front Immunol. 2017;8:626. https://doi.org/10.3389/fimmu.2017.00626.
118. Calvente CJ, Tameda M, Johnson CD, Del Pilar H, Lin YC, Adronikou N, et al. Neutrophils contribute to spontaneous resolution of liver inflammation and fibrosis via microRNA-223. J Clin Invest. 2019;129:4091–109. https://doi.org/10.1172/JCI122258.
119. Yang W, Tao Y, Wu Y, Zhao X, Ye W, Zhao D, et al. Neutrophils promote the development of reparative macrophages mediated by ROS to orchestrate liver repair. Nat Commun. 2019;10:1076. https://doi.org/10.1038/s41467-019-09046-8.
120. Horckmans M, Ring L, Duchene J, Santovito D, Schloss MJ, Drechsler M, et al. Neutrophils orchestrate post-myocardial infarction healing by polarizing macrophages towards a reparative phenotype. Eur Heart J. 2017;38:187–97. https://doi.org/10.1093/eurheartj/ehw002.
121. Hossain M, Kubes P. Innate immune cells orchestrate the repair of sterile injury in the liver and beyond. Eur J Immunol. 2019;49:831–41. https://doi.org/10.1002/eji.201847485.
122. Nakamura K, Kageyama S, Kupiec-Weglinski JW. The evolving role of neutrophils in liver transplant ischemia-reperfusion injury. Curr Transplant Rep. 2019;6:78–89. https://doi.org/10.1007/s40472-019-0230-4.
123. Meszaros AT, Hofmann J, Buch ML, Cardini B, Dunzendorfer-Matt T, Nardin F, et al. Mitochondrial respiration during normothermic liver machine perfusion predicts clinical outcome. EBioMedicine. 2022;85:104311. https://doi.org/10.1016/j.ebiom.2022.104311.
124. Hofmann J, Otarashvili G, Meszaros A, Ebner S, Weissenbacher A, Cardini B, et al. Restoring mitochondrial function while avoiding redox stress: the key to preventing ischemia/reperfusion injury in machine perfused liver grafts? Int J Mol Sci. 2020;21. https://doi.org/10.3390/ijms21093132.
125. Mitra K, Wunder C, Roysam B, Lin G, Lippincott-Schwartz J. A hyperfused mitochondrial state achieved at G1-S regulates cyclin E buildup and entry into S phase. Proc Natl Acad Sci USA. 2009;106:11960–5. https://doi.org/10.1073/pnas.0904875106.
126. Schrepfer E, Scorrano L. Mitofusins, from mitochondria to metabolism. Mol Cell. 2016;61:683–94. https://doi.org/10.1016/j.molcel.2016.02.022.
127. Margineantu DH, Gregory Cox W, Sundell L, Sherwood SW, Beechem JM, Capaldi RA. Cell cycle dependent morphology changes and associated mitochondrial DNA redistribution in mitochondria of human cell lines. Mitochondrion. 2002;1:425–35. https://doi.org/10.1016/s1567-7249(02)00006-5.
128. Wu G. Amino acids: metabolism, functions, and nutrition. Amino Acids. 2009;37:1–17. https://doi.org/10.1007/s00726-009-0269-0.
129. Tsun ZY, Possemato R. Amino acid management in cancer. Semin Cell Dev Biol. 2015;43:22–32. https://doi.org/10.1016/j.semcdb.2015.08.002.
130. Lukey MJ, Katt WP, Cerione RA. Targeting amino acid metabolism for cancer therapy. Drug Discov Today. 2017;22:796–804. https://doi.org/10.1016/j.drudis.2016.12.003.
131. Felig P, Pozefsky T, Marliss E, Cahill GF. Alanine: key role in gluconeogenesis. Science. 1970;167:1003–4. https://doi.org/10.1126/science.167.3920.1003.
132. Meijer AJ. Amino acids as regulators and components of nonproteinogenic pathways. J Nutr. 2003;133:2057S–62S. https://doi.org/10.1093/jn/133.6.2057S.

133. McCommis KS, Chen Z, Fu X, McDonald WG, Colca JR, Kletzien RF, et al. Loss of mitochondrial pyruvate carrier 2 in the liver leads to defects in gluconeogenesis and compensation via pyruvate-alanine cycling. Cell Metab. 2015;22:682–94. https://doi.org/10.1016/j.cmet.2015.07.028.
134. Wolf PL. Biochemical diagnosis of liver disease. Indian J Clin Biochem. 1999;14:59–90. https://doi.org/10.1007/BF02869152.
135. Kim WR, Flamm SL, Di Bisceglie AM, Bodenheimer HC. Serum activity of alanine aminotransferase (ALT) as an indicator of health and disease. Hepatology. 2008;47:1363–70. https://doi.org/10.1002/hep.22109.
136. Maezono K, Kajiwara K, Mawatari K, Shinkai A, Torii K, Maki T. Alanine protects liver from injury caused by F-galactosamine and CCl4. Hepatology. 1996;24:185–91. https://doi.org/10.1002/hep.510240130.
137. Maezono K, Mawatari K, Kajiwara K, Shinkai A, Maki T. Effect of alanine on D-galactosamine-induced acute liver failure in rats. Hepatology. 1996;24:1211–6. https://doi.org/10.1053/jhep.1996.v24.pm0008903400.
138. Brosnan ME, Brosnan JT. Hepatic glutamate metabolism: a tale of 2 hepatocytes. Am J Clin Nutr. 2009;90:857S–61S. https://doi.org/10.3945/ajcn.2009.27462Z.
139. Wu G, Fang YZ, Yang S, Lupton JR, Turner ND. Glutathione metabolism and its implications for health. J Nutr. 2004;134:489–92. https://doi.org/10.1093/jn/134.3.489.
140. Zeb A, Rahman SU. Protective effects of dietary glycine and glutamic acid toward the toxic effects of oxidized mustard oil in rabbits. Food Funct. 2017;8:429–36. https://doi.org/10.1039/c6fo01329e.
141. Wang L, Hou Y, Yi D, Li Y, Ding B, Zhu H, et al. Dietary supplementation with glutamate precursor α-ketoglutarate attenuates lipopolysaccharide-induced liver injury in young pigs. Amino Acids. 2015;47:1309–18. https://doi.org/10.1007/s00726-015-1966-5.
142. Brosnan JT. Amino acids, then and now–a reflection on Sir Hans Krebs' contribution to nitrogen metabolism. IUBMB Life. 2001;52:265–70. https://doi.org/10.1080/152165401317291101.
143. Yanni AE, Agrogiannis G, Nomikos T, Fragopoulou E, Pantopoulou A, Antonopoulou S, et al. Oral supplementation with L-aspartate and L-glutamate inhibits atherogenesis and fatty liver disease in cholesterol-fed rabbit. Amino Acids. 2010;38:1323–31. https://doi.org/10.1007/s00726-009-0340-x.
144. Leng W, Liu Y, Shi H, Li S, Zhu H, Pi D, et al. Aspartate alleviates liver injury and regulates mRNA expressions of TLR4 and NOD signaling-related genes in weaned pigs after lipopolysaccharide challenge. J Nutr Biochem. 2014;25:592–9. https://doi.org/10.1016/j.jnutbio.2014.01.010.
145. Wheeler M, Stachlewitz RF, Yamashina S, Ikejima K, Morrow AL, Thurman RG. Glycine-gated chloride channels in neutrophils attenuate calcium influx and superoxide production. FASEB J. 2000;14:476–84. https://doi.org/10.1096/fasebj.14.3.476.
146. Carini R, Bellomo G, Grazia De Cesaris M, Albano E. Glycine protects against hepatocyte killing by KCN or hypoxia by preventing intracellular Na+ overload in the rat. Hepatology. 1997;26:107–12. https://doi.org/10.1002/hep.510260114.
147. Weinberg JM, Davis JA, Abarzua M, Rajan T. Cytoprotective effects of glycine and glutathione against hypoxic injury to renal tubules. J Clin Invest. 1987;80:1446–54. https://doi.org/10.1172/JCI113224.
148. Lee DY, Kim EH. Therapeutic effects of amino acids in liver diseases: current studies and future perspectives. J Cancer Prev. 2019;24:72–8. https://doi.org/10.15430/JCP.2019.24.2.72.
149. Rivera CA, Bradford BU, Hunt KJ, Adachi Y, Schrum LW, Koop DR, et al. Attenuation of CCl(4)-induced hepatic fibrosis by GdCl(3) treatment or dietary glycine. Am J Physiol Gastrointest Liver Physiol. 2001;281:G200–7. https://doi.org/10.1152/ajpgi.2001.281.1.G200.
150. Senthilkumar R, Viswanathan P, Nalini N. Effect of glycine on oxidative stress in rats with alcohol induced liver injury. Pharmazie. 2004;59:55–60.
151. Rentsch M, Puellmann K, Sirek S, Iesalnieks I, Kienle K, Mueller T, et al. Benefit of Kupffer cell modulation with glycine versus Kupffer cell depletion after liver transplantation in the

rat: effects on postischemic reperfusion injury, apoptotic cell death graft regeneration and survival. Transpl Int. 2005;18:1079–89. https://doi.org/10.1111/j.1432-2277.2005.00185.x.
152. Yin M, Ikejima K, Arteel GE, Seabra V, Bradford BU, Kono H, et al. Glycine accelerates recovery from alcohol-induced liver injury. J Pharmacol Exp Ther. 1998;286:1014–9.
153. Yan SL, Wu ST, Yin MC, Chen HT, Chen HC. Protective effects from carnosine and histidine on acetaminophen-induced liver injury. J Food Sci. 2009;74:H259–65. https://doi.org/10.1111/j.1750-3841.2009.01330.x.
154. Xu H, Sakakibara S, Morifuji M, Salamatulla Q, Aoyama Y. Excess dietary histidine decreases the liver copper level and serum alanine aminotransferase activity in Long-Evans Cinnamon rats. Br J Nutr. 2003;90:573–9. https://doi.org/10.1079/bjn2003939.
155. Mardinoglu A, Agren R, Kampf C, Asplund A, Uhlen M, Nielsen J. Genome-scale metabolic modelling of hepatocytes reveals serine deficiency in patients with non-alcoholic fatty liver disease. Nat Commun. 2014;5:3083. https://doi.org/10.1038/ncomms4083.
156. Sim WC, Yin HQ, Choi HS, Choi YJ, Kwak HC, Kim SK, et al. L-serine supplementation attenuates alcoholic fatty liver by enhancing homocysteine metabolism in mice and rats. J Nutr. 2015;145:260–7. https://doi.org/10.3945/jn.114.199711.
157. Zhang L, Huang X, Meng Z, Dong B, Shiah S, Moore DD, et al. Significance and mechanism of CYP7a1 gene regulation during the acute phase of liver regeneration. Mol Endocrinol. 2009;23:137–45. https://doi.org/10.1210/me.2008-0198.
158. Staudinger JL, Goodwin B, Jones SA, Hawkins-Brown D, MacKenzie KI, LaTour A, et al. The nuclear receptor PXR is a lithocholic acid sensor that protects against liver toxicity. Proc Natl Acad Sci USA. 2001;98:3369–74. https://doi.org/10.1073/pnas.051551698.
159. Fan M, Wang X, Xu G, Yan Q, Huang W. Bile acid signaling and liver regeneration. Biochim Biophys Acta. 2015;1849:196–200. https://doi.org/10.1016/j.bbagrm.2014.05.021.
160. Ueda J, Chijiiwa K, Nakano K, Zhao G, Tanaka M. Lack of intestinal bile results in delayed liver regeneration of normal rat liver after hepatectomy accompanied by impaired cyclin E-associated kinase activity. Surgery. 2002;131:564–73. https://doi.org/10.1067/msy.2002.123008.
161. Otao R, Beppu T, Isiko T, Mima K, Okabe H, Hayashi H, et al. External biliary drainage and liver regeneration after major hepatectomy. Br J Surg. 2012;99:1569–74. https://doi.org/10.1002/bjs.8906.
162. Barone M, Francavilla A, Polimeno L, Ierardi E, Romanelli D, Berloco P, et al. Modulation of rat hepatocyte proliferation by bile salts: in vitro and in vivo studies. Hepatology. 1996;23:1159–66. https://doi.org/10.1053/jhep.1996.v23.pm0008621149.
163. Columbano A, Ledda-Columbano GM. Mitogenesis by ligands of nuclear receptors: an attractive model for the study of the molecular mechanisms implicated in liver growth. Cell Death Differ. 2003;10(Suppl 1):S19–21. https://doi.org/10.1038/sj.cdd.4401113.
164. Fernández-Barrena MG, Monte MJ, Latasa MU, Uriarte I, Vicente E, Chang HC, et al. Lack of Abcc3 expression impairs bile-acid induced liver growth and delays hepatic regeneration after partial hepatectomy in mice. J Hepatol. 2012;56:367–73. https://doi.org/10.1016/j.jhep.2011.05.031.
165. Uriarte I, Santamaria E, López-Pascual A, Monte MJ, Argemí J, Latasa MU, et al. New insights into the regulation of bile acids synthesis during the early stages of liver regeneration: a human and experimental study. Biochim Biophys Acta Mol basis Dis. 2024;1870:167166. https://doi.org/10.1016/j.bbadis.2024.167166.
166. Alvarez-Sola G, Uriarte I, Latasa MU, Jimenez M, Barcena-Varela M, Santamaría E, et al. Bile acids, FGF15/19 and liver regeneration: from mechanisms to clinical applications. Biochim Biophys Acta Mol basis Dis. 2018;1864:1326–34. https://doi.org/10.1016/j.bbadis.2017.06.025.
167. Kong B, Sun R, Huang M, Chow MD, Zhong XB, Xie W, et al. Fibroblast growth factor 15-dependent and bile acid-independent promotion of liver regeneration in mice. Hepatology. 2018;68:1961–76. https://doi.org/10.1002/hep.30041.
168. Oscarsson E, Håkansson Å, Andrén Aronsson C, Molin G, Agardh D. Effects of probiotic bacteria. Front Nutr. 2021;8:680771. https://doi.org/10.3389/fnut.2021.680771.

169. Briani F, Bagli M, Venturi G, Bacchion F, Mugnolo A. Inclisiran: early LDL-C target achievement in a real-life population. Atheroscler Plus. 2025;59:54–8. https://doi.org/10.1016/j.athplu.2025.01.001.
170. Tilg H, Adolph TE, Trauner M. Gut-liver axis: pathophysiological concepts and clinical implications. Cell Metab. 2022;34:1700–18. https://doi.org/10.1016/j.cmet.2022.09.017.
171. Meijnikman AS, Nieuwdorp M, Schnabl B. Endogenous ethanol production in health and disease. Nat Rev Gastroenterol Hepatol. 2024;21:556–71. https://doi.org/10.1038/s41575-024-00937-w.
172. Li N, Hua J. Immune cells in liver regeneration. Oncotarget. 2017;8:3628–39. https://doi.org/10.18632/oncotarget.12275.
173. Di-Iacovo N, Pieroni S, Piobbico D, Castelli M, Scopetti D, Ferracchiato S, et al. Liver regeneration and immunity: a tale to tell. Int J Mol Sci. 2023;24. https://doi.org/10.3390/ijms24021176.
174. Cressman DE, Greenbaum LE, DeAngelis RA, Ciliberto G, Furth EE, Poli V, et al. Liver failure and defective hepatocyte regeneration in interleukin-6-deficient mice. Science. 1996;274:1379–83. https://doi.org/10.1126/science.274.5291.1379.
175. Inoue H, Ogawa W, Ozaki M, Haga S, Matsumoto M, Furukawa K, et al. Role of STAT-3 in regulation of hepatic gluconeogenic genes and carbohydrate metabolism in vivo. Nat Med. 2004;10:168–74. https://doi.org/10.1038/nm980.
176. Caligiuri A, Gentilini A, Pastore M, Gitto S, Marra F. Cellular and molecular mechanisms underlying liver fibrosis regression. Cells. 2021;10. https://doi.org/10.3390/cells10102759.
177. Dooley S, ten Dijke P. TGF-β in progression of liver disease. Cell Tissue Res. 2012;347:245–56. https://doi.org/10.1007/s00441-011-1246-y.
178. Tanaka M, Miyajima A. Liver regeneration and fibrosis after inflammation. Inflamm Regen. 2016;36:19. https://doi.org/10.1186/s41232-016-0025-2.
179. Ding BS, Cao Z, Lis R, Nolan DJ, Guo P, Simons M, et al. Divergent angiocrine signals from vascular niche balance liver regeneration and fibrosis. Nature. 2014;505:97–102. https://doi.org/10.1038/nature12681.
180. Ramachandran P, Pellicoro A, Vernon MA, Boulter L, Aucott RL, Ali A, et al. Differential Ly-6C expression identifies the recruited macrophage phenotype, which orchestrates the regression of murine liver fibrosis. Proc Natl Acad Sci USA. 2012;109:E3186–95. https://doi.org/10.1073/pnas.1119964109.
181. Yagi S, Hirata M, Miyachi Y, Uemoto S. Liver regeneration after hepatectomy and partial liver transplantation. Int J Mol Sci. 2020;21. https://doi.org/10.3390/ijms21218414.
182. Zuñiga-Aguilar E, Ramírez-Fernández O. Fibrosis and hepatic regeneration mechanism. Transl Gastroenterol Hepatol. 2022;7:9. https://doi.org/10.21037/tgh.2020.02.21.
183. Michalopoulos GK. Liver regeneration after partial hepatectomy: critical analysis of mechanistic dilemmas. Am J Pathol. 2010;176:2–13. https://doi.org/10.2353/ajpath.2010.090675.
184. Brunnthaler L, Pereyra D, Brenner M, Santol J, Herrmann L, Schrottmaier WC, et al. Intrahepatic neutrophil accumulation and extracellular trap formation are associated with posthepatectomy liver failure. Hepatol Commun. 2024;8. https://doi.org/10.1097/HC9.0000000000000348.
185. Sparrelid E, Olthof PB, Dasari BVM, Erdmann JI, Santol J, Starlinger P, et al. Current evidence on posthepatectomy liver failure: comprehensive review. BJS Open. 2022;6. https://doi.org/10.1093/bjsopen/zrac142.
186. Riauka R, Ignatavicius P, Barauskas G. Hypophosphatemia as a prognostic tool for posthepatectomy liver failure: a systematic review. World J Gastrointest Surg. 2023;15:249–57. https://doi.org/10.4240/wjgs.v15.i2.249.
187. Niederwieser T, Braunwarth E, Dasari BVM, Pufal K, Szatmary P, Hackl H, et al. Early postoperative arterial lactate concentrations to stratify risk of post-hepatectomy liver failure. Br J Surg. 2021;108:1360–70. https://doi.org/10.1093/bjs/znab338.

188. Baumgartner R, Engstrand J, Rajala P, Grip J, Ghorbani P, Sparrelid E, et al. Comparing the accuracy of prediction models to detect clinically relevant post-hepatectomy liver failure early after major hepatectomy. Br J Surg. 2024;111. https://doi.org/10.1093/bjs/znad433.
189. Gyoeri GP, Pereyra D, Braunwarth E, Ammann M, Jonas P, Offensperger F, et al. The 3-60 criteria challenge established predictors of postoperative mortality and enable timely therapeutic intervention after liver resection. Hepatobiliary Surg Nutr. 2019;8:111–24. https://doi.org/10.21037/hbsn.2019.02.01.
190. Santol J, Ammann M, Reese T, Kern AE, Laferl V, Oldhafer F, et al. Comparison of the LiMAx test vs. the APRI+ALBI score for clinical utility in preoperative risk assessment in patients undergoing liver surgery - a European multicenter study. Eur J Surg Oncol. 2024;50:108048. https://doi.org/10.1016/j.ejso.2024.108048.
191. Rassam F, Olthof PB, Takkenberg B, Besselink MG, Busch OR, Erdmann JI, et al. Functional assessment of liver regeneration after major hepatectomy. Hepatobiliary Surg Nutr. 2022;11:530–8. https://doi.org/10.21037/hbsn-20-866.
192. Wang L, Xie L, Zhang N, Zhu W, Zhou J, Pan Q, et al. Predictive value of intraoperative Indocyanine green clearance measurement on postoperative liver function after anatomic major liver resection. J Gastrointest Surg. 2020;24:1342–51. https://doi.org/10.1007/s11605-019-04262-5.
193. Nakajima T, Ikuta S, Aihara T, Ikuta L, Matsuki G, Fujikawa M, et al. Intraoperatively measured prehepatectomy portal vein pressure as a useful predictor of posthepatectomy liver failure. Langenbecks Arch Surg. 2024;409:314. https://doi.org/10.1007/s00423-024-03508-4.
194. Kaffarnik MF, Lock JF, Vetter H, Ahmadi N, Lojewski C, Malinowski M, et al. Early diagnosis of sepsis-related hepatic dysfunction and its prognostic impact on survival: a prospective study with the LiMAx test. Crit Care. 2013;17:R259. https://doi.org/10.1186/cc13089.
195. Rahbari NN, Garden OJ, Padbury R, Brooke-Smith M, Crawford M, Adam R, et al. Posthepatectomy liver failure: a definition and grading by the International Study Group of Liver Surgery (ISGLS). Surgery. 2011;149:713–24. https://doi.org/10.1016/j.surg.2010.10.001.
196. van Keulen AM, Buettner S, Besselink MG, Busch OR, van Gulik TM, IJzermans JNM, et al. Primary and secondary liver failure after major liver resection for perihilar cholangiocarcinoma. Surgery. 2021;170:1024–30. https://doi.org/10.1016/j.surg.2021.04.013.
197. Primavesi F, Maglione M, Cipriani F, Denecke T, Oberkofler CE, Starlinger P, et al. E-AHPBA-ESSO-ESSR Innsbruck consensus guidelines for preoperative liver function assessment before hepatectomy. Br J Surg. 2023;110:1331–47. https://doi.org/10.1093/bjs/znad233.

Microbiota and Liver–Gut Axis in Liver Regeneration

2

Luigi Colecchia, Giovanni Marasco, and Giovanni Barbara

2.1 Gut–Liver Axis in Health

The gastrointestinal mucosa is a semi-permeable barrier that serves a variety of key functions, such as digestion and absorption of nutrients, immune defense and secretion of enzymes and hormones [1]. Moving from the innermost luminal layer to the outer basolateral layer the intestinal barrier is composed of gut microbiota, mucus layer, epithelial cells monolayer, and an immune cell within the lamina propria [2].

The gut microbiota comprises over 100 trillion microorganisms, including bacteria, fungi, viruses, and archaea [3]. It is highly dynamic, exhibiting substantial intra- and inter-individual variation over time as a result of a variety of factors, including, among others, kind of delivery at birth, diet, physical activity, medications, and intestinal transit time [4]. Along the gastrointestinal tract, overall bacterial abundance and diversity tend to increase, likely due to the different conditions found in the lumen. In fact, there is a significant gradient of decreased partial oxygen concentration and increased pH and mucus thickness, limiting growth in the stomach, and favoring it in the gut [5]. Gut microbiota performs critical functions for its host in a profoundly symbiotic relationship, including assisting with efficient nutrient extraction, modulating hormonal pathways through microbial-derived metabolites, metabolizing drugs and xenobiotics, priming host immunity, and competing with pathogens in the gut lumen for nutrient uptake [6].

The mucus layer covers the luminal surface of the gastrointestinal tract and serves as the primary defense against mechanical, chemical, and biological threats [7]. The mucus barrier in the colon is made up of two layers: the outer layer is colonized by bacteria, while the inner layer is nearly devoid of bacteria due to the small

L. Colecchia · G. Marasco · G. Barbara (✉)
Department of Medical and Surgical Sciences, University of Bologna, Bologna, Italy

IRCCS Azienda Ospedaliero-Universitaria di Bologna, Bologna, Italy
e-mail: giovanni.barbara@unibo.it

L. Aldrighetti et al. (eds.), *Liver Regeneration Techniques In Hepatic Surgery*,
https://doi.org/10.1007/978-3-032-10997-2_2

size of the meshes that make it up that do not allow the passage of bacteria and the presence of antimicrobial molecules such as IgA [1].

The intestinal epithelial cell (IEC) barrier, situated beneath the mucus layer, consists of a monolayer of cells, including enterocytes, goblet cells, tuft cells, and enterochromaffin cells [8]. The functions of IECs depend on intercellular connections established by the apical junctional complex, comprising tight junctions, adherens junctions, and desmosomes [9]. These protein complexes close the gaps between epithelial cells, only allowing the passage of small molecules. In fact, molecules present in the gut have the ability to traverse the intestinal epithelial monolayer by either passing between cells (transcellular route) or the intercellular space (paracellular route) [9]. The immunologic defense systems within the intraepithelial compartment, lamina propria, and mesenteric lymph nodes form the subsequent barrier. Additionally, the gut vascular barrier serves to prevent the translocation of viable microbes from the lamina propria into the portal circulation [10]. Under healthy conditions, the intestinal barrier prevents the passage of microbes into the lamina propria. Therefore, most gut microbiota–hosts interactions occur indirectly through the mediation of their metabolic products [11]. Proper permeability of this barrier is fundamental for the appropriate functioning of the gut–liver axis, as an increased permeability of the gut mucosal epithelial barrier increases metabolites and bacterial translocation in several clinical conditions [12]. Intestinal epithelial cells and mononuclear phagocytes can detect bacteria or their products and produce pro-inflammatory cytokines. Neutrophils, mast cells, and macrophages sense pro-inflammatory cytokines and release proteases that reduce the integrity of the IEC barrier inducing the opening of protease-activated receptors or by direct cleavage of intercellular junction proteins [9].

The liver is the first organ to encounter microbial metabolites, which are crucial for the liver's immune and metabolic functions, and viable bacteria, which may pass the intestinal barrier. Specifically, liver Kupffer cells, localized in the periportal area, serve as a critical protective barrier by phagocytosing viable bacteria and translocated microbial products [13].

The liver engages in direct communication with the gut via the biliary system. Bile, a solution rich in IgA, bicarbonate, antimicrobial molecules, and bile acids (BAs), is produced and released by hepatocytes [4]. Bile acids serve multiple functions, including aiding in the digestion and absorption of lipids and lipid-soluble vitamins, and affecting the composition of gut microbiota [4]. An illustrative and exemplificative dual relationship between the gut and liver is represented by the enterohepatic circulation of biliary acids [14]. BAs biosynthesis starts from cholesterol modifications by cholesterol 7α-hydroxylase (classic pathway) or sterol 27-hydroxylase (alternative pathway), forming the primary BAs cholic acid and chenodeoxycholic acid. Primary BAs are conjugated with glycine or with taurine, resulting in the formation of bile salts that are released into the duodenum upon meal consumption, where they are subsequently metabolized by the gut microbiota along the gastrointestinal tract. Approximately 95% of BAs are reabsorbed through both passive and active transport before reaching the terminal ileum and subsequently the liver. The residual BAs proceed to the colon, which hosts the predominant gut microbiota, enabling the synthesis of key secondary BAs, namely deoxycholic acid and lithocholic acid, through dihydroxylation and subsequent passive reabsorption [15]. The primary functions of gut microbiota in BAs metabolism include deconjugation and dihydroxylation of BAs. Deconjugation is the process by which the amino acid moiety, either glycine or taurine, attached to BAs is removed, mitigating BAs' toxicity for the host. Bacteria derive advantages from this process by utilizing the released amino acids for energy and nutrient acquisition [15]. Dihydroxylation is a biochemical process performed by gut microbiota that involves the removal of hydroxyl groups from the steroid backbone of BAs. This transformation converts primary BAs into secondary BAs, which play a crucial role in lipid digestion, immune modulation, and metabolic regulation [15].

In summary, the gastrointestinal mucosa is essential for digestion, nutrient absorption, immune defense, and hormone secretion. It includes gut microbiota, mucus, epithelial cells, and immune cells. The gut microbiota aids in nutrient extraction, hormone modulation, drug metabolism, and immunity. The mucus layer protects against threats, while the epithelial cell barrier regulates molecule passage. The liver processes microbial metabolites and communicates with the gut via bile. Bile acids, modified by gut microbiota, are reabsorbed, highlighting the gut–liver axis's importance in health. Proper barrier permeability is crucial to prevent clinical several clinical conditions.

2.2 Gut Microbiota Changes During Liver Regeneration

In healthy conditions, the predominant gut microbial phyla include *Firmicutes*, *Bacteroidetes*, *Actinobacteria*, *Proteobacteria*, *Fusobacteria*, and *Verrucomicrobia*, with *Firmicutes* and *Bacteroidetes* comprising 90% of the gut microbiota [3]. The *Firmicutes* phylum comprises about 200 distinct genera, including *Lactobacillus*, *Bacillus*, *Clostridium*, *Enterococcus*, and *Ruminicoccus* [3]. The *Clostridium* genus constitutes 95% of the *Firmicutes* phylum [3]. *Bacteroidetes* comprises major genera, including *Bacteroides* and *Prevotella* [16]. Similar compositions can also be observed in mice gut microbiota, with *Firmicutes* being more represented than *Bacteroidetes* in adult mice [17].

In the context of liver regeneration, studies in mice demonstrated that liver cell proliferation post-partial hepatectomy (PH) was associated with profound changes in the composition of gut microbiota over all the phases of liver regeneration [18, 19]. It was found that the abundance of *Bacteroidetes*, specifically *S24-7* and *Rikenellaceae*, increased steadily in the days after PH, while *Firmicutes* such as *Clostridiales*, *Lachnospiraceae*, and *Ruminococcaceae* decreased reciprocally during liver regeneration [18, 19].

Although studies in mice lead to consistent results, gut microbiota analysis during liver cell proliferation in rats showed fluctuating changes according to the phase of liver regeneration. The abundance of *Bacteroidetes* first decreased at 12 h post-PH, then gradually returned to baseline levels at 48 h and finally decreased steadily from day 3 [20]. These changes could facilitate liver regeneration by increasing gut mucosal epithelial barrier permeability, affecting metabolite release, and other pathways needed to support the hepatocyte cell cycle [21]. However, further studies in mice and especially in humans are needed to assess the dynamic changes of microbiota during acute liver events that lead to liver regeneration.

2.3 Gut Microbiota Influences Liver Regeneration

Several studies have demonstrated a pivotal role of gut microbiota in liver regeneration first in mice and in humans. After PH in rodents, most of the liver mass is restored within 7–8 days, with complete restoration achieved within 3 weeks [22]. Initial studies demonstrated reduced liver regeneration rates following PH in germ-free (GF) mice [23, 24]. For example, liver/body weight ratio, mitotic count, and hepatocyte proliferative index at 72 h after PH were all reduced in GF mice with respect to control groups. Interestingly, the authors compared the results with a third population of GF mice recolonized with normal gut microbiota, finding comparable results to that of control subjects [23]. Subsequent studies assessed liver regeneration rates in antibiotic-treated mice compared to healthy controls, finding similar results to the ones observed in GF mice [25, 26]. The effects of altering gut microbiota with antibiotics were also observed when three homogeneous populations of mice that had all been administered an antibiotic cocktail one week before PH were compared according to postoperative intervention. The control group received bottled water, the second group antibiotics, and the third group received both antibiotics and probiotics (*Bifidobacterium* and *Lactobacillus*) for a duration of 2 weeks. Liver proliferation was diminished in mice treated with postoperative antibiotics compared to controls and mice supplemented with probiotics [27]. Similarly, it was shown that after PH, in antibiotic-pre-treated mice, fecal microbiota transplantation (FMT), compared to placebo, resulted in improved liver regeneration and decreased postoperative mortality [28]. Studies in rats showed similar results, with reduced liver regeneration characterized by delayed hepatocyte proliferation observed following PH in rats that underwent simultaneous bowel resection [29].

The earliest study in humans performed in a Western country [30] was a randomized double-blind trial in which 19 patients who underwent right hepatectomy were compared according to the postoperative treatment received after liver resection: one group received a combination of probiotics, prebiotics, and four fibers (beta-glucan, inulin, pectin, and resistant starch), while the other group received only fibers for 10 days. Although the study was limited by the low sample size and the relatively high number of complications related to the procedure, liver function capacity was higher in the patients treated with probiotics and prebiotics. Other studies comparing the effects of probiotics before or after PH evaluated the PH-related complications instead of the liver functional reserve, as indirect marker of regeneration. For this purpose, a systematic review and meta-analysis [31] included 205 participants (103 receiving probiotics vs. 102 controls) and concluded that patients treated with probiotics experienced lower postoperative infection rates, reduced hospitalization stays, and reduced the antibiotic usage.

2.4 Gut Microbiota-Derived Molecules Influence Liver Regeneration

The recognition of the critical role of gut microbiota in liver regeneration has increased over time, along with the knowledge of the multiple regenerative mechanisms in which gut microbiota is implicated. The main gut microbiota-derived molecules involved, which are going to be addressed in this section, are lipopolysaccharides (LPS), gut microbiota-modified BAs, short-chain fatty acids (SCFA), and tryptophan derivatives.

2.4.1 Lipopolysaccharides

One of the most important and researched gut microbiota-derived molecules are LPS, produced by enteric gram-negative bacteria. Under healthy conditions, low-grade portal venous LPS can be phagocytosed and detoxified by Kupffer cells in the liver [32]. Partial hepatectomy or liver chemical injury leads to relatively increased local concentration of LPS in the liver that extensively bind Toll-like receptor 4 (TLR-4) present in non-hepatocyte parenchymal liver cells (i.e., stellate cells and Kupffer cells), leading to NF-κB activation and production of tumor necrosis factor α and interleukin-6 (IL-6) [33]. IL-6 signaling via the soluble IL-6 receptor binding stimulates hepatic stellate cells to generate hepatocyte growth factor (HGF) [22, 34]. HGF collaborates with various extrahepatic factors, including triiodothyronine (T3), insulin, and epidermal growth factor, which are also induced by the presence of LPS in the general blood circulation, enabling remnant hepatocytes to proliferate [22]. This inflammation-driven regeneration shuts down when the liver sufficiently regenerates to restore the phagocytic function of LPS by Kupffer cells [34]. As a matter of fact, it was observed that limiting gut-derived LPS through gut bacterial depletion or endotoxin neutralization significantly hindered liver regeneration, a condition that was reversed by the administration of exogenous LPS supplements [35].

2.4.2 Bile Acids

The role of BAs in liver regeneration is ambivalent following PH since excessive intrahepatic BAs levels directly injure hepatocytes while reduced levels were proven to significantly hamper liver regeneration [36]. After an acute event such as PH, BA levels increase significantly in relation to the remnant liver, leading to cholestatic injury. Protective mechanisms include reduction in BAs basolateral uptake and production, alongside an increase in basolateral efflux and biliary excretion [21]. Gut microbiota is a key player in this protective mechanism as it can modify the aqueous solubility of the BAs pool. In fact, in eubiotic conditions, gut microbiota normally deconjugates BAs, making them largely permeable to the gut membrane and allowing their recirculation to the liver via portal flow [36]. The main bacteria involved in deconjugation are *Clostridia*, part of the *Firmicutes* phyla. It can be speculated that during liver regeneration reduced *Firmicutes* (especially *Clostridia*) lead to reduced deconjugation of BAs and consequent reduction of their reabsorption from the gut (Fig. 2.1). This mechanism regulates the ratio of intrahepatic BAs levels to remnant liver mass.

Nonetheless, BAs are essential for normal liver regeneration; in fact, it was shown that patients undergoing major hepatectomy without external biliary drainage exhibit superior liver regeneration compared to those with external biliary drainage [37]. Secondary BAs serve as the most effective agonists of the Taketa G-protein-coupled receptor 5 (TGR5) [15]. TGR5 induces the synthesis and secretion of intestinal glucagon-like peptide-1, which stimulates insulin secretion. Thyroid hormone and insulin, in conjunction with other growth factors, induce hepatocyte proliferation [15]. Therefore, the reduction of secondary BAs caused by dysbiosis reduces the activation of TGR5 and, consequently, reduces liver regeneration.

2.4.3 Short-Chain Fatty Acids

Short-chain fatty acids, most commonly acetate, propionate, and butyrate, are metabolites generated in the colon by bacterial fermentation of nondigestible carbohydrates [38]. *Firmicutes* are the main producers of butyrate, which is primarily metabolized in the intestinal epithelium, while *Bacteroidetes* generate acetate and propionate, which reach the liver where they are metabolized [32]. SCFAs facilitate liver regeneration by preserving the integrity of the gut mucosal epithelial barrier since they function as a nutrient source for colonocytes [38]. Additionally, SCFAs that reach the liver activate signaling pathways, which promote the hepatocyte cell cycle, facilitating hepatic regeneration [39]. Furthermore, during liver regeneration, SCFAs might enhance hepatic gluconeogenesis and improve the metabolic phenotype by increasing the postprandial release of the gut hormone GLP-1 and the peptide YY, known to induce hepatic regeneration [38].

2.4.4 Tryptophan

Tryptophan is an essential amino acid absorbed in the small intestine. Part of tryptophan that reaches the colon is metabolized by gut microbiota into indole and its derivatives [40]. These molecules were found to enhance intestinal barrier function by facilitating goblet cell differentiation and mucus production. Indoles can also modulate GLP-1 secretion, contributing to liver regeneration [21].

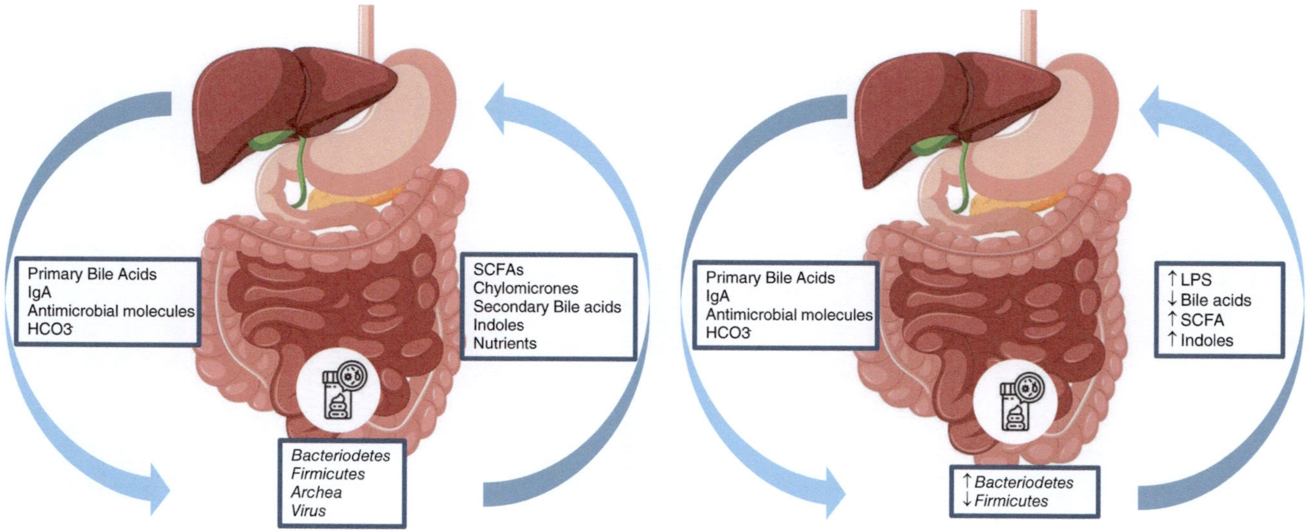

Fig. 2.1 Gut–liver axis in health and during liver regeneration. *Left panel*: In healthy conditions, gut and brain communicate via the gut–liver axis: the bidirectional relationship mediated through the portal vein, which transports nutrients, metabolites, and microbial products from the gut to the liver and the bile, which transport primary bile acids, IgA, antimicrobial other molecules, and bicarbonate ($HCO3^-$). *Right panel*: In the context of liver regeneration after liver insult, the relationship changes, and the substantial change in the composition of gut microbiota leads to increased permeability of the intestinal epithelial barrier, which leads to increased lipopolysaccharides (LPS), short-chain fatty acids (SCFA), and indole passage and reduced bile acid recirculation

2.5 Conclusion

Overall, the bidirectional relationship between the gut and the liver is crucial for the homeostasis of the entire organism. The liver is continuously exposed to compounds originating from the gut, such as microbial metabolites, which have a major impact on liver health and function. At the same time, the liver can actively modify the composition and functions of gut microbiota via the continuous flow of BAs in the enterohepatic circulation.

Although studies in humans are scant, evidence from studies in mice and rats shows that during liver regeneration there are significant changes in the composition of gut microbiota related to *Bacteroidetes* increase and *Firmicutes* decrease. Further research is needed to understand how these changes specifically correlate to liver regeneration phases. However, both preclinical and clinical studies show that the gut microbiota can influence liver regeneration after liver injury. Although limited in sample size and methodology, pivotal studies on gut microbiota modulation have shown a beneficial effect. More evidence on gut microbiota modulation will lead to the development of possible therapeutic options to support liver regeneration.

References

1. Barbara G, Barbaro MR, Fuschi D, et al. Inflammatory and microbiota-related regulation of the intestinal epithelial barrier. Front Nutr. 2021;8:718356. https://doi.org/10.3389/fnut.2021.718356.
2. Song C, Chai Z, Chen S, Zhang H, Zhang X, Zhou Y. Intestinal mucus components and secretion mechanisms: what we do and do not know. Exp Mol Med. 2023;55(4):681–91. https://doi.org/10.1038/s12276-023-00960-y.
3. Hou K, Wu ZX, Chen XY, et al. Microbiota in health and diseases. Signal Transduct Target Ther. 2022;7(1):1–28. https://doi.org/10.1038/s41392-022-00974-4.
4. Hsu CL, Schnabl B. The gut–liver axis and gut microbiota in health and liver disease. Nat Rev Microbiol. 2023;21(11):719–33. https://doi.org/10.1038/s41579-023-00904-3.
5. McCallum G, Tropini C. The gut microbiota and its biogeography. Nat Rev Microbiol. 2024;22(2):105–18. https://doi.org/10.1038/s41579-023-00969-0.
6. Fan Y, Pedersen O. Gut microbiota in human metabolic health and disease. Nat Rev Microbiol. 2020;19(1):55–71. https://doi.org/10.1038/s41579-020-0433-9.
7. Barbaro MR, Cremon C, Marasco G, et al. Molecular mechanisms underlying loss of vascular and epithelial integrity in irritable bowel syndrome. Gastroenterology. 2024;167:1152–66. https://doi.org/10.1053/j.gastro.2024.07.004.
8. Kurashima Y, Kiyono H. Mucosal ecological network of epithelium and immune cells for gut homeostasis and tissue healing. Annu Rev Immunol. 2017;35:119–47. https://doi.org/10.1146/ANNUREV-IMMUNOL-051116-052424.
9. Anderson JM, Van Itallie CM. Physiology and function of the tight junction. Cold Spring Harb Perspect Biol. 2009;1(2):a002584. https://doi.org/10.1101/CSHPERSPECT.A002584.
10. Di Tommaso N, Santopaolo F, Gasbarrini A, Ponziani FR. The gut–vascular barrier as a new protagonist in intestinal and extraintestinal diseases. Int J Mol Sci. 2023;24(2):1470. https://doi.org/10.3390/IJMS24021470.
11. König J, Wells J, Cani PD, et al. Human intestinal barrier function in health and disease. Clin Transl Gastroenterol. 2016;7(10):e196. https://doi.org/10.1038/ctg.2016.54.

12. Albillos A, de Gottardi A, Rescigno M. The gut-liver axis in liver disease: pathophysiological basis for therapy. J Hepatol. 2020;72(3):558–77. https://doi.org/10.1016/j.jhep.2019.10.003.
13. McDonald B, Zucoloto AZ, Yu IL, et al. Programing of an intravascular immune firewall by the gut microbiota protects against pathogen dissemination during infection. Cell Host Microbe. 2020;28(5):660–668.e4. https://doi.org/10.1016/J.CHOM.2020.07.014.
14. Fleishman JS, Kumar S. Bile acid metabolism and signaling in health and disease: molecular mechanisms and therapeutic targets. Signal Transduct Target Ther. 2024;9(1):97. https://doi.org/10.1038/s41392-024-01811-6.
15. Fuchs CD, Simbrunner B, Baumgartner M, Campell C, Reiberger T, Trauner M. Bile acid metabolism and signaling in liver disease. J Hepatol. 2025;82(1):134–53. https://doi.org/10.1016/j.jhep.2024.09.032.
16. Rinninella E, Raoul P, Cintoni M, et al. What is the healthy gut microbiota composition? A changing ecosystem across age, environment, diet, and diseases. Microorganisms. 2019;7(1):14. https://doi.org/10.3390/MICROORGANISMS7010014.
17. Chu M, Zhang X. Bacterial atlas of mouse gut microbiota. Cell Microbiol. 2022;2022:1–21. https://doi.org/10.1155/2022/5968814.
18. Liu HX, Santos Rocha C, Dandekar S, Wan YJY. Functional analysis of the relationship between intestinal microbiota and the expression of hepatic genes and pathways during the course of liver regeneration. J Hepatol. 2016;64:641–50.
19. Sun R, Fei F, Jin D, et al. The integrated analysis of gut microbiota and metabolome revealed steroid hormone biosynthesis is a critical pathway in liver regeneration after 2/3 partial hepatectomy. Front Pharmacol. 2024;15:1407401. https://doi.org/10.3389/fphar.2024.1407401.
20. Bao Q, Yu L, Chen D, Li L. Variation in the gut microbial community is associated with the progression of liver regeneration. Hepatol Res. 2020;50(1):121–36. https://doi.org/10.1111/HEPR.13424.
21. Xu Z, Jiang N, Xiao Y, Yuan K, Wang Z. The role of gut microbiota in liver regeneration. Front Immunol. 2022;13:1003376. https://doi.org/10.3389/fimmu.2022.1003376.
22. Michalopoulos GK, Bhushan B. Liver regeneration: biological and pathological mechanisms and implications. Nat Rev Gastroenterol Hepatol. 2021;18(1):40–55. https://doi.org/10.1038/S41575-020-0342-4.
23. Amin AR, Hairulhisyam NM, Aqilah RNF, et al. Impact of gut recolonization on liver regeneration: hepatic matrisome gene expression after partial hepatectomy in mice. Int J Mol Sci. 2023;24(13):10774. https://doi.org/10.3390/IJMS241310774.
24. Cornell RP, Liljequist BL, Bartizal KF. Depressed liver regeneration after partial hepatectomy of germ–free, athymic and lipopolysaccharide–resistant mice. Hepatology. 1990;11(6):916–22. https://doi.org/10.1002/hep.1840110603.
25. Wu X, Sun R, Chen Y, et al. Oral ampicillin inhibits liver regeneration by breaking hepatic innate immune tolerance normally maintained by gut commensal bacteria. Hepatology. 2015;62(1):253–64. https://doi.org/10.1002/HEP.27791.
26. Yin Y, Sichler A, Ecker J, et al. Gut microbiota promote liver regeneration through hepatic membrane phospholipid biosynthesis. J Hepatol. 2023;78(4):820–35. https://doi.org/10.1016/j.jhep.2022.12.028.
27. Leng L, Ma J, Lv L, et al. Serum proteome profiling provides a deep understanding of the "gut-liver axis" in relation to liver injury and regeneration. Acta Biochim Biophys Sin Shanghai. 2021;53(3):372–80. https://doi.org/10.1093/abbs/gmab001.
28. Meyerovich G, Klausner JM, Cohen SJ, Lubezky N. Manipulation of intestinal microbiome composition affects liver regeneration after 70% hepatectomy in a murine model. HPB. 2020;22:S7–8. https://doi.org/10.1016/J.HPB.2020.04.794.
29. Miyazaki M, Kohda S, Itoh H, et al. Inhibition of hepatic regeneration after 70% partial hepatectomy by simultaneous resection of the bowel in rats. Eur Surg Res. 1995;27(6):396–405. https://doi.org/10.1159/000129426.
30. Rayes N, Pilarski T, Stockmann M, Bengmark S, Neuhaus P, Seehofer D. Effect of pre- and probiotics on liver regeneration after resection: a randomised, double-blind pilot study. Benef Microbes. 2012;3(3):237–44. https://doi.org/10.3920/BM2012.0006.

31. Gan Y, Su S, Li B, Fang C. Efficacy of probiotics and prebiotics in prevention of infectious complications following hepatic resections: systematic review and meta-analysis. J Gastrointestin Liver Dis. 2019;28:205–11. https://doi.org/10.15403/jgld-182.
32. Zheng Z, Wang B. The gut-liver axis in health and disease: the role of gut microbiota-derived signals in liver injury and regeneration. Front Immunol. 2021;12:775526. https://doi.org/10.3389/fimmu.2021.775526.
33. Barchetta I, Cimini FA, Sentinelli F, et al. Reduced lipopolysaccharide-binding protein (LBP) levels are associated with non-alcoholic fatty liver disease (NAFLD) and adipose inflammation in human obesity. Int J Mol Sci. 2023;24(24):17174. https://doi.org/10.3390/ijms242417174.
34. Taub R. Liver regeneration: from myth to mechanism. Nat Rev Mol Cell Biol. 2004;5(10):836–47. https://doi.org/10.1038/nrm1489.
35. Cornell RP. Restriction of gut-derived endotoxin impairs DNA synthesis for liver regeneration. Am J Phys Regul Integr Comp Phys. 1985;249(5):R563–9. https://doi.org/10.1152/ajpregu.1985.249.5.R563.
36. Liu HX, Keane R, Sheng L, Yvonne Wan YJ. Implications of microbiota and bile acid in liver injury and regeneration. J Hepatol. 2015;63(6):1502–10.
37. Otao R, Beppu T, Isiko T, et al. External biliary drainage and liver regeneration after major hepatectomy. Br J Surg. 2012;99(11):1569–74. https://doi.org/10.1002/bjs.8906.
38. Morrison DJ, Preston T. Formation of short chain fatty acids by the gut microbiota and their impact on human metabolism. Gut Microbes. 2016;7(3):189–200. https://doi.org/10.1080/19490976.2015.1134082.
39. Koh A, De Vadder F, Kovatcheva-Datchary P, Bäckhed F. From dietary fiber to host physiology: short-chain fatty acids as key bacterial metabolites. Cell. 2016;165(6):1332–45. https://doi.org/10.1016/J.CELL.2016.05.041/ASSET/95008553-7832-494E-9FD9-91A065597DE1/MAIN.ASSETS/GR4.JPG.
40. Platten M, Nollen EAA, Röhrig UF, Fallarino F, Opitz CA. Tryptophan metabolism as a common therapeutic target in cancer, neurodegeneration and beyond. Nat Rev Drug Discov. 2019;18(5):379–401. https://doi.org/10.1038/s41573-019-0016-5.

3 Metabolic Factors Affecting Liver Regeneration

Markus Ammann and Patrick Starlinger

3.1 Introduction

Liver regeneration is a tightly regulated process involving hepatocyte and non-parenchymal cell proliferation, along with extracellular matrix remodeling. This process is triggered by stimuli such as partial hepatectomy, toxic injury, or viral infection, as demonstrated in liver regeneration models [1]. The metabolic demands are substantial, requiring hepatic metabolism to reorganize in order to sustain both cellular proliferation and essential liver functions [2].

This chapter explores the metabolic factors influencing liver regeneration, with a focus on glucose, lipid, and amino acid metabolism, as well as mitochondrial function. We will examine how these pathways are altered during regeneration and discuss potential metabolic interventions to enhance recovery. Given its central metabolic role, the liver must balance with the increased energy and biosynthetic needs of proliferating cells. The balance of glucose homeostasis, lipid, and protein synthesis is maintained through intricate signaling networks integrating metabolic cues with growth factor signaling and cell cycle regulation [3].

Clinically, impaired regenerative capacity in chronic liver disease can lead to liver failure, emphasizing the need for therapies that enhance regeneration [4]. In liver surgery and transplantation, optimizing metabolic conditions may improve outcomes. Liver regeneration is not merely an increase in energy production but rather a sophisticated metabolic reprogramming tailored to the needs of regenerating tissue.

M. Ammann
Department of General, Visceral and Vascular Surgery, University Clinic Wiener Neustadt, Wiener Neustadt, Austria

P. Starlinger (✉)
Department of Hepatobiliary and Pancreas Surgery, Mayo Clinic, Rochester, MN, USA
e-mail: Starlinger.patrick@mayo.edu

L. Aldrighetti et al. (eds.), *Liver Regeneration Techniques In Hepatic Surgery*,
https://doi.org/10.1007/978-3-032-10997-2_3

3.2 Role of Metabolism in Liver Regeneration

Liver regeneration is closely linked to its metabolic functions. As the central organ for metabolic homeostasis, the liver must coordinate metabolic shifts to support regeneration while maintaining homeostasis. This requires significant *metabolic reprogramming* to meet the energy and biosynthetic demands of proliferating hepatocytes. Glucose-derived carbons are redirected toward *macromolecule synthesis* rather than *ATP production*, similar to the Warburg effect in tumor cells, which is essential for cell proliferation [2]. Moreover, optimal *mitochondrial function* is critical for successful regeneration [5]. The liver's unique architecture, characterized by a *metabolic zonation* and a distinct metabolic profile of hepatocytes along the periportal-pericentral gradient, plays a crucial role in shaping the regenerative process [6, 7]. Several key *metabolic sensors and signaling pathways* integrate metabolic cues with the regenerative response [8]:

1. *AMPK* (AMP-activated protein kinase): regulates metabolism and cell growth in response to energy availability.
2. *mTOR* (mammalian target of rapamycin): responds to nutrient and growth factors, controlling protein synthesis and proliferation.
3. *SIRT1* (Sirtuin 1): links metabolism to epigenetic regulation via NAD + -dependent deacetylation.
4. *PPARα* (peroxisome proliferator-activated receptor alpha): regulates fatty acid oxidation and is important for the metabolic adaptations during early regeneration.
5. *PGC-1α* (PPARγ coactivator 1- α): coordinates mitochondrial biogenesis and metabolic adaptation during regeneration.

Additionally, cellular metabolism has also been linked to *epigenetic regulations* affecting histone acetylation [9] and DNA methylation [10] (Fig. 3.1).

3.3 Glucose Metabolism and Liver Regeneration

In most mammalian tissues, glucose is primarily catabolized via glycolysis, producing pyruvate as a key ATP-generating pathway. Inside mitochondria, the pyruvate dehydrogenase complex converts it into acetyl-CoA, which then enters the tricarboxylic acid (TCA) cycle, condensing with oxaloacetate to generate ATP (GPT), along with NADH and FADH2, serving as electron carriers for oxidative phosphorylation (OXPHOS) [11].

During fasting, the liver plays a central role in maintaining glucose homeostasis by supplying glucose through glycogenolysis and gluconeogenesis.

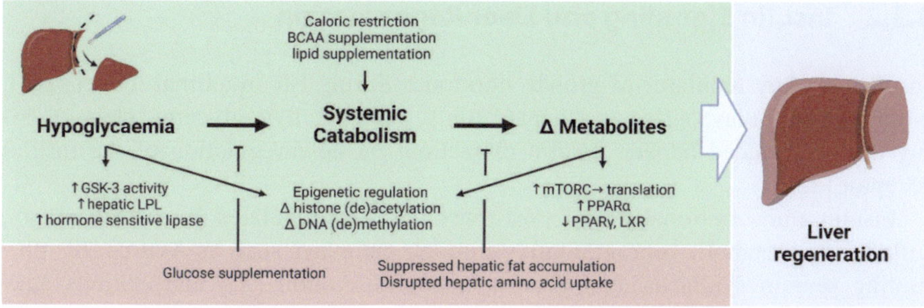

Fig. 3.1 Metabolic concept of liver regeneration. Hypoglycemia plays a critical role in inducing systemic catabolism, promoting lipid and amino acid mobilization, which influences epigenetic regulation and activates key metabolic pathways involved in cell proliferation. Counteracting hypoglycemia or fat accumulation negatively impacts liver regeneration. BCAA, branched-chain amino acids; GSK-3, glycogen synthase kinase-3; LPL, lipoprotein lipase; mTORC, mechanistic target of rapamycin complex; PPARα, peroxisome proliferator-activated receptor α; PPARγ, peroxisome proliferator-activated receptor γ; LXR, liver X receptor. (Graphic created with BioRender.com)

3.3.1 Alterations of Glucose Metabolism During Liver Regeneration

Following liver resection, mice develop hypoglycemia within hours due to the loss of hepatic glycogen stores and gluconeogenic capacity [12], leading to an upregulation of hepatic gluconeogenesis, while glycolytic activity is suppressed. This hypoglycemic state has been repeatedly shown to be essential for liver regeneration [2]. (Figure 3.1) Key metabolic reprogramming events include

- *Downregulation of glycolysis:* Inhibition of glucokinase (GK), the rate-limiting enzyme of glycolysis [13], and inhibition of liver-specific phosphofructokinase-1 (L-PFK), thereby reducing glycolytic flux and prioritizing gluconeogenesis [14]. Additionally, there is a shift from liver-type pyruvate kinase (PK-L) to its less-active M2 isoform (PK-M2), slowing the final step of glycolysis, diverting glucose-derived carbon from ATP production toward macromolecule precursor synthesis (similar to the Warburg effect) [15, 16].
- *Glycogen depletion:* Glycogen synthase kinase 3 (GSK3) suppresses glycogen synthesis, thereby contributing to postoperative hypoglycemia [2]. Additionally, GSK3 regulates the Wnt/β-catenin pathway, crucial for liver regeneration initiation [17], and phosphorylates transcription factors and cell cycle regulators involved in the process [18].
- *Upregulation of the pentose phosphate pathway (PPP):* Induction of PPP via increased expression of glucose-6-phosphate dehydrogenase (G6PD) and transketolase is supplying ribose-5-phosphate for nucleotide synthesis and DNA replication, [19] as well as NADPH and glutathione, for oxidative stress response [20]. The metabolic shift from glucose to PPP is facilitated by nuclear erythroid 2-related factor 2 (Nrf2) [21].

3.3.2 Insulin Signaling and Liver Regeneration

Insulin is a key regulator of growth hormones during LR in animal models [22]. Notably, insulin levels rise post-hepatectomy, even in a hypoglycemic state, possibly due to reduced hepatic insulin extraction via downregulation of the insulin receptor [22].

Insulin transcriptionally and post-translationally regulates liver metabolism, influencing metabolic reprogramming through pathways such as Akt/mTOR, promoting protein synthesis, cell growth, and proliferation [23] and exhibits anti-apoptotic and anti-inflammatory effects [24].

3.4 Lipid Metabolism in Liver Regeneration

Lipid metabolism plays a crucial role in liver regeneration (LR), providing energy, membrane components, and signaling molecules. Post-hepatectomy, hepatic lipid metabolism undergoes profound shifts, including increased lipid mobilization, trafficking, oxidation, and synthesis [25]. These changes result in transient regeneration-associated steatosis (TRAS), stemming from import of mobilized peripheral lipid stores, which is regulated by circulating cytokines and metabolites [26]. (Figure 3.1) Importantly, the dynamic nature of both lipid accumulation and its timely resolution are critical for effective regeneration [26, 27].

3.4.1 Lipid Droplets and Transient Hepatic Steatosis in Liver Regeneration

Lipid droplets (LDs), once regarded as passive storage organelles, are now recognized as dynamic structures essential for liver regeneration (LR). During early LR, hepatocytes transiently accumulate LDs, which seems critical given their prevention impairs LR [2]. This transient regeneration-associated steatosis (TRAS) reflects a complex, time-dependent metabolic adaptation, serving as [28, 29]

- *Energy reservoirs*: storing triglycerides (TG) for lipolysis, providing fatty acids for β-oxidation.
- *Membrane precursors*: supplying phospholipids and cholesterol for hepatocyte proliferation.
- *Signaling platforms*: interacting with mitochondria and the endoplasmic reticulum to regulate metabolic pathways.

Peripherally derived fatty acids, mobilized from hypoglycemia-induced adipose tissue lipolysis, increase in plasma, during TRAS [12], elevating hepatic TG and cholesterol levels [30–32]. Although TRAS is widely considered necessary for LR, results from genetic and conditional models have been inconsistent, with outcomes varying based on whether import (Caveolin-1), storage (Plin2), or mobilization (TM6SF2, PNPLA3) was disrupted [26].

The regulation of fatty acid synthesis and lipogenesis during LR remains unclear as some studies report downregulation [33], while others observe increased expression of key lipogenic enzymes, including acetyl-CoA carboxylase (ACC) and fatty acid synthase (FASN) [31, 34] (Fig. 3.2).

Failure in lipid accumulation but also delayed TRAS resolution due to compromised β-oxidation impairs LR [35].

3.4.2 Fatty Acid Oxidation and Energy Production

Fatty acid oxidation is the primary source of energy (ATP) in the early stage of LR [28]. Mitochondrial β-oxidation is upregulated [8], generating acetyl-CoA, which

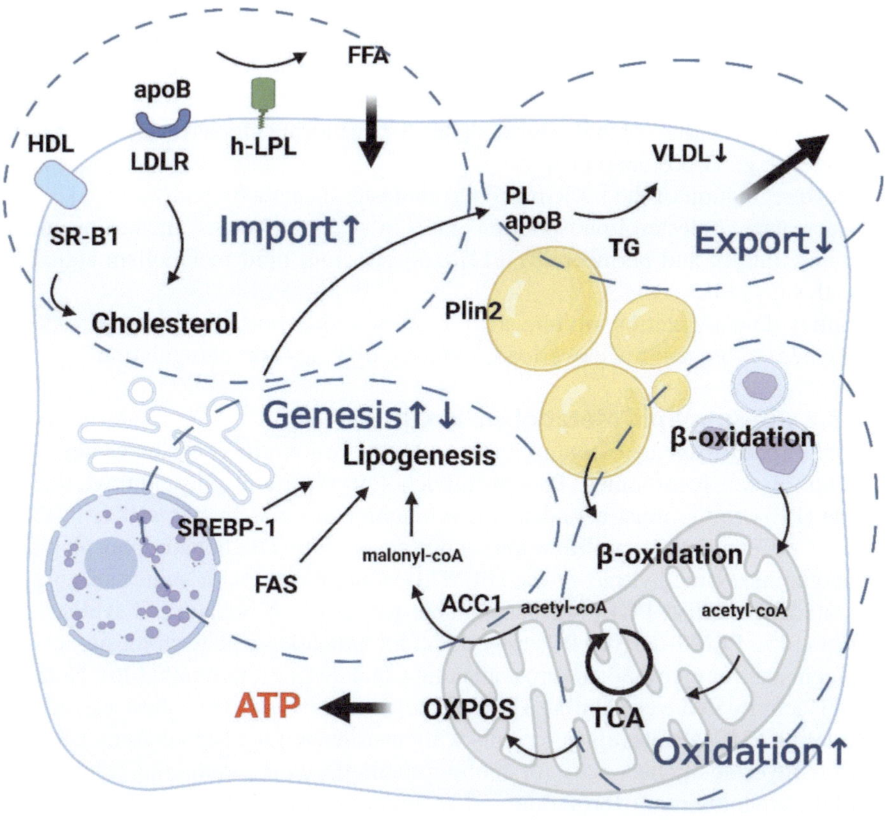

Fig. 3.2 Theoretical concept or TRAS formation. Hepatic lipid accumulation results from increased lipid import and reduced export. While the regulation of de novo fatty acid synthesis remains unclear, it is likely timepoint- and context-dependent. Lipid oxidation is upregulated to enhance ATP production during liver regeneration. (Graphic created with BioRender.com)

enters the TCA cycle. The transcription factor peroxisome proliferator-activated receptor alpha (PPARα) plays a central regulatory role by inducing lipid catabolism genes, including carnitine palmitoyl transferase 1A (CPT1) [5] and acyl-CoA dehydrogenases (ACAD) [41]. Additionally, PGC-1α promotes peroxisomal β-oxidation by upregulating acyl-CoA oxidase 1 (ACOX1) and peroxisomal bifunctional enzyme (PBFE) [36, 37].

3.4.3 Cholesterol, Phospholipid, and Lipoprotein Metabolism

3.4.3.1 Cholesterol Metabolism in LR

The liver plays a central role in cholesterol homeostasis, serving as the primary site of cholesterol biosynthesis and excretion [38]. Cholesterol is essential for membrane structure and bile acid synthesis. During LR, cholesterol metabolism undergoes several key alterations [39]:

- Intrahepatic cholesterol increases with decreased circulating levels.
- Downregulated 3-hydroxy-3-methylglutaryl-coenzyme A reductase (HMG-CoA R) gene expression and cholesterol synthesis, and shifting toward the mevalonate pathway, providing prenyl intermediates for anchoring signal transduction molecules (e.g., G-proteins) [40].
- Downregulation of the LXR-mediated cholesterol catabolic pathway [41].
- Decreased cholesterol/phospholipid ratio in cell membranes, increasing membrane fluidity and permeability [42], and affecting lipid metabolism signaling pathways [43].
- Initial downregulation of bile acid synthesis via cholesterol 7α-hydroxylase (Cyp7a) to prevent toxic overload, followed by long-term upregulation.

3.4.3.2 Phospholipid Metabolism in LR

Phospholipids (PLs) are essential for hepatocyte proliferation, serving as key components of cell membranes. Phosphatidylcholine (PC) and phosphatidylethanolamine (PE) are the most abundant PL in mammalian membranes and critical for cellular differentiation, proliferation, and regeneration. The hepatic phosphatidylethanolamine N-methyltransferase (PEMT) pathway is a major source of polyunsaturated PC (PUFA-PC) [44], accountable for ~30% of hepatic PC synthesis in rodents [45]. PEMT-derived PCs are critical for arachidonic acid synthesis, serving as precursors for eicosanoids (prostaglandins, leukotrienes, lipoxins) [46]. Notably, PEMT activity decreases during LR [47], supported by our data, showing reduced circulating PUFA-PC levels in patients with insufficient post-hepatectomy LR [48].

PCs are critically necessary for apolipoprotein B (apoB)-containing lipoproteins (VLDL, chylomicrons) formation and secretion [49, 50]. Reduced PC synthesis leading to lipid retention in hepatocytes [51], and alterations in hepatic PL composition have been linked to impaired LR [52].

3.4.3.3 Lipoprotein Metabolism in LR

Lipoprotein metabolism is closely integrated with lipid mobilization, storage, and utilization during LR. Notably, lipoprotein lipase, typically absent in the liver, is expressed after partial hepatectomy to hydrolyze TGs from circulating very low-density lipoproteins (VLDL) and chylomicrons [53].

ApoA1, the major protein constituent of high-density lipoproteins (HDL), facilitates cholesterol ester uptake from peripheral tissues via ATP-binding cassette transporter A1 (ABCA1) and lecithin-cholesterol acyltransferase (LCAT), during reverse cholesterol transport [54] and regulates mitochondrial energy metabolism [55], and biogenesis [56]. In line with this, our data show significant reductions in circulating HDL during human LR [57].

ApoB is produced in two isoforms: apoB-100 (liver) and apoB-48 (intestine). After liver resection, circulating apoB levels decline [58] associated with reduced lipid export via VLDL [59]. Initially, VLDL secretion declines but later surges to prevent pathological steatosis [60]. Mutations affecting VLDL secretion (e.g., TM6SF2, PNPLA3) impair LR [61].

The hepatic LDL receptor (LDLR), facilitating apoB-containing lipoprotein uptake, is upregulated during LR [71], enabling cholesterol import from the periphery [12]. LDLR knockout disrupts early cytokine expression (IL-6, TNFα, HGF), essential for LR initiation, and alters PL metabolism, particularly PC synthesis, impairing hepatocyte proliferation [62].

3.4.4 Sphingolipid Metabolism in Liver Regeneration

Sphingolipids are essential components of cell membranes and key regulators of cellular signaling, playing a critical role in immune regulation, cell proliferation, survival, and apoptosis by acting as auto- and paracrine mediators [63].

During LR, sphingolipid synthesis is upregulated, altering the balance between sphingomyelin, ceramide, sphingosine-1-phosphate (S1P) [64]., collectively influencing hepatocyte proliferation, survival, and apoptosis [63], S1P, for example, interacts with HGF and promotes IL-6 production by liver sinusoidal endothelial cells (LSECs), enhancing hepatocyte proliferation [65].

3.5 Amino Acid Metabolism and Protein Synthesis

Amino acid (AA) metabolism and protein synthesis are essential for liver regeneration (LR), providing critical building blocks for cell growth and proliferation. The liver plays a central role in AA metabolism, serving as the primary site for systemic protein synthesis and degradation, additionally utilizing AAs for gluconeogenesis during periods of starvation and LR.

Beyond being necessary for protein synthesis, AA availability is crucial for regulating cell proliferation via activation of the mTOR pathway [66] and its downstream target, S6 kinase [67], further promoting cell cycle progression by enhancing the translation of key proteins, such as cyclin D1 [68].

3.5.1 Role of Amino Acids in Regeneration

Amino acid (AA) metabolism is crucial during LR, with several key changes observed:

- *Branched-chain amino acids (BCAA)*: leucine, isoleucine, and valine support LR [69] by stimulating protein synthesis and cell growth via the mTOR pathway [66] (Fig. 3.1).
- *Tryptophan,* once converted to serotonin (delivered by platelets through tryptophan hydroxylase), supports LR [70], repeatedly demonstrated, also in the human setting [71].
- *Glutamine* serves as a fuel source and precursor for nucleotide synthesis. Uptake and utilization of glutamine are increased during LR [72]. Glutaminase activity increases, converting glutamine into glutamate, further processed into α-ketoglutarate (α-KG) can enter the TCA cycle [73].
- *Arginine,* as a precursor for nitric oxide (NO) formation, promotes LR through vasodilation and increases hepatic blood flow [74].

3.5.2 Urea Cycle and Nitrogen Balance

The urea cycle is essential for maintaining nitrogen balance during LR. Increased protein catabolism is paralleled by ammonia production. During the early stages of LR, there is a transient decrease in the activity of urea cycle enzymes, leading to the accumulation of AA necessary for protein synthesis [75]. However, a tight regulation is necessary to prevent ammonia toxicity, which can compromise LR [2].

3.5.3 Hepatic Protein Synthesis during Liver Regeneration

Protein synthesis is markedly upregulated during LR, with significant increases in ribosomal RNA synthesis and polyribosome formation, in order to produce new cellular components, enzymes, and growth factors required for LR. Several factors regulate hepatic protein synthesis during LR:

- *Growth factors:* HGF and epidermal growth factor (EGF) stimulate protein synthesis and cell proliferation [76].
- *Cytokines:* IL-6 and TNF-α are key in initiating the regenerative response and modulating protein synthesis [76].
- *Hormones:* insulin and glucagon regulate AA uptake and protein synthesis via the insulin/AKT pathway [77].

- *Nutrient-sensing pathways*: the mTOR pathway integrates signals from growth factors, AA, and energy status to regulate protein synthesis and cell proliferation [78].

In response to AA starvation, the general control nonderepressible 2 (GCN2) kinase regulates efficient protein synthesis according to AA availability [79].

3.6 Mitochondrial Function and Energy Metabolism

Mitochondrial function and flexibility are pivotal in LR, providing ATP via OXPHOS during heightened metabolic demands in LR. Studies have demonstrated that mitochondrial DNA content and expression of genes involved in OXPHOS increase significantly following partial hepatectomy [36]. Impairment of mitochondrial function, such as complex I inhibition, can severely hinder LR by reducing ATP availability [80].

Oxidative stress associated with LR can affect mitochondrial function and dynamics [81]. While a certain level of ROS is necessary for activating regenerative signaling pathways, excessive ROS production can cause mitochondrial damage and impair regeneration [82].

Metabolic flexibility, the ability to switch between different fuel sources, is essential for successful LR and is regulated via AMPK [83], PGC-1α, and Sirtuins [8].

Recent studies suggested a quality control process for mitochondria during LR. Mitochondria with malfunctioning electron chain transport (ECT) are inhibited from generating acetyl-CoA by blocking pyruvate dehydrogenase 4 (PDK4) and Acyl-CoA synthetase short-chain family member 2 (ACSS2). This results in the accumulation of long-chain fatty acids, preventing the breakdown of carbohydrates and acetyl-CoA synthesis from pyruvate, affecting energy production, epigenetic regulation of chromatin acetylation, and membrane lipid production [5] and ultimately sequestration via mitophagy, removing damaged mitochondria [84].

3.7 Metabolic Dysfunction-Associated Steatotic Liver Disease (MASLD)

Liver regeneration (LR) can be significantly affected by underlying liver diseases that alter hepatic metabolism. Understanding how these pathological conditions impact regenerative capacity is essential for developing targeted therapies and improving patient outcomes.

Metabolic dysfunction-associated steatotic liver disease (MASLD) is the most prevalent liver disease and represents a major public health concern, affecting approximately 25% of the Western population. Of these, 25% progress to the more advanced stage of metabolic dysfunction-associated steatohepatitis (MASH), which involves significant inflammation and can lead to fibrosis and cirrhosis [85].

While transient steatosis (TRAS) occurs during normal LR, chronic hepatic steatosis is commonly associated with impaired LR after partial hepatectomy in most experimental models. However, conclusions must be drawn with caution as different genetic and pharmacological/nutritional models were used to induce the steatotic phenotype, which may not directly translate to the human genesis of MASLD [86].

Interestingly, the model most closely resembling human MASH formation is a Western diet-fed model, where mice develop steatosis, insulin resistance, and diabetes depending on the duration of exposure (6–26 weeks). Remarkably, mice with short-term exposure displayed improved LR compared to standard-diet fed mice [87], underscoring the impact of magnitude and duration of chronic steatosis linked to the detrimental effect on LR.

A meta-analysis by Meijer et al. revealed steatosis in humans associated with postoperative morbidity, but mortality was increased only in advanced stage of macrovesicular steatosis of >30% [88]. Whether detrimental outcomes are due to postoperative liver failure or complications linked to metabolic syndrome-associated predispositions remains unclear.

It is important to acknowledge that the histological phenotype of steatosis in human liver resection specimens is multifactorial, including metabolic syndrome, chemotherapy-associated liver injury (CALI), other noxious agents (including alcoholic steatohepatitis, ALD), or combinations of these (MASH+ASH = MetALD). It is possible that the steatotic phenotype from chronic liver injury represents both the effector of liver injury from lipotoxicity and steatosis associated with chronic repair mechanisms.

Steatotic livers seem more vulnerable to ischemia/reperfusion injury, which can occur during liver resections (e.g., Pringle maneuver) and liver transplantation, [89] due to incompletely oxidized substrates from mitochondrial dysfunction and ROS formation, [90] impairing critical metabolic pathways and triggering inflammatory cascades, heightening the risk of overall operative morbidity [91].

Given the presumed link between liver steatosis and impaired LR, several interventions aimed at reducing hepatic lipid content to improve postoperative outcomes have been explored.

These include lifestyle management (dietary measures and physical exercise) and pharmacological interventions such as GLP-1 analogs or pioglitazone [92]. However, in the context of liver surgery, these interventions may not succeed within the short time frame between planning and execution of liver resections. Metabolic preconditioning has been successfully used to reduce perioperative complications in nonhepatic surgeries, but its applicability to liver surgery, given the specific complications arising from impaired LR, has not been supported by data and can only be extrapolated from experimental models. Notably, in one study, reducing hepatic lipid content in mice undergoing partial hepatectomy by administering GLP-1 analogs impaired LR [93].

Current evidence does not support steatosis as a direct cause of impaired liver regeneration. Rather, it may serve as a nonspecific marker of underlying disease.

Whether improving steatosis alone, without addressing associated metabolic and cardiovascular risk factors, yields benefits remains unclear.

3.8 Interventional Considerations

3.8.1 Glucose Administration

Postoperative hypoglycemia is a critical factor influencing LR. Both oral and parenteral glucose supplementation have been reported detrimental in experimental models of liver resection and caloric restriction was identified to trigger hepatocyte proliferation. The role of insulin in LR has been debated, with studies dating back to the 1970s presenting contrasting results on whether insulin acts as a promoter or inhibitor of regeneration. The effects of insulin may depend on the specific context in which it is administered [2].

3.8.2 Lipid Substitution

It has been shown that both parenteral and oral substitutions of various lipid formulations enhance LR in experimental hepatectomy models. Parenteral lipid emulsions and carnitine, which facilitates the uptake of acyl-groups into mitochondria, have been demonstrated to accelerate LR [69]. Additionally, dietary supplementation with palmitate and carnitine has been shown to augment LR in toxin-induced injury models [94].

3.8.3 Choline Supplementation

Choline depletion in animal diets induces fatty liver formation, often used as a model for liver disease [95]. While choline substitution has been proven to reverse fatty liver formation in this model, its effect on improving LR in humans is less clear. However, it has been shown to improve MASLD and prevent progression to MASH and cirrhosis and can influence DNA methylation [96].

3.8.4 Amino Acid Supplementation

BCAAs are known to regulate mTOR signaling [97] and stimulate the secretion of HGF from hepatic stellate cells (HSC), promoting liver cell proliferation [98]. One study found that administering BCAAs as part of an emulsion of lipids and dextrose after liver resections for hepatocellular carcinoma (HCC) reduced postoperative complications. Another study reported improved physical performance in patients who received BCAA supplementation for 1 year postoperatively [99]. Additionally, supplementation with BCAAs prior to portal vein embolization (PVE) followed by major hepatic resection resulted in improved liver function after resection over the subsequent 6 months [100].

Glutamine supplementation has been shown to enhance liver regeneration in experimental models by increasing mitosis, promoting cell proliferation, and protein synthesis, thereby improving liver function [101]. L-arginine supplementation boosting NO production has also been shown beneficial in rodent LR [102].

3.8.5 Statins and Fibrates

Inhibition of the rate-limiting step in cholesterol synthesis, 5-hydroxy-3-methylglu taryl-coenzyme A (HMG-CoA) reductase, by statins has been speculated to improve LR. Statins not only impact cholesterol metabolism but also increase LDLR expression in the liver, reduce mevalonate and isoprenoid levels, and modulate intracellular signaling proteins. Additionally, statins promote hepatic angiogenesis and modulate the acute phase response by influencing margination, chemotaxis, and improving microcirculation by preventing microthrombi formation [103]. Studies in mouse partial hepatectomy models have shown low-dose statins improve LR [104]. In humans, statins have been associated with better disease-free survival after hepatocellular carcinoma (HCC) resection in cirrhosis [105]. Furthermore, perioperative statin use was shown to reduce the risk of post-hepatectomy liver failure (PHLF) [103].

Fibrates, which are PPARα agonists and widely used to treat hyperlipidemia [106], have effects beyond lipid regulation, including the modulation of hepatic glucose and bile acid homeostasis, oxidative stress, and inflammatory responses [107]. One experimental study demonstrated that fibrates modulate PPARα interaction with YAP-TEAD transcriptional activity, a key regulator of cell proliferation [108, 109]. However, in the context of postoperative LR, fibrates can hinder the formation of transient hepatic regenerative activity (TRAS) and have been shown to impede LR [2]. In humans, fibrates have been shown to improve liver function in patients with underlying liver disease [110], although their effects in surgical cohorts have yet to be tested.

3.8.6 PCSK9 Inhibitors

Protein convertase subtilisin/kexin type 9 (PCSK9) inhibition has been identified as a promising treatment for both alcoholic [111] and nonalcoholic fatty liver disease [112]. Mechanistically, PCSK9 promotes the degradation of LDLR. Systemic or hepatocyte-specific knockdown of PCSK9 reduces plasma cholesterol levels but increases liver lipid content. PCSK9 inhibition enhances LDL-cholesterol uptake and decreases circulating LDL cholesterol levels. The mechanisms underlying PCSK9 inhibition are multifaceted and its effects on LR are complex. It increases fatty acid transport, inhibits VLDL production, and decreases hepatic lipogenesis, ultimately reducing plasma hyperlipidemia and hepatic steatosis [26]. Although these effects may be beneficial for LR, studies in mouse models have shown that PCSK9 knockout impairs LR [113]. The net impact of PCSK9 inhibition on LR requires further investigation.

3.8.7 GLP-1 and GLP-2

Glucagon-like peptide-1 (GLP-1) and glucagon-like peptide-2 (GLP-2) are incretin hormones secreted by enteroendocrine L-cells. GLP-1 has long been utilized in diabetes therapy for its role in promoting insulin secretion. More recently, it has been indicated for obesity treatment, reducing body weight and hepatic lipid content through its effects on lipid metabolism. Mechanistically, GLP-1 decreases lipid absorption, chylomicron formation, lipogenesis, and VLDL production, ultimately lowering circulating triglycerides, cholesterol, and LDL levels, thereby reducing hepatic lipid content and cardiovascular risk. However, these metabolic changes have been linked to impaired LR. A study in rodents found that perioperative GLP-1 analog administration reduced LR after partial hepatectomy [93]. Similarly, our human cohort data associated elevated preoperative endogenous GLP-1 levels with poorer outcomes and increased PHLF risk [48].

Conversely, GLP-2, secreted in parallel with GLP-1 in response to the same stimuli, exerts opposing effects on lipid metabolism. It enhances lipid absorption, ApoB48 production, chylomicron and VLDL formation, and circulating lipid pools, including triglycerides and cholesterol, contributing to hepatic steatosis. In rodent hepatectomy models, GLP-2 supplementation increased hepatocyte proliferation [114]. Additionally, GLP-2 supports intestinal barrier function, exhibits immunomodulatory properties, enhances portal venous flow via NO formation, and influences bile acid homeostasis [57]. In our human study, postoperative endogenous GLP-2 secretion increased after liver resection, particularly in cases of PHLF, suggesting a potential rescue mechanism during liver failure, representing a potential therapeutic target. Moreover, GLP-2 supplementation has been reported to mitigate hepatic injury associated with long-term parenteral nutrition in short bowel syndrome [115].

3.9 Future Perspectives

Liver regeneration relies on highly conserved metabolic mechanisms, underscored by alternative fluxes in conditions of specific substrate accumulation. This is evident in the persistence of liver regeneration-associated hepatic steatosis, even when key pathways are pharmacologically inhibited or genetically disrupted. Studies in models with liver-specific deletions (e.g., glucocorticoid receptors, liver fatty acid-binding protein, intestine-specific microsomal transfer protein, caveolin-1, leptin, etc.) demonstrate that single impairment not always fully abrogates LR. Instead, multiple metabolic pathways operate in parallel, enabling alternative routes to compensate for disrupted fluxes, which complicates the interpretation of single-gene knockout models.

To ensure translational relevance, liver regeneration models should closely reflect human physiology. Emerging technologies, such as spatial metabolomics, enhance our ability to dissect metabolic alterations in a zonation-dependent manner. Identifying targetable metabolic pathways through such approaches may improve therapeutic strategies.

A fundamental feature of metabolic reprogramming during regeneration is its transient nature. As our understanding of these dynamics advances, metabolic parameters will become integral to liver function assessment and prognostic tools, aiding in patient stratification for liver surgery.

References

1. Michalopoulos GK. Principles of liver regeneration and growth homeostasis. Compr Physiol. 2013;3(1):485–513.
2. Huang J, Rudnick DA. Elucidating the metabolic regulation of liver regeneration. Am J Pathol. 2014;184(2):309–21.
3. Tao Y, Wang M, Chen E, Tang H. Liver regeneration: analysis of the main relevant signaling molecules. Mediat Inflamm. 2017;2017:4256352.
4. Forbes SJ, Newsome PN. Liver regeneration – mechanisms and models to clinical application. Nat Rev Gastroenterol Hepatol. 2016;13(8):473–85.
5. Wang X, Menezes CJ, Jia Y, Xiao Y, Venigalla SSK, Cai F, et al. Metabolic inflexibility promotes mitochondrial health during liver regeneration. Science. 2024;384(6701):eadj4301.
6. Chembazhi UV, Bangru S, Hernaez M, Kalsotra A. Cellular plasticity balances the metabolic and proliferation dynamics of a regenerating liver. Genome Res. 2021;31(4):576–91.
7. Santos AA, Delgado TC, Marques V, Ramirez-Moncayo C, Alonso C, Vidal-Puig A, et al. Spatial metabolomics and its application in the liver. Hepatology. 2024;79(5):1158–79.
8. Abu Shelbayeh O, Arroum T, Morris S, Busch KB. PGC-1alpha is a master regulator of mitochondrial lifecycle and ROS stress response. Antioxidants (Basel). 2023;12(5):1075.
9. Huang J, Barr E, Rudnick DA. Characterization of the regulation and function of zinc-dependent histone deacetylases during rodent liver regeneration. Hepatology. 2013;57(5):1742–51.
10. Chen L, Zeng Y, Yang H, Lee TD, French SW, Corrales FJ, et al. Impaired liver regeneration in mice lacking methionine adenosyltransferase 1A. FASEB J. 2004;18(7):914–6.
11. Han HS, Kang G, Kim JS, Choi BH, Koo SH. Regulation of glucose metabolism from a liver-centric perspective. Exp Mol Med. 2016;48(3):e218.
12. Rudnick DA, Davidson NO. Functional relationships between lipid metabolism and liver regeneration. Int J Hepatol. 2012;2012:549241.
13. Brouwers M, Jacobs C, Bast A, Stehouwer CDA, Schaper NC. Modulation of Glucokinase regulatory protein: a double-edged sword? Trends Mol Med. 2015;21(10):583–94.
14. Pilkis SJ, Claus TH. Hepatic gluconeogenesis/glycolysis: regulation and structure/function relationships of substrate cycle enzymes. Annu Rev Nutr. 1991;11:465–515.
15. Chatzipanagiotou S, Nath A, Vogt B, Jungermann K. Alteration in the capacities as well as in the zonal and cellular distributions of pyruvate kinase L and M2 in regenerating rat liver. Biol Chem Hoppe Seyler. 1985;366(3):271–80.
16. Christofk HR, Vander Heiden MG, Harris MH, Ramanathan A, Gerszten RE, Wei R, et al. The M2 splice isoform of pyruvate kinase is important for cancer metabolism and tumour growth. Nature. 2008;452(7184):230–3.
17. Yin Y, Kong D, He K, Xia Q. Aurora kinase a regulates liver regeneration through macrophages polarization and Wnt/beta-catenin signalling. Liver Int. 2022;42(2):468–78.

18. Kockeritz L, Doble B, Patel S, Woodgett JR. Glycogen synthase kinase-3--an overview of an over-achieving protein kinase. Curr Drug Targets. 2006;7(11):1377–88.
19. Kowalik MA, Columbano A, Perra A. Emerging role of the pentose phosphate pathway in hepatocellular carcinoma. Front Oncol. 2017;7:87.
20. Chan BKY, Elmasry M, Forootan SS, Russomanno G, Bunday TM, Zhang F, et al. Pharmacological activation of Nrf2 enhances functional liver regeneration. Hepatology. 2021;74(2):973–86.
21. Tan VWT, Salmi TM, Karamalakis AP, Gillespie A, Ong AJS, Balic JJ, et al. SLAM-ITseq identifies that Nrf2 induces liver regeneration through the pentose phosphate pathway. Dev Cell. 2024;59(7):898–910e6.
22. Kotsis T, Nastos C, Stamatis K, Chondroudaki I, Pafiti A, Frangou M, et al. Insulin metabolism and assessment of hepatic insulin extraction during liver regeneration. A study in a rat model. J Investig Surg. 2020;33(1):69–76.
23. Titchenell PM, Chu Q, Monks BR, Birnbaum MJ. Hepatic insulin signalling is dispensable for suppression of glucose output by insulin in vivo. Nat Commun. 2015;6:7078.
24. Fisette A, Hassanain M, Metrakos P, Doi SA, Salman A, Schricker T, et al. High-dose insulin therapy reduces postoperative liver dysfunction and complications in liver resection patients through reduced apoptosis and altered inflammation. J Clin Endocrinol Metab. 2012;97(1):217–26.
25. Zhang L, Li Y, Wang Y, Qiu Y, Mou H, Deng Y, et al. mTORC2 facilitates liver regeneration through sphingolipid-induced PPAR-alpha-fatty acid oxidation. Cell Mol Gastroenterol Hepatol. 2022;14(6):1311–31.
26. Hu Y, Wang R, Liu J, Wang Y, Dong J. Lipid droplet deposition in the regenerating liver: a promoter, inhibitor, or bystander? Hepatol Commun. 2023;7(10):e0267.
27. Hall Z, Chiarugi D, Charidemou E, Leslie J, Scott E, Pellegrinet L, et al. Lipid remodeling in hepatocyte proliferation and hepatocellular carcinoma. Hepatology. 2021;73(3):1028–44.
28. Kachaylo E, Tschuor C, Calo N, Borgeaud N, Ungethum U, Limani P, et al. PTEN Down-regulation promotes beta-oxidation to fuel hypertrophic liver growth after hepatectomy in mice. Hepatology. 2017;66(3):908–21.
29. Fernandez-Rojo MA, Restall C, Ferguson C, Martel N, Martin S, Bosch M, et al. Caveolin-1 orchestrates the balance between glucose and lipid-dependent energy metabolism: implications for liver regeneration. Hepatology. 2012;55(5):1574–84.
30. Newberry EP, Kennedy SM, Xie Y, Luo J, Stanley SE, Semenkovich CF, et al. Altered hepatic triglyceride content after partial hepatectomy without impaired liver regeneration in multiple murine genetic models. Hepatology. 2008;48(4):1097–105.
31. Ou-Yang Q, Lin XM, Zhu YJ, Zheng B, Li L, Yang YC, et al. Distinct role of nuclear receptor corepressor 1 regulated de novo fatty acids synthesis in liver regeneration and hepatocarcinogenesis in mice. Hepatology. 2018;67(3):1071–87.
32. Shteyer E, Liao Y, Muglia LJ, Hruz PW, Rudnick DA. Disruption of hepatic adipogenesis is associated with impaired liver regeneration in mice. Hepatology. 2004;40(6):1322–32.
33. Zhao Y, Tran M, Wang L, Shin DJ, Wu J. PDK4-deficiency reprograms intrahepatic glucose and lipid metabolism to facilitate liver regeneration in mice. Hepatol Commun. 2020;4(4):504–17.
34. Liu Y, Jiang L, Sun C, Ireland N, Shah YM, Liu Y, et al. Insulin/Snail1 axis ameliorates fatty liver disease by epigenetically suppressing lipogenesis. Nat Commun. 2018;9(1):2751.
35. Qu X, Wen Y, Jiao J, Zhao J, Sun X, Wang F, et al. PARK7 deficiency inhibits fatty acid beta-oxidation via PTEN to delay liver regeneration after hepatectomy. Clin Transl Med. 2022;12(9):e1061.
36. Lamanilao GG, Dogan M, Patel PS, Azim S, Patel DS, Bhattacharya SK, et al. Key hepatoprotective roles of mitochondria in liver regeneration. Am J Physiol Gastrointest Liver Physiol. 2023;324(3):G207–G18.
37. Bagattin A, Hugendubler L, Mueller E. Transcriptional coactivator PGC-1alpha promotes peroxisomal remodeling and biogenesis. Proc Natl Acad Sci USA. 2010;107(47):20376–81.

38. Goldstein JL, Brown MS. Regulation of the mevalonate pathway. Nature. 1990;343(6257):425–30.
39. Delgado-Coello B, Briones-Orta MA, Macias-Silva M, Mas-Oliva J. Cholesterol: recapitulation of its active role during liver regeneration. Liver Int. 2011;31(9):1271–84.
40. Arai M, Yokosuka O, Chiba T, Imazeki F, Kato M, Hashida J, et al. Gene expression profiling reveals the mechanism and pathophysiology of mouse liver regeneration. J Biol Chem. 2003;278(32):29813–8.
41. Lo Sasso G, Celli N, Caboni M, Murzilli S, Salvatore L, Morgano A, et al. Down-regulation of the LXR transcriptome provides the requisite cholesterol levels to proliferating hepatocytes. Hepatology. 2010;51(4):1334–44.
42. Tomassoni ML, Albi E, Magni MV. Changes of nuclear membrane fluidity during rat liver regeneration. Biochem Mol Biol Int. 1999;47(6):1049–59.
43. Smart EJ, Graf GA, McNiven MA, Sessa WC, Engelman JA, Scherer PE, et al. Caveolins, liquid-ordered domains, and signal transduction. Mol Cell Biol. 1999;19(11):7289–304.
44. Vance DE. Physiological roles of phosphatidylethanolamine N-methyltransferase. Biochim Biophys Acta. 2013;1831(3):626–32.
45. DeLong CJ, Shen YJ, Thomas MJ, Cui Z. Molecular distinction of phosphatidylcholine synthesis between the CDP-choline pathway and phosphatidylethanolamine methylation pathway. J Biol Chem. 1999;274(42):29683–8.
46. Alba MM, Ebright B, Hua B, Slarve I, Zhou Y, Jia Y, et al. Eicosanoids and other oxylipins in liver injury, inflammation and liver cancer development. Front Physiol. 2023;14:1098467.
47. Houweling M, Cui Z, Tessitore L, Vance DE. Induction of hepatocyte proliferation after partial hepatectomy is accompanied by a markedly reduced expression of phosphatidylethanolamine N-methyltransferase-2. Biochim Biophys Acta. 1997;1346(1):1–9.
48. Ammann M, Jonas JP, Pereyra D, Santol J, Hackl H, Kalchbrenner T, et al. Plasma GLP-1 and metabolic dynamics during human liver regeneration and their association with posthepatectomy liver failure. Hepatobiliary Surg Nutr. 2025;14(1):49–65.
49. Skipski VP, Barclay M, Barclay RK, Fetzer VA, Good JJ, Archibald FM. Lipid composition of human serum lipoproteins. Biochem J. 1967;104(2):340–52.
50. Martinez-Una M, Varela-Rey M, Mestre D, Fernandez-Ares L, Fresnedo O, Fernandez-Ramos D, et al. S-Adenosylmethionine increases circulating very-low density lipoprotein clearance in non-alcoholic fatty liver disease. J Hepatol. 2015;62(3):673–81.
51. Agren JJ, Kurvinen JP, Kuksis A. Isolation of very low density lipoprotein phospholipids enriched in ethanolamine phospholipids from rats injected with triton WR 1339. Biochim Biophys Acta. 2005;1734(1):34–43.
52. van der Veen JN, Kennelly JP, Wan S, Vance JE, Vance DE, Jacobs RL. The critical role of phosphatidylcholine and phosphatidylethanolamine metabolism in health and disease. Biochim Biophys Acta Biomembr. 2017;1859(9 Pt B):1558–72.
53. Sabugal R, Robert MQ, Julve J, Auwerx J, Llobera M, Peinado-Onsurbe J. Hepatic regeneration induces changes in lipoprotein lipase activity in several tissues and its re-expression in the liver. Biochem J. 1996;318(Pt 2):597–602.
54. Thomas MJ, Bhat S, Sorci-Thomas MG. Three-dimensional models of HDL apoA-I: implications for its assembly and function. J Lipid Res. 2008;49(9):1875–83.
55. Ruan X, Li Z, Zhang Y, Yang L, Pan Y, Wang Z, et al. Apolipoprotein A-I possesses an anti-obesity effect associated with increase of energy expenditure and up-regulation of UCP1 in brown fat. J Cell Mol Med. 2011;15(4):763–72.
56. Li CX, Chen LL, Li XC, Ng KT, Yang XX, Lo CM, et al. ApoA-1 accelerates regeneration of small-for-size fatty liver graft after transplantation. Life Sci. 2018;215:128–35.
57. Ammann M, Santol J, Pereyra D, Kalchbrenner T, Wuerger T, Laengle J, et al. Glucagon-like peptide-1 and glucagon-like peptide-2 regulation during human liver regeneration. Sci Rep. 2023;13(1):15980.
58. Maldonado V, Chan L, Melendez J, Rincon AR, Zhu HJ, Panduro A. Regulation of apo B mRNA expression in liver and intestine during liver regeneration induced by CCl4. Biochim Biophys Acta. 1994;1211(1):1–6.

59. Andreo U, Guo L, Chirieac DV, Tuyama AC, Montenont E, Brodsky JL, et al. Insulin-stimulated degradation of apolipoprotein B100: roles of class II phosphatidylinositol-3-kinase and autophagy. PLoS One. 2013;8(3):e57590.
60. Heeren J, Scheja L. Metabolic-associated fatty liver disease and lipoprotein metabolism. Mol Metab. 2021;50:101238.
61. Abshagen K, Degenhardt B, Liebig M, Wendt A, Genz B, Schaeper U, et al. Liver-specific Repin1 deficiency impairs transient hepatic steatosis in liver regeneration. Sci Rep. 2018;8(1):16858.
62. Pauta M, Rotllan N, Vales F, Fernandez-Hernando A, Allen RM, Ford DA, et al. Impaired liver regeneration in Ldlr−/− mice is associated with an altered hepatic profile of cytokines, growth factors, and lipids. J Hepatol. 2013;59(4):731–7.
63. Nojima H, Shimizu H, Murakami T, Shuto K, Koda K. Critical roles of the sphingolipid metabolic pathway in liver regeneration, hepatocellular carcinoma progression and therapy. Cancers (Basel). 2024;16(5):850.
64. Nojima H, Freeman CM, Gulbins E, Lentsch AB. Sphingolipids in liver injury, repair and regeneration. Biol Chem. 2015;396(6–7):633–43.
65. Nowatari T, Murata S, Nakayama K, Sano N, Maruyama T, Nozaki R, et al. Sphingosine 1-phosphate has anti-apoptotic effect on liver sinusoidal endothelial cells and proliferative effect on hepatocytes in a paracrine manner in human. Hepatol Res. 2015;45(11):1136–45.
66. Lee DY, Kim EH. Therapeutic effects of amino acids in liver diseases: current studies and future perspectives. J Cancer Prev. 2019;24(2):72–8.
67. Sancak Y, Peterson TR, Shaul YD, Lindquist RA, Thoreen CC, Bar-Peled L, et al. The rag GTPases bind raptor and mediate amino acid signaling to mTORC1. Science. 2008;320(5882):1496–501.
68. Son SM, Park SJ, Stamatakou E, Vicinanza M, Menzies FM, Rubinsztein DC. Leucine regulates autophagy via acetylation of the mTORC1 component raptor. Nat Commun. 2020;11(1):3148.
69. Holecek M. Nutritional modulation of liver regeneration by carbohydrates, lipids, and amino acids: a review. Nutrition. 1999;15(10):784–8.
70. Solhi R, Lotfinia M, Gramignoli R, Najimi M, Vosough M. Metabolic hallmarks of liver regeneration. Trends Endocrinol Metab. 2021;32(9):731–45.
71. Starlinger P, Assinger A, Haegele S, Wanek D, Zikeli S, Schauer D, et al. Evidence for serotonin as a relevant inducer of liver regeneration after liver resection in humans. Hepatology. 2014;60(1):257–66.
72. Yoo HC, Yu YC, Sung Y, Han JM. Glutamine reliance in cell metabolism. Exp Mol Med. 2020;52(9):1496–516.
73. Delgado TC, de Las HJ, Martinez-Chantar ML. Understanding gut-liver axis nitrogen metabolism in fatty liver disease. Front Endocrinol (Lausanne). 2022;13:1058101.
74. Yan Y, Chen Q, Dai X, Xiang Z, Long Z, Wu Y, et al. Amino acid metabolomics and machine learning for assessment of post-hepatectomy liver regeneration. Front Pharmacol. 2024;15:1345099.
75. Brebnor LD, Balinsky JB. Changes in activities of urea cycle enzymes in early stages of liver regeneration after partial hepatectomy in rats. Life Sci. 1983;32(12):1391–400.
76. Su AI, Guidotti LG, Pezacki JP, Chisari FV, Schultz PG. Gene expression during the priming phase of liver regeneration after partial hepatectomy in mice. Proc Natl Acad Sci USA. 2002;99(17):11181–6.
77. Ma X, Huang T, Chen X, Li Q, Liao M, Fu L, et al. Molecular mechanisms in liver repair and regeneration: from physiology to therapeutics. Signal Transduct Target Ther. 2025;10(1):63.
78. Fouraschen SM, de Ruiter PE, Kwekkeboom J, de Bruin RW, Kazemier G, Metselaar HJ, et al. mTOR signaling in liver regeneration: rapamycin combined with growth factor treatment. World J Transplant. 2013;3(3):36–47.
79. Levy JL, Mirek ET, Rodriguez EM, Tolentino MJ, Zalma BA, Roepke TA, et al. GCN2 drives diurnal patterns in the hepatic integrated stress response and maintains circadian rhythms in

whole body metabolism during amino acid insufficiency. Am J Physiol Endocrinol Metab. 2024;327(4):E563–E76.
80. Goikoetxea-Usandizaga N, Serrano-Macia M, Delgado TC, Simon J, Fernandez Ramos D, Barriales D, et al. Mitochondrial bioenergetics boost macrophage activation, promoting liver regeneration in metabolically compromised animals. Hepatology. 2022;75(3):550–66.
81. Frances DE, Ronco MT, Ingaramo PI, Monti JA, Pisani GB, Parody JP, et al. Role of reactive oxygen species in the early stages of liver regeneration in streptozotocin-induced diabetic rats. Free Radic Res. 2011;45(10):1143–53.
82. Bai H, Fang CW, Shi Y, Zhai S, Jiang A, Li YN, et al. Mitochondria-derived H(2)O(2) triggers liver regeneration via FoxO3a signaling pathway after partial hepatectomy in mice. Cell Death Dis. 2023;14(3):216.
83. Viollet B, Guigas B, Leclerc J, Hebrard S, Lantier L, Mounier R, et al. AMP-activated protein kinase in the regulation of hepatic energy metabolism: from physiology to therapeutic perspectives. Acta Physiol (Oxf). 2009;196(1):81–98.
84. Ecker J, Brunner S, Janssen KP. Metabolic inflexibility of mitochondria: beneficial for the fitness of regenerating liver cells. Signal Transduct Target Ther. 2024;9(1):233.
85. Peng C, Stewart AG, Woodman OL, Ritchie RH, Qin CX. Non-alcoholic Steatohepatitis: a review of its mechanism, Models and Medical Treatments. Front Pharmacol. 2020;11:603926.
86. Vacca M, Kamzolas I, Harder LM, Oakley F, Trautwein C, Hatting M, et al. An unbiased ranking of murine dietary models based on their proximity to human metabolic dysfunction-associated steatotic liver disease (MASLD). Nat Metab. 2024;6(6):1178–96.
87. Sydor S, Gu Y, Schlattjan M, Bechmann LP, Rauen U, Best J, et al. Steatosis does not impair liver regeneration after partial hepatectomy. Lab Investig. 2013;93(1):20–30.
88. de Meijer VE, Kalish BT, Puder M, Ijzermans JN. Systematic review and meta-analysis of steatosis as a risk factor in major hepatic resection. Br J Surg. 2010;97(9):1331–9.
89. Chu MJ, Hickey AJ, Phillips AR, Bartlett AS. The impact of hepatic steatosis on hepatic ischemia-reperfusion injury in experimental studies: a systematic review. Biomed Res Int. 2013;2013:192029.
90. Cheng Z, Ristow M. Mitochondria and metabolic homeostasis. Antioxid Redox Signal. 2013;19(3):240–2.
91. Rodimova S, Mozherov A, Elagin V, Karabut M, Shchechkin I, Kozlov D, et al. Effect of hepatic pathology on liver regeneration: the Main metabolic mechanisms causing impaired hepatic regeneration. Int J Mol Sci. 2023;24(11):9112.
92. Peloso A, Tihy M, Moeckli B, Rubbia-Brandt L, Toso C. Clearing steatosis prior to liver surgery for colorectal metastasis: a narrative review and case illustration. Nutrients. 2022;14(24):5340.
93. Fontana J, Kucera O, Mezera V, Andel M, Cervinkova Z. Glucagon-like peptide-1 analogues exenatide and liraglutide exert inhibitory effect on the early phase of liver regeneration after partial hepatectomy in rats. Physiol Res. 2017;66(5):833–44.
94. Chanda S, Mehendale M. Role of nutritional fatty acid and L-carnitine in the final outcome of thioacetamide hepatotoxicity. FASEB J. 1994;8(13):1061–8.
95. Rizki G, Arnaboldi L, Gabrielli B, Yan J, Lee GS, Ng RK, et al. Mice fed a lipogenic methionine-choline-deficient diet develop hypermetabolism coincident with hepatic suppression of SCD-1. J Lipid Res. 2006;47(10):2280–90.
96. Mehedint MG, Zeisel SH. Choline's role in maintaining liver function: new evidence for epigenetic mechanisms. Curr Opin Clin Nutr Metab Care. 2013;16(3):339–45.
97. Lo EKK, Felicianna, Xu JH, Zhan Q, Zeng Z, El-Nezami H. The emerging role of branched-chain amino acids in liver diseases. Biomedicine. 2022;10(6):1444.
98. Tomiya T, Inoue Y, Yanase M, Arai M, Ikeda H, Tejima K, et al. Leucine stimulates the secretion of hepatocyte growth factor by hepatic stellate cells. Biochem Biophys Res Commun. 2002;297(5):1108–11.
99. Marchesini G, Marzocchi R, Noia M, Bianchi G. Branched-chain amino acid supplementation in patients with liver diseases. J Nutr. 2005;135(6 Suppl):1596S–601S.

100. Beppu T, Nitta H, Hayashi H, Imai K, Okabe H, Nakagawa S, et al. Effect of branched-chain amino acid supplementation on functional liver regeneration in patients undergoing portal vein embolization and sequential hepatectomy: a randomized controlled trial. J Gastroenterol. 2015;50(12):1197–205.
101. Skullman S, Wiren M, Chu M, Permert J, Garlick PJ, McNurlan MA, et al. Effects of graded glutamine intake on liver protein metabolism following partial hepatectomy. Eur J Gastroenterol Hepatol. 1995;7(9):881–6.
102. Kurokawa T, An J, Tsunekawa K, Shimomura Y, Kazama S, Ishikawa N, et al. Effect of L-arginine supplement on liver regeneration after partial hepatectomy in rats. World J Surg Oncol. 2012;10:99.
103. Dasari BVM, Pathanki A, Hodson J, Roberts KJ, Marudanayagam R, Mirza DF, et al. Propensity-matched analysis of the influence of perioperative statin therapy on outcomes after liver resection. BJS Open. 2019;3(4):509–15.
104. Colakoglu T, Nursal TZ, Ezer A, Kayaselcuk F, Parlakgumus A, Belli S, et al. Effects of different doses of statins on liver regeneration through angiogenesis and possible relation between these effects and acute phase responses. Transplant Proc. 2010;42(9):3823–7.
105. Kargiotis K, Athyros VG, Giouleme O, Katsiki N, Katsiki E, Anagnostis P, et al. Resolution of non-alcoholic steatohepatitis by rosuvastatin monotherapy in patients with metabolic syndrome. World J Gastroenterol. 2015;21(25):7860–8.
106. McKeage K, Keating GM. Fenofibrate: a review of its use in dyslipidaemia. Drugs. 2011;71(14):1917–46.
107. Ghonem NS, Assis DN, Boyer JL. Fibrates and cholestasis. Hepatology. 2015;62(2):635–43.
108. Fan S, Gao Y, Zhao P, Xie G, Zhou Y, Yang X, et al. Fenofibrate-promoted hepatomegaly and liver regeneration are PPARalpha-dependent and partially related to the YAP pathway. Acta Pharm Sin B. 2024;14(7):2992–3008.
109. Starlinger P, Brunnthaler L, Watkins R, Pereyra D, Stift J, Finsterbusch M, et al. Tyrosine phosphorylation of YAP-1 in biliary epithelial cells mediates posthepatectomy liver regeneration and is affected by serotonin. J Cell Biochem. 2023;124(5):687–700.
110. Gandhi N, Lenton R, Bhartia M, Abbas A, Raju J, Ramachandran S. Effect of fibrate treatment on liver function tests in patients with the metabolic syndrome. Springerplus. 2014;3:14.
111. Lee JS, Mukhopadhyay P, Matyas C, Trojnar E, Paloczi J, Yang YR, et al. PCSK9 inhibition as a novel therapeutic target for alcoholic liver disease. Sci Rep. 2019;9(1):17167.
112. Han L, Wu L, Yin Q, Li L, Zheng X, Du S, et al. A promising therapy for fatty liver disease: PCSK9 inhibitors. Phytomedicine. 2024;128:155505.
113. Zaid A, Roubtsova A, Essalmani R, Marcinkiewicz J, Chamberland A, Hamelin J, et al. Proprotein convertase subtilisin/kexin type 9 (PCSK9): hepatocyte-specific low-density lipoprotein receptor degradation and critical role in mouse liver regeneration. Hepatology. 2008;48(2):646–54.
114. El-Jamal N, Erdual E, Neunlist M, Koriche D, Dubuquoy C, Maggiotto F, et al. Glugacon-like peptide-2: broad receptor expression, limited therapeutic effect on intestinal inflammation and novel role in liver regeneration. Am J Physiol Gastrointest Liver Physiol. 2014;307(3):G274–85.
115. Lim DW, Wales PW, Josephson JK, Nation PN, Wizzard PR, Sergi CM, et al. Glucagon-Like peptide 2 improves cholestasis in parenteral nutrition–associated liver disease. JPEN J Parenter Enteral Nutr. 2016;40(1):14–21.

4 Pathogenesis of Postoperative Liver Failure

Tim Reese and Karl J. Oldhafer

4.1 Introduction

Postoperative liver failure (POLF) is a serious and potentially fatal complication following major liver surgery, characterized by the inability of the liver to maintain essential metabolic, synthesis, and detoxification functions [1, 2]. Despite significant advances in liver surgery in recent decades, POLF remains a major clinical challenge, with a reported incidence of 1–20%, depending on the extent of resection and the presence of underlying liver disease [3, 4]. Advances in imaging modalities, functional and volumetric liver assessments, and perioperative optimization have improved patient outcomes significantly. Nevertheless, POLF remains a multifactorial condition influenced by pre-existing liver disease, the extent of resection, and the complex interplay of surgical, hemodynamic, and molecular factors [4]. The high morbidity and mortality associated with POLF highlight the urgent need for a deeper understanding of its pathogenesis and the development of effective prevention and treatment strategies [1, 4].

4.2 Pathophysiology

The pathogenesis of POLF is characterized by a multifaceted interplay of cellular, molecular, and hemodynamic factors that collectively compromise the liver's capacity to meet the metabolic, synthetic, and detoxification demands. Central to this

T. Reese
Division of Surgery and Oncology, Department of Clinical Science, Intervention and Technology, Karolinska Institutet, Karolinska University Hospital, Stockholm, Sweden

K. J. Oldhafer (✉)
Department of Surgery, Division of Hepatobiliary and Pancreatic Surgery, Asklepios Hospital Barmbek, Semmelweis University Campus Hamburg, Hamburg, Germany
e-mail: k.oldhafer@asklepios.com

L. Aldrighetti et al. (eds.), *Liver Regeneration Techniques In Hepatic Surgery*,
https://doi.org/10.1007/978-3-032-10997-2_4

process are mechanisms such as small-for-size syndrome (SFSS), ischemia–reperfusion injury (IRI), impaired liver regeneration, portal hypertension, mitochondrial dysfunction, and immune dysregulation.

The liver's remarkable regenerative capacity is critical for recovery after major resection [5]. However, this capacity is often impaired in the setting of POLF, particularly in patients with underlying liver disease such as fibrosis, steatosis, or cirrhosis. Liver regeneration occurs in distinct phases, beginning with the priming of hepatocytes by cytokines such as interleukin-6 (IL-6) and tumor necrosis factor-alpha (TNF-α). These cytokines activate transcription factors like signal transducer and activator of transcription 3 (STAT3), which initiate hepatocyte proliferation. Subsequent phases involve growth factors, including hepatocyte growth factor (HGF) and epidermal growth factor (EGF), which stimulate DNA replication and cell cycle progression through pathways such as phosphatidylinositol-3-kinase (PI3K)/Akt and mitogen-activated protein kinase [5, 6]. However, chronic liver conditions, hemodynamic, or metabolic factors disrupt these processes, limiting regenerative signaling and increasing the risk of POLF.

4.2.1 Small-for-Size Syndrome or Insufficient Future Liver Remnant

One of the primary contributors to POLF is SFSS (first described in the setting of liver transplantation [7]), which occurs when the future liver remnant (FLR) is too small to sustain the body's metabolic needs [8, 9]. Basically, there is an imbalance between the needs of the human body with the remaining liver volume and portal venous flow (see below), which leads to decompensation of liver function [2]. In this situation, the liver cannot sustain the patients' needs and regenerative process is impaired or even inhibited. The smaller the residual liver, the higher the probability of developing PHLF [4, 8–10]. Preoperative contrast-enhanced computed tomography scans can be used to calculate the FLR and relate it to the total liver volume. Alternatively, the FLR can be calculated on the basis of the calculated liver volume (so-called standardized FLR (sFLR)) [8]. Inadequate FLR is defined as less than 25 or 30% of total liver volume in healthy or chemotherapy-treated individuals or less than 40% in those with chronic liver disease.

4.2.2 Portal Hyperperfusion and Hypertension

Following major hepatectomy, a sudden increase in portal hyperperfusion and hypertension in the remaining liver tissue leads to excessive shear stress, causing sinusoidal endothelial cell damage [11]. Normally, the sinusoidal endothelial cells release nitric oxide and other growth factors in order to begin the regenerative cascade [12]; however, in patients developing a postoperative portal hypertension, the sinusoidal structure is severely damaged [13]. This disrupts hepatic microcirculation and amplifies hepatocyte apoptosis and necrosis. The loss of sinusoidal endothelial cells results in impaired metabolic and immune homeostasis, while increased oxidative stress from blood flow perpetuates cellular injury [11, 14]. The hepatic arterial buffer response, a compensatory mechanism to maintain liver perfusion, is often inadequate or absent in the context of portal hypertension, further impairing the remaining liver function [13, 15]. The literature shows that post-liver resection, an overwhelming increase in portal pressure can result in deleterious effects on liver regeneration and patient outcome [16–18].

4.2.3 Ischemia–Reperfusion Injury

Liver surgery inherently involves episodes of hypoxic and ischemic damage to the hepatic parenchyma, primarily due to vascular occlusion, mechanical manipulation, and parenchymal transection. During ischemia, the interruption of oxygen supply halts mitochondrial electron transport, resulting in ATP depletion, intracellular acidosis, and cellular edema [19]. Upon restoration of blood flow, the reintroduction of oxygen into hypoxic tissue triggers a surge in reactive oxygen species (ROS) production. This oxidative burst contributes to hepatocellular apoptosis and necrosis, endothelial dysfunction, and sterile inflammation [20].

Ischemia–reperfusion (I/R) injury is typically divided into two distinct phases: an acute phase, lasting approximately 3 h post-reperfusion, and a late phase, extending up to 48 h. The acute phase is characterized by mitochondrial dysfunction and the generation of ROS within hepatocytes, Kupffer cells, and sinusoidal endothelial cells. Oxidative stress activates Kupffer cells via Toll-like receptor 4 (TLR4) signaling. Activated Kupffer cells further amplify ROS production, leading to the degradation of IκB, the inhibitor of nuclear factor kappa B (NF-κB). Freed from inhibition, NF-κB translocates into the nucleus, where it drives the expression of pro-inflammatory cytokines such as IL-1β, IL-6, and TNF-α [21].

These cytokines stimulate the expression of adhesion molecules and complement components, promoting the recruitment of neutrophils and $CD4^+$ T cells to the liver. These immune cells are key effectors of the late phase of I/R injury. Neutrophils exacerbate liver injury through the release of ROS, matrix metalloproteinases (MMPs), and proteases, all of which contribute to hepatocyte necrosis and parenchymal damage [22].

Patients of advanced age or those with underlying hepatic steatosis or cirrhosis exhibit decreased tolerance to vascular occlusion and are more susceptible to I/R injury. Importantly, ischemia–reperfusion injury also impairs liver regeneration, further complicating postoperative recovery and long-term outcomes.

4.2.4 Mitochondrial Dysfunction

Mitochondria play a central role in liver regeneration after liver resection, supporting not only the energetic demands of hepatocyte proliferation but also regulating key checkpoints of the regenerative process. Their function is especially critical in the early postoperative period when the remnant liver must rapidly restore volume and function.

In the G1/S transition, hepatocyte mitochondria adopt a hyperfused network morphology, significantly increasing ATP production and enabling progression through the cell cycle. This morphological change facilitates cyclin E1 accumulation and supports biosynthetic activity [23, 24]. Mitochondrial dysfunction at this stage impairs regeneration and has been associated with delayed recovery and postoperative liver failure [25]. Mitochondria are also involved in the controlled termination of regeneration [23].

Because mitochondria are not passive energy providers but active regulators of liver regeneration, maintaining mitochondrial integrity may improve postoperative outcomes and should be considered a target in perioperative management in the future.

4.2.5 Immune Dysregulation

Immune dysregulation plays a significant role in the progression of POLF. The release of significant quantities of inflammatory mediators by various cell types, including natural killer cells, dendritic cells, Kupffer cells, and neutrophils is a key element of the process of hepatocyte proliferation [26]. In case of POLF, neutrophils are excessively recruited to the liver, where they contribute to tissue damage through degranulation and the formation of neutrophil extracellular traps [27].

Kupffer cells have been shown to play a pivotal role in the process of immune surveillance and the maintenance of responses within the hepatic system [28, 29]. They have been shown to be responsible for the capture and subsequent phagocytosis of antigens and bacteria derived from the gastrointestinal tract. In addition to this, they have also been observed to play a vital role in the regulation of immune responses to antigens that are otherwise harmless. In circumstances where their functionality is compromised due to tissue injury, such as that resulting from liver resection, Kupffer cells play a critical role in the regeneration process. Notably, Kupffer cells are recognized as the primary innate immune cells to become activated through the process of recognition and subsequent to lipopolysaccharides and uptake of DAMPs, via Toll-like receptors located on their cell surface [28]. This results in the release of pro- and anti-inflammatory molecules, which in turn stimulates the migration of immune cells to the liver, thus regulating the body's immune response.

An elevated bacterial load in the liver, consequent to hepatic inflow occlusion and diminished toxin clearance, results in the inhibition of Kupffer cell function [30, 31]. The disturbance of Kupffer cell function can lead to a process of apoptosis and irreversible necrosis [32]. An augmented systemic inflammatory response (SIRS) can ultimately result in PHLF and multiorgan failure [33]. An overwhelming immune response may be triggered through excessive bleeding or hepatic inflow or outflow exclusion. Hepatic ischemia and reperfusion lead to activation of the liver's innate immune system. While this is intended to facilitate liver regeneration, an excessive immune response can exacerbate liver injury [34].

4.3 Risk Factors

Several factors predispose patients to POLF.

4.3.1 Patient Related

Age and Sex As individuals age, a decline in the production of acute-phase proteins may contribute to impaired regeneration [35]. Alternatively, the loss of fenestration in the sinusoidal space that occurs with age could result in the inhibition of liver regeneration [4].

It has been demonstrated that males are predisposed to a heightened risk of developing a POPF [36], and the stimulatory effect of estradiol on liver regeneration has been well-documented [37]. This effect was also demonstrated by a faster hypertrophy of the liver in female patients compared to male patients [38]. However, this effect was not observed in postmenopausal women.

Nutritional and Metabolic Status Nutritional status plays a pivotal role in determining postoperative outcomes, including the risk of POLF [39]. Malnutrition, often characterized by hypoalbuminemia, low muscle mass, and deficiencies in micronutrients, is an independent risk factor for poor liver regeneration and increased surgical morbidity [40, 41]. Sarcopenia, the loss of skeletal muscle mass and strength, has emerged as a critical prognostic factor in patients undergoing liver surgery [42, 43]. This condition reflects not only inadequate nutritional intake but also systemic inflammation and metabolic dysregulation commonly associated with chronic liver disease [42, 44]. Advancements in body composition assessment have improved the ability to detect nutritional deficits preoperatively. Techniques such as bioelectrical impedance analysis (BIA), dual-energy X-ray absorptiometry (DEXA), and computed tomography (CT)-based muscle mass measurement provide evaluations of sarcopenia and nutritional reserves [45]. These tools are particularly valuable in identifying at-risk patients who might otherwise appear well-nourished based on traditional parameters such as body mass index (BMI). Preoperative nutritional optimization, such as immunonutrition, can reduce the risk of POLF [46]; however, recent studies failed to show a beneficial effect [47, 48]. Strategies include high-protein dietary supplementation, correction of vitamin and mineral deficiencies, and tailored exercise programs to improve muscle mass and functional capacity. Emerging evidence suggests that supplementation with branched-chain amino acids (BCAAs) may enhance liver regeneration and reduce postoperative complications [49, 50]. One of the few studies to investigate the mechanism of reduced muscle mass with reduced liver regeneration is the study by Hagiwara et al. [49], which showed slower and lower liver regeneration in mice with muscle atrophy. Muscle atrophic mice showed a significant decrease in liver glycogen and BCAA after regeneration, but the slower and lower regeneration could be reversed by oral administration of BCAA.

Patients suffering from diabetes have been shown to have a significantly elevated risk of POLF [51, 52]. The underlying pathophysiology of this condition involves impaired liver regeneration, a consequence of elevated oxidative stress and reduced growth factors [53]. Insulin depletions have also been demonstrated to impair liver regeneration [4]. Recent studies are focusing on the potential of therapeutic interventions that aim to induce a state of hyperinsulinemia and normoglycemia to enhance the regenerative response in the liver [54, 55].

Sepsis It has been observed that liver dysfunction can facilitate bacterial translocation and infection. Moreover, sepsis plays a pivotal role in the death of patients with liver dysfunction following hepatectomy [56]. Sepsis directly or indirectly assaults the cells involved in the regenerative process and therefore inhibiting the regenerative process [57].

4.3.2 Liver Related

Pre-existing Liver Disease Pre-existing liver disease, such as cirrhosis, nonalcoholic steatohepatitis (NASH), or cholestasis, significantly increases the risk of POLF. These conditions impair the liver's regenerative capacity and reduce functional hepatic reserve. Optimizing the liver condition preoperatively, including control of ascites and nutritional supplementation, can mitigate some risks [31, 58].

Steatosis Steatosis has been demonstrated to induce hemodynamic changes in the liver sinusoids, thus engendering an elevated risk of ischemia–reperfusion injury [59], leading to impaired liver regeneration, because of increased hepatocellular lipid peroxidation [60].

Chemotherapy Irinotecan and platinum-based chemotherapies can cause liver injury and affect liver regeneration and can cause steatohepatitis [61, 62]. Patients on oxaliplatin-containing regimens are more likely to develop sinusoidal obstruction syndrome and biliary complications [63].

Cholestasis It has been demonstrated that cholestasis can diminish hepatic regeneration. For instance, following PVE, the hypertrophy of a nonembolized lobe is impeded in patients with cholestasis [64, 65]. When there is a significant dilation of the biliary tract, it can compress the portal vein, resulting in a hepatic artery buffer response [66]. It has been shown that cholestasis affects the production of several factors associated with the liver regeneration process, such as c-myc, which is inhibited in cholestasis [67]. Other factors associated with liver regeneration, such as EGF and IL6, are decreased in a cholestatic liver [68, 69]. Additionally, bile acid accumulation, accompanied by disrupted bile acid signaling, particularly through the farnesoid X receptor (FXR) and Takeda G protein-coupled receptor 5 (TGR5) [70], further hinders the proliferative response. Furthermore, the absence of enterohepatic circulation during biliary obstruction has been demonstrated to have a detrimental effect on hepatic regeneration. External biliary drainage in obstructive jaundice has been shown to significantly suppress liver regeneration [71, 72].

Fibrosis/Cirrhosis As fibrosis extent increases, so does the risk of mortality. Co-morbidities like portal hypertension, jaundice, and coagulopathy, common in high-grade fibrosis or cirrhosis, further increase this risk. Reduced liver function and reserve, a feature of chronic liver disease, result in impaired postoperative liver regeneration [4, 14].

4.3.3 Surgery Related

Extent of Resection The extent of liver resection is one of the most critical surgical factors influencing the risk of POLF. There is a well-established correlation between the volume of resected liver tissue and the likelihood of impaired postoperative hepatic function. Resections involving more than 70–75% of the total liver volume are associated with a markedly increased risk of POLF, particularly when the future liver remnant (FLR) is insufficient to meet metabolic and synthetic demands [73, 74].

In patients with normal liver parenchyma, an FLR of ≥25–30% is generally considered adequate. However, in patients with compromised liver function—such as those with steatosis, fibrosis, cirrhosis, or chemotherapy-associated liver injury—a larger FLR of ≥40% is often necessary [75, 76]. This highlights the need for individualized planning based on both anatomical and functional liver reserve.

Importantly, FLR volume alone is not a reliable surrogate for functional capacity. Therefore, it is increasingly recommended to combine cross-sectional imaging (e.g., CT or MRI volumetry) with quantitative liver function tests. Tools such as the LiMAx® test, indocyanine green (ICG) clearance, or 99mTc-mebrofenin hepatobiliary scintigraphy provide functional insights that significantly improve risk stratification [77, 78].

To address insufficient FLR, preoperative strategies like portal vein embolization (PVE) or associating liver partition and portal vein ligation for staged hepatectomy (ALPPS) can be employed to induce hypertrophy of the remnant liver. These methods, while effective, must be carefully weighed against potential complications, and selected based on patient-specific liver function and oncological context [41, 79, 80].

Ensuring adequate FLR volume and function remains a cornerstone of safe liver surgery. Failure to do so is one of the primary drivers of POLF, a condition associated with significant perioperative morbidity and mortality.

Vascular Occlusion Prolonged vascular occlusion remains an essential technique in liver surgery, particularly during complex resections, where minimizing blood loss is critical. Techniques such as the Pringle maneuver and total vascular exclusion (TVE) are widely employed for temporary inflow and outflow control. However, extended periods of ischemia significantly exacerbate ischemia–reperfusion injury, contributing to hepatocellular damage and increasing the risk of POLF (see above).

To mitigate the adverse consequences of IRI, several protective strategies have been developed and validated. Intermittent clamping, in which short periods of ischemia are alternated with brief reperfusion intervals, has been shown to reduce hepatocellular injury and improve postoperative outcomes compared to continuous clamping [81].

Moreover, hypothermic strategies—either systemic or localized to the liver—have been demonstrated to attenuate the metabolic demand during ischemia and blunt the inflammatory response during reperfusion, particularly in experimental models and selected clinical settings [82, 83].

The choice and timing of vascular occlusion techniques must be individualized based on the extent of resection, the underlying hepatic parenchyma (e.g., fibrosis, steatosis, cirrhosis), and the patient's overall functional reserve. A tailored approach combining protective strategies offers the best balance between minimizing blood loss and reducing the risk of IRI-related complications [84].

Blood loss and coagulopathy present additional intraoperative challenges. Excessive blood loss can lead to secondary ischemic injury and massive transfusions may dilute clotting factors, further compromising liver function [85]. To address this, modern surgical techniques prioritize blood conservation [86], advanced hemostatic devices, low central venous pressure (CVP), and hemodynamic monitoring. Maintaining low CVP during parenchymal transection reduces venous congestion and minimizes blood loss [87, 88]. Additionally, close intraoperative monitoring of portal pressures and systemic hemodynamics enables timely adjustments to optimize perfusion of the remnant liver [18]. By integrating these intraoperative strategies, surgeons can significantly reduce the physiological stress on the liver and improve postoperative outcomes. This highlights the importance of a multidisciplinary approach, combining surgical expertise, anesthetic management, and advanced technologies to minimize the risk of POLF.

4.4 Conclusion

POLF remains a critical challenge in hepatic surgery, with profound implications for patient survival and quality of life. Its pathogenesis is driven by a complex interplay of molecular, hemodynamic, and surgical factors, necessitating a multidisciplinary approach to its prevention and management.

Significant progress has been made in understanding the mechanisms underlying POLF, particularly in the areas of ischemia–reperfusion injury, impaired liver regeneration, and portal hypertension. Advances in preoperative risk stratification, including the use of functional liver tests, volumetric imaging, and personalized predictive models, have allowed for better patient selection and optimization. Techniques such as portal vein embolization (PVE) and hepatic vein embolization (HVE) have expanded the boundaries of safe resection, while intraoperative innovations have enhanced surgical safety.

Despite these advancements, POLF continues to carry high morbidity and mortality rates, particularly in patients with pre-existing liver disease or extensive resections. The biggest problem with POLF is treatment, as this is only symptomatic [2,

3] and often cannot influence the actual course of the disease. Postoperative care remains pivotal, with a focus on early detection through biomarker monitoring. Emerging technologies, including molecular therapies targeting liver regeneration and new strategies for mitigating ischemia–reperfusion injury, hold promise for further reducing the burden of POLF.

References

1. Baumgartner R, Gilg S, Björnsson B, Hasselgren K, Ghorbani P, Sauter C, et al. Impact of post-hepatectomy liver failure on morbidity and short- and long-term survival after major hepatectomy. BJS Open. 2022;6(4):zrac097.
2. Bekheit M, Grundy L, Salih AK, Bucur P, Vibert E, Ghazanfar M. Post-hepatectomy liver failure: a timeline centered review. Hepatobiliary Pancreat Dis Int. 2023;S1499–3872(23):00035–8.
3. Qadan M, Garden JO, Corvera CU, Visser BC. Management of postoperative hepatic failure. J Am Coll Surg. 2016 Feb;222(2):195–208.
4. Sparrelid E, Olthof PB, Dasari BVM, Erdmann JI, Santol J, Starlinger P, et al. Current evidence on posthepatectomy liver failure: comprehensive review. BJS Open. 2022;6(6):zrac142.
5. Forbes SJ, Newsome PN. Liver regeneration – mechanisms and models to clinical application. Nat Rev Gastroenterol Hepatol. 2016;13(8):473–85.
6. Maspero M, Yilmaz S, Cazzaniga B, Raj R, Ali K, Mazzaferro V, et al. The role of ischaemia-reperfusion injury and liver regeneration in hepatic tumour recurrence. JHEP Rep. 2023 Nov;5(11):100846.
7. Ito T, Kiuchi T, Yamamoto H, Oike F, Ogura Y, Fujimoto Y, et al. Changes in portal venous pressure in the early phase after living donor liver transplantation: pathogenesis and clinical implications. Transplantation. 2003;75(8):1313–7.
8. Dixon M, Cruz J, Sarwani N, Gusani N. The future liver remnant: definition, evaluation, and management. Am Surg. 2021 Feb;87(2):276–86.
9. Guglielmi A, Ruzzenente A, Conci S, Valdegamberi A, Iacono C. How much remnant is enough in liver resection? Dig Surg. 2012;29(1):6–17.
10. Shoup M, Gonen M, D'Angelica M, Jarnagin WR, DeMatteo RP, Schwartz LH, et al. Volumetric analysis predicts hepatic dysfunction in patients undergoing major liver resection. J Gastrointest Surg. 2003;7(3):325–30.
11. Xu H, Qiu X, Wang Z, Wang K, Tan Y, Gao F, et al. Role of the portal system in liver regeneration: from molecular mechanisms to clinical management. Liver Res. 2024 Mar;8(1):1–10.
12. Matsumoto K, Yoshitomi H, Rossant J, Zaret KS. Liver Organogenesis Promoted by Endothelial Cells Prior to Vascular Function. Science. 2001;294(5542):559–63.
13. Kohler A, Moller PW, Frey S, Tinguely P, Candinas D, Obrist D, et al. Portal hyperperfusion after major liver resection and associated sinusoidal damage is a therapeutic target to protect the remnant liver. American Journal of Physiology-Gastrointestinal and Liver. Physiology. 2019;317(3):G264–74.
14. Ray S, Mehta NN, Golhar A, Nundy S. Post hepatectomy liver failure—a comprehensive review of current concepts and controversies. Ann Med Surg. 2018 Oct;34:4–10.
15. Demetris AJ, Kelly DM, Eghtesad B, Fontes P, Wallis Marsh J, Tom K, et al. Pathophysiologic observations and histopathologic recognition of the portal hyperperfusion or small-for-size syndrome. Am J Surg Pathol. 2006 Aug;30(8):986–93.
16. van Mierlo KMC, Schaap FG, Dejong CHC, Olde Damink SWM. Liver resection for cancer: new developments in prediction, prevention and management of postresectional liver failure. J Hepatol. 2016 Dec;65(6):1217–31.
17. Allard MA, Adam R, Bucur PO, Termos S, Cunha AS, Bismuth H, et al. Posthepatectomy portal vein pressure predicts liver failure and mortality after major liver resection on noncirrhotic liver. Ann Surg. 2013;258(5):822–9. discussion 829–830

18. Bogner A, Reissfelder C, Striebel F, Mehrabi A, Ghamarnejad O, Rahbari M, et al. Intraoperative increase of portal venous pressure is an immediate predictor of posthepatectomy liver failure after major hepatectomy: a prospective study. Ann Surg. 2021;274(1):e10–7.
19. Wu MY, Yiang GT, Liao WT, Tsai APY, Cheng YL, Cheng PW, et al. Current Mechanistic Concepts in Ischemia and Reperfusion Injury. Cell Physiol Biochem. 2018;46(4):1650–67.
20. Jiménez-Castro MB, Cornide-Petronio ME, Gracia-Sancho J, Peralta C. Inflammasome-mediated inflammation in liver ischemia-reperfusion injury. Cells. 2019;8(10):1131.
21. Llacuna L, Marí M, Lluis JM, García-Ruiz C, Fernández-Checa JC, Morales A. Reactive oxygen species mediate liver injury through parenchymal nuclear factor-κB inactivation in prolonged ischemia/reperfusion. Am J Pathol. 2009;174(5):1776–85.
22. Jaeschke H. Mechanisms of Liver Injury. II. Mechanisms of neutrophil-induced liver cell injury during hepatic ischemia-reperfusion and other acute inflammatory conditions. Am J Physiol Gastrointest Liver Physiol. 2006 Jun;290(6):G1083–8.
23. Lamanilao GG, Dogan M, Patel PS, Azim S, Patel DS, Bhattacharya SK, et al. Key hepatoprotective roles of mitochondria in liver regeneration. Am J Physiol Gastrointest Liver Physiol. 2023;324(3):G207–18.
24. Mitra K, Wunder C, Roysam B, Lin G, Lippincott-Schwartz J. A hyperfused mitochondrial state achieved at G1-S regulates cyclin E buildup and entry into S phase. Proc Natl Acad Sci U S A. 2009;106(29):11960–5.
25. Budai A, Horváth G, Tretter L, Radák Z, Koltai E, Bori Z, et al. Mitochondrial function after associating liver partition and portal vein ligation for staged hepatectomy in an experimental model. Br J Surg. 2019 Jan;106(1):120–31.
26. Zhao Y, Zhao S, Liu S, Ye W, Chen W, dong. Kupffer cells, the limelight in the liver regeneration. Int Immunopharmacol. 2025 Jan;146:113808.
27. Brunnthaler L, Pereyra D, Brenner M, Santol J, Herrmann L, Schrottmaier WC, et al. Intrahepatic neutrophil accumulation and extracellular trap formation are associated with posthepatectomy liver failure. Hepatol Commun [Internet]. 2024;8(1) [cited 2025 Mar 31]. Available from: https://journals.lww.com/10.1097/HC9.0000000000000348
28. Markose D, Kirkland P, Ramachandran P, Henderson NC. Immune cell regulation of liver regeneration and repair. J Immunol Regen Med. 2018 Sep;2:1–10.
29. Di-Iacovo N, Pieroni S, Piobbico D, Castelli M, Scopetti D, Ferracchiato S, et al. Liver regeneration and immunity: a tale to tell. IJMS. 2023;24(2):1176.
30. Sakamoto T, Liu Z, Murase N, Ezure T, Yokomuro S, Poli V, et al. Mitosis and apoptosis in the liver of interleukin-6-deficient mice after partial hepatectomy. Hepatology. 1999 Feb;29(2):403–11.
31. Taub R. Liver regeneration: from myth to mechanism. Nat Rev. Mol Cell Biol. 2004 Oct;5(10):836–47.
32. Brenner C, Galluzzi L, Kepp O, Kroemer G. Decoding cell death signals in liver inflammation. J Hepatol. 2013 Sep;59(3):583–94.
33. Schmidt SC, Hamann S, Langrehr JM, Höflich C, Mittler J, Jacob D, et al. Preoperative high-dose steroid administration attenuates the surgical stress response following liver resection: results of a prospective randomized study. J Hepatobiliary Pancreat Surg. 2007;14(5):484–92.
34. Jaeschke H. Molecular mechanisms of hepatic ischemia-reperfusion injury and preconditioning. Am J Physiol Gastrointest Liver Physiol. 2003;284(1):G15–26.
35. Furrer K, Rickenbacher A, Tian Y, Jochum W, Bittermann AG, Käch A, et al. Serotonin reverts age-related capillarization and failure of regeneration in the liver through a VEGF-dependent pathway. Proc Natl Acad Sci U S A. 2011;108(7):2945–50.
36. Mullen JT, Ribero D, Reddy SK, Donadon M, Zorzi D, Gautam S, et al. Hepatic insufficiency and mortality in 1059 noncirrhotic patients undergoing major hepatectomy. J Am Coll Surg. 2007;204(5):854–62. discussion 862–864
37. Yokoyama Y, Schwacha MG, Samy TSA, Bland KI, Chaudry IH. Gender dimorphism in immune responses following trauma and hemorrhage. Immunol Res. 2002;26(1–3):63–76.

38. Birrer DL, Linecker M, López-López V, Brusadin R, Navarro-Barrios Á, Reese T, et al. Sex disparities in outcomes following major liver surgery – new powers of estrogen? Ann Surg. 2022 Jul;276:875–81.
39. Lee DU, Wang E, Fan GH, Hastie DJ, Addonizio EA, Chou H, et al. Malnutrition as a risk factor of adverse postoperative outcomes in patients undergoing hepatic resection: analysis of US hospitals. Br J Nutr. 2022;128(4):675–83.
40. Skullman S, Wirén M, Garlick PJ, McNurlan MA, Larsson J. Protein synthesis in regenerating rat liver during malnutrition. J Hepatol. 1994 Aug;21(2):174–81.
41. Reese T, Galavics C, Schneider M, Brüning R, Oldhafer KJ. Sarcopenia influences the kinetic growth rate after ALPPS. Surgery. 2022;S0039–6060(22):00252–5.
42. Berardi G, Antonelli G, Colasanti M, Meniconi R, Guglielmo N, Laurenzi A, et al. Association of sarcopenia and body composition with short-term outcomes after liver resection for malignant tumors. JAMA Surg. 2020;155(11):e203336.
43. Denbo JW, Kim BJ, Vauthey JN, Tzeng CW, Ma J, Huang SY, et al. Overall body composition and sarcopenia are associated with poor liver hypertrophy following portal vein embolization. J Gastrointest Surg. 2021 Feb;25(2):405–10.
44. Cruz-Jentoft AJ, Sayer AA. Sarcopenia. Lancet. 2019;393(10191):2636–46.
45. Sheptulina AF, Lyusina EO, Mamutova EM, Yafarova AA, Kiselev AR, Drapkina OM. Bioelectrical impedance analysis demonstrates reliable agreement with dual-energy X-ray absorptiometry in identifying reduced skeletal muscle mass in patients with metabolic dysfunction-associated steatotic liver disease and hypertension. Diagnostics (Basel). 2024;14(20):2301.
46. Joliat GR, Kobayashi K, Hasegawa K, Thomson JE, Padbury R, Scott M, et al. Guidelines for perioperative care for liver surgery: Enhanced Recovery After Surgery (ERAS) society recommendations 2022. World J Surg. 2023 Jan;47(1):11–34.
47. Russell K, Zhang HG, Gillanders LK, Bartlett AS, Fisk HL, Calder PC, et al. Preoperative immunonutrition in patients undergoing liver resection: a prospective randomized trial. World J Hepatol. 2019;11(3):305–17.
48. Linecker M, Botea F, Aristotele Raptis D, Nicolaescu D, Limani P, Alikhanov R, et al. Perioperative omega-3 fatty acids fail to confer protection in liver surgery: results of a multicentric, double-blind, randomized controlled trial. J Hepatol. 2020 Mar;72(3):498–505.
49. Hagiwara K, Watanabe A, Harimoto N, Araki K, Yokobori T, Muranushi R, et al. Liver regeneration after hepatectomy is significantly suppressed in a muscular atrophy mouse model. J Hepatobiliary Pancreat Sci. 2024 Mar;31(3):152–61.
50. Beppu T, Nitta H, Hayashi H, Imai K, Okabe H, Nakagawa S, et al. Effect of branched-chain amino acid supplementation on functional liver regeneration in patients undergoing portal vein embolization and sequential hepatectomy: a randomized controlled trial. J Gastroenterol. 2015 Dec;50(12):1197–205.
51. Little SA, Jarnagin WR, DeMatteo RP, Blumgart LH, Fong Y. Diabetes is associated with increased perioperative mortality but equivalent long-term outcome after hepatic resection for colorectal cancer. J Gastrointest Surg. 2002;6(1):88–94.
52. Luo J, Xu L, Li L, Zhang J, Zhang M, Xu M. Diabetes mellitus and postoperative blood glucose value help predict posthepatectomy liver failure in patients with hepatocellular carcinoma. J Gastrointest Oncol. 2021 Oct;12(5):2377–87.
53. Mendes-Braz M, Martins JO. Diabetes mellitus and liver surgery: the effect of diabetes on oxidative stress and inflammation. Mediators Inflamm. 2018;2018:1–11.
54. Hassanain M, Metrakos P, Fisette A, Doi SAR, Schricker T, Lattermann R, et al. Randomized clinical trial of the impact of insulin therapy on liver function in patients undergoing major liver resection. Br J Surg. 2013;100(5):610–8.
55. Fisette A, Hassanain M, Metrakos P, Doi SAR, Salman A, Schricker T, et al. High-dose insulin therapy reduces postoperative liver dysfunction and complications in liver resection patients through reduced apoptosis and altered inflammation. J Clin Endocrinol Metab. 2012 Jan;97(1):217–26.

56. Capussotti L, Viganò L, Giuliante F, Ferrero A, Giovannini I, Nuzzo G. Liver dysfunction and sepsis determine operative mortality after liver resection. J Br Surg. 2009 Jan;96(1):88–94.
57. Nesseler N, Launey Y, Aninat C, Morel F, Mallédant Y, Seguin P. Clinical review: the liver in sepsis. Crit Care. 2012;16(5):235.
58. Clavien PA, Petrowsky H, DeOliveira ML, Graf R. Strategies for safer liver surgery and partial liver transplantation. N Engl J Med. 2007;356(15):1545–59.
59. Reddy SK, Marsh JW, Varley PR, Mock BK, Chopra KB, Geller DA, et al. Underlying steatohepatitis, but not simple hepatic steatosis, increases morbidity after liver resection: a case-control study. Hepatology. 2012 Dec;56(6):2221–30.
60. Veteläinen R, van Vliet AK, van Gulik TM. Severe steatosis increases hepatocellular injury and impairs liver regeneration in a rat model of partial hepatectomy. Ann Surg. 2007 Jan;245(1):44–50.
61. Mehta NN, Ravikumar R, Coldham CA, Buckels JAC, Hubscher SG, Bramhall SR, et al. Effect of preoperative chemotherapy on liver resection for colorectal liver metastases. Eur J Surg Oncol. 2008 Jul;34(7):782–6.
62. Vauthey JN, Pawlik TM, Ribero D, Wu TT, Zorzi D, Hoff PM, et al. Chemotherapy regimen predicts steatohepatitis and an increase in 90-day mortality after surgery for hepatic colorectal metastases. J Clin Oncol. 2006;24(13):2065–72.
63. Rubbia-Brandt L, Audard V, Sartoretti P, Roth AD, Brezault C, Le Charpentier M, et al. Severe hepatic sinusoidal obstruction associated with oxaliplatin-based chemotherapy in patients with metastatic colorectal cancer. Ann Oncol. 2004 Mar;15(3):460–6.
64. Imamura H, Shimada R, Kubota M, Matsuyama Y, Nakayama A, Miyagawa S, et al. Preoperative portal vein embolization: an audit of 84 patients. Hepatology. 1999 Apr;29(4):1099–105.
65. Yokoyama Y, Nagino M, Nimura Y. Mechanisms of hepatic regeneration following portal vein embolization and partial hepatectomy: a review. World J Surg. 2007 Feb;31(2):367–74.
66. Kanda H, Nimura Y, Yasui A, Uematsu T, Kamiya S, Machiki Y, et al. Hepatic blood flow after acute biliary obstruction and drainage in conscious dogs. Hepatogastroenterology. 1996;43(7):235–40.
67. Tracy TF, Bailey PV, Goerke ME, Sotelo-Avila C, Weber TR. Cholestasis without cirrhosis alters regulatory liver gene expression and inhibits hepatic regeneration. Surgery. 1991;110(2):176–82. discussion 182–183
68. Bissig KD, Marti U, Solioz M, Forestier M, Zimmermann H, Lüthi M, et al. Epidermal growth factor is decreased in liver of rats with biliary cirrhosis but does not act as paracrine growth factor immediately after hepatectomy. J Hepatol. 2000 Aug;33(2):275–81.
69. Fujiwara Y, Shimada M, Yamashita Y, Adachi E, Shirabe K, Takenaka K, et al. Cytokine characteristics of jaundice in mouse liver. Cytokine. 2001 Feb;13(3):188–92.
70. Fan M, Wang X, Xu G, Yan Q, Huang W. Bile acid signaling and liver regeneration. Biochimica et Biophysica Acta (BBA) – Gene Regul Mech. 2015 Feb;1849(2):196–200.
71. Iyomasa S, Terasaki M, Kuriki H, Nimura Y, Shionoya S, Kojima K, et al. Decrease in regeneration capacity of rat liver after external biliary drainage. Eur Surg Res. 1992;24(5):265–72.
72. Olthof PB, Coelen RJS, Wiggers JK, Besselink MGH, Busch ORC, van Gulik TM. External biliary drainage following major liver resection for perihilar cholangiocarcinoma: impact on development of liver failure and biliary leakage. HPB (Oxford). 2016 Apr;18(4):348–53.
73. Piccus R, Joshi K, Hodson J, Bartlett D, Chatzizacharias N, Dasari B, et al. Significance of predicted future liver remnant volume on liver failure risk after major hepatectomy: a case matched comparative study. Front Surg. 2023;10:1174024.
74. Yamamoto R, Sugiura T, Okamura Y, Ito T, Yamamoto Y, Ashida R, et al. Utility of remnant liver volume for predicting posthepatectomy liver failure after hepatectomy with extrahepatic bile duct resection. BJS Open. 2021 Jan 8;5(1):zraa049.
75. Umemura K, Shimizu A, Notake T, Kubota K, Hosoda K, Yasukawa K, et al. Minimum proportion of future liver remnant in safe major hepatopancreatoduodenectomy. Ann Gastroenterol Surg. 2025 Jan;9(1):188–98.
76. Reese T, Gilg S, Böcker J, Wagner KC, Vali M, Engstrand J, et al. Impact of the future liver remnant volume before major hepatectomy. Eur J Surg Oncol. 2024 Nov;50(11):108660.

77. Stockmann M, Lock JF, Riecke B, Heyne K, Martus P, Fricke M, et al. Prediction of postoperative outcome after hepatectomy with a new bedside test for maximal liver function capacity. Ann Surg. 2009 Jul;250(1):119–25.
78. Makridis G, Reese T, Zádori ZS, Suling AI, Stark M, Horling K, et al. Is an intraoperative liver function assessment possible? Application of the 13C-methacetin-breath-test during major liver resections—a pilot study. HPB. 2023;26:91–101. S1365182X23019287
79. Schnitzbauer AA, Lang SA, Goessmann H, Nadalin S, Baumgart J, Farkas SA, et al. Right portal vein ligation combined with in situ splitting induces rapid left lateral liver lobe hypertrophy enabling 2-staged extended right hepatic resection in small-for-size settings. Ann Surg. 2012 Mar;255(3):405–14.
80. Ratti F, Serenari M, Avolio A, Batignani G, Boggi U, Brolese A, et al. Cornerstones and divergencies in the implementation and use of liver hypertrophy techniques: results from a nationwide survey for the set-up of the prospective registry. Updates Surg. 2024 Sep;76(5):1783–96.
81. Belghiti J, Noun R, Malafosse R, Jagot P, Sauvanet A, Pierangeli F, et al. Continuous versus intermittent portal triad clamping for liver resection: a controlled study. Ann Surg. 1999 Mar;229(3):369–75.
82. Dinant S, Roseboom HJ, Levi M, Van Vliet AK, Van Gulik TM. Hypothermic in situ perfusion of the porcine liver using Celsior or Ringer-lactate solution. Langenbecks Arch Surg. 2009 Jan;394(1):143–50.
83. Azoulay D, Salloum C, Allard MA, Serrablo A, Moussa M, Romano P, et al. Complex hepatectomy under total vascular exclusion of the liver preserving the caval flow with portal hypothermic perfusion and temporary portacaval shunt: a proof of concept. Ann Surg Oncol. 2024 Oct;31(10):6485–94.
84. Rahbari NN, Wente MN, Schemmer P, Diener MK, Hoffmann K, Motschall E, et al. Systematic review and meta-analysis of the effect of portal triad clamping on outcome after hepatic resection. British Journal of Surgery. 2008;95(4):424–32.
85. Clevenger B, Mallett SV. Transfusion and coagulation management in liver transplantation. World J Gastroenterol. 2014;20(20):6146–58.
86. Martel G, Carrier FM, Wherrett C, Lenet T, Mallette K, Brousseau K, et al. Hypovolaemic phlebotomy in patients undergoing hepatic resection at higher risk of blood loss (PRICE-2): a randomised controlled trial. Lancet Gastroenterol Hepatol. 2025 Feb;10(2):114–24.
87. Hughes MJ, Ventham NT, Harrison EM, Wigmore SJ. Central venous pressure and liver resection: a systematic review and meta-analysis. HPB (Oxford). 2015 Oct;17(10):863–71.
88. Stephanos M, Stewart CMB, Mahmood A, Brown C, Hajibandeh S, Hajibandeh S, et al. Low versus standard central venous pressure during laparoscopic liver resection: a systematic review, meta-analysis and trial sequential analysis. Ann Hepatobiliary Pancreat Surg. 2024;28(2):115–24.

Diagnosis and Classification of Posthepatectomy Liver Failure

5

Emrullah Birgin, Jan Heil, and Nuh N. Rahbari

Abbreviations

APRI-ALBI	Aspartate aminotransferase to platelet ratio index albumin bilirubin grade
CRP	C-reactive protein
ICG	Indocyanine green
INR	International normalized ratio
ISGLS	International Study Group of Liver Surgery
MELD	Model for end-stage liver disease
PHLF	Posthepatectomy liver failure

5.1 Introduction

Posthepatectomy liver failure (PHLF) is the most severe perioperative morbidity after liver resection, with mortality rates up to 30% [1–3]. In recent decades, the risk of PHLF has decreased due to meticulous preoperative preparation, parenchymal-sparing surgery, minimally invasive approaches, innovations in regenerative liver surgery, and improved perioperative care [4–6]. Simultaneously, indications for liver surgery were considerably extended, including patients with advanced liver disease, multimorbidity, and frailty, which in turn increases the risk of PHLF. Therefore, an internationally accepted definition is mandatory to diagnose

E. Birgin · J. Heil · N. N. Rahbari (✉)
Department of General and Visceral Surgery, Ulm University Hospital, Ulm, Germany
e-mail: Emrullah.birgin@uniklinik-ulm.de; Jan.heil@uniklinik-ulm.de; nuh.rahbari@uniklinik-ulm.de

L. Aldrighetti et al. (eds.), *Liver Regeneration Techniques In Hepatic Surgery*, https://doi.org/10.1007/978-3-032-10997-2_5

and classify PHLF for comparing clinical study outcomes and mitigate the consequences of PHLF for patients.

5.2 Terminology

In 2011, the International Study Group of Liver Surgery (ISGLS) defined PHLF as an acquired deterioration of liver function due to an insufficient functional reserve of the liver remnant following hepatectomy [7]. Moreover, the ISGLS proposed the terminology *posthepatectomy* rather than *postoperative liver failure* to specifically refer to liver surgery-associated liver failure. Since the *diagnosis of PHLF* cannot be made without a strict definition of PHLF excluding clinical conditions and outcomes affected by PHLF, the ISGLS provided a set of applicable criteria to characterize PHLF with different severity grades. However, some *prediction models* used in liver surgery are incorrectly applied as definitions and diagnoses of PHLF. These prediction models were initially developed to assess *postoperative mortality after liver surgery*, not to provide a definition and grading of PHLF as compared to the ISGLS definition. The most popular risk prediction models include the *50–50 criteria* [i.e., reduction of the prothrombin time (PT) by 50% and increase of a serum bilirubin by 50% on postoperative day 5] [8], the *3–60 criteria* (i.e., increase of C-reactive protein (CRP) level at >3 mg/dl and an antithrombin III level of <60% on postoperative day 1) [9], and the postoperative *hyperbilirubinemia of > 7 mg/dl* model after liver surgery [10]. Accordingly, various other definitions of liver failure circulated before 2011 and continue to be applied in the literature based on arbitrary defined postoperative laboratory values of bilirubin, international normalized ratio (INR), prothrombin time (PTT), aminotransferase, or arterial lactate without considering the severity of PHLF and the patient's clinical condition [11–17]. Thus, a universally accepted and validated definition, as provided by the ISGLS, remains essential for comparing outcomes between studies and ensuring consistency in scientific communication.

5.3 Liver Function Tests

Various liver function tests are available to assess the postoperative decline of liver function. Laboratory analyses provide valuable and rapid data on liver cell injury (such as alanine–aminotransferase, aspartate–aminotransferase), hepatic synthesis (such as albumin and INR), and excretory function (such as bilirubin, gamma-glutamyl transferase, alkaline phosphatase). Consequently, a combination of these parameters is often used in risk assessment models of postoperative mortality such as the Child–Turcotte–Pugh score (which combines albumin, bilirubin, and INR), the MELD score (incorporating bilirubin, creatinine, and INR) and the APRI-ALBI score (combining aspartate aminotransferase to platelet ratio index and albumin–bilirubin grade), respectively. The indocyanine green (ICG) retention test at 15 min is another widely used tool—particularly in Asian centers—for assessment of global hepatic function reserve but may be influenced by confounders such as histological findings and intrahepatic shunts, which can decrease the validity of ICG clearance [18]. Another test to evaluate the global hepatic function is the LiMAx® test (^{13}C-Methacetin breath test) [19]. This test has been predominantly used in selective German centers. However, it has shown limited effectiveness in predicting PHLF compared to other assessment tools and lacks prospective studies involving substantial patient cohorts [20, 21]. Moreover, imaging-based studies (such as contrast-enhanced magnetic resonance imaging or liver scintigraphy using ^{99m}Technetium-labeled iminodiacetic acids) with volumetric assessments of the future liver remnant are reliable tools for evaluating regional hepatic function reserve. Altogether, these various tests are primarily used to evaluate the extent of liver injury in the *preoperative* setting [22, 23]. However, the diagnosis of PHLF ultimately relies on robust, simple, and reliable diagnostic tests in the *postoperative* period.

5.4 Diagnosis and Definition of PHLF

In recent decades, several studies have evaluated the value of liver function assessment based on biochemical tests. However, studies using imaging or ICG retention tests to diagnose PHLF are scarce owing to their limited availability in routine clinical practice and the decreasing incidence of PHLF in recent years. Elevated serum transaminase levels are highly sensitive indicators of liver injury; however, their utility in identifying liver failure during the postoperative period remains controversial [24, 25]. Postoperative transient elevations of serum transaminases are often attributed to ischemia–reperfusion injury from intraoperative application of portal triad occlusion (i.e., the Pringle maneuver), which has been reported not to be associated with a compromised postoperative liver function [26, 27]. Similarly, a decrease in perioperative serum albumin levels may correlate with worse postoperative outcomes, but large-scale cohort studies with validated cutoff values for determining PHLF are lacking [28]. Furthermore, serum albumin levels are highly susceptible to other clinical conditions, such as renal failure or malnutrition. Parameters of liver cholestasis, such as serum gamma-glutamyl transferase or alkaline phosphatase, can also be elevated postoperatively due to liver regeneration. Nevertheless, some studies have demonstrated that postoperative elevations of two biochemical tests initially described in the Child–Pugh system—INR and serum bilirubin–are significantly associated with posthepatectomy mortality [7, 8]. Therefore, INR and serum bilirubin levels are frequently utilized as biochemical indicators to diagnose PHLF.

5.5 The ISGLS Definition of PHLF

In 2010, the ISGLS developed a consensus-based definition of PHLF. This process involved a systematic literature review, a consensus meeting, and a validation study [7]. A review of 52 different definitions of PHLF published between 2003 and 2009 was conducted and scrutinized in detail. The results revealed various definitions of PHLF with arbitrary cutoff values of different biochemical tests. Consequently, a new cohort study was conducted involving 835 patients who underwent partial hepatectomy [2]. For the first time in history, the natural progression of posthepatectomy biochemical values was systematically assessed through serial laboratory measurements. The study revealed that patients with elevated levels of serum bilirubin and/or INR on or after postoperative day 5, as well as those requiring postoperative clotting factors, experienced significantly higher rates of postoperative morbidity and mortality. Other potential causes for changes in bilirubin and INR levels, such as biliary obstruction, use of anticoagulants, or administration of vitamin K, were excluded. Additionally, other biochemical parameters like serum albumin, transaminase, gamma-glutamyl transferase, and alkaline phosphatase levels were not associated significantly with adverse postoperative outcomes. Therefore, the ISGLS included serum bilirubin and INR as part of the biochemical tests along with the need for postoperative clotting factors on or after postoperative day 5 to define PHLF. It is important to acknowledge that the ISGLS definition of PHLF was based on actual patient data and required the combination of two liver function tests. Finally, the ISGLS proposed the definition of PHLF as a "postoperatively acquired deterioration in the ability of the liver to maintain its synthetic, excretory, and detoxifying functions, which are characterized by an increased INR and concomitant hyperbilirubinemia on or after postoperative day 5" and validated this definition in a study involving 576 patients [7]. It is important that the ISGLS deliberately decided to avoid the use of fixed cutoff values to define increased INR and concomitant hyperbilirubinemia but rather referred to the cutoff values of the respective laboratories at the individual centers. This helped significantly to increase the applicability of the definition across centers, countries, and continents.

5.6 Severity of Postoperative Liver Failure According to the ISGLS Criteria

PHLF is a complex condition impacting multiple organ systems. PHLF resolution depends on liver regeneration after surgery, but effective monitoring methods are lacking [29]. Detecting and treating liver failure symptoms is vital to prevent multiorgan failure and death. The most relevant PHLF symptoms are depicted in Fig. 5.1 and include

- *Central nervous system-related symptoms* due to elevated levels of ammonia, causing hepatic encephalopathy.

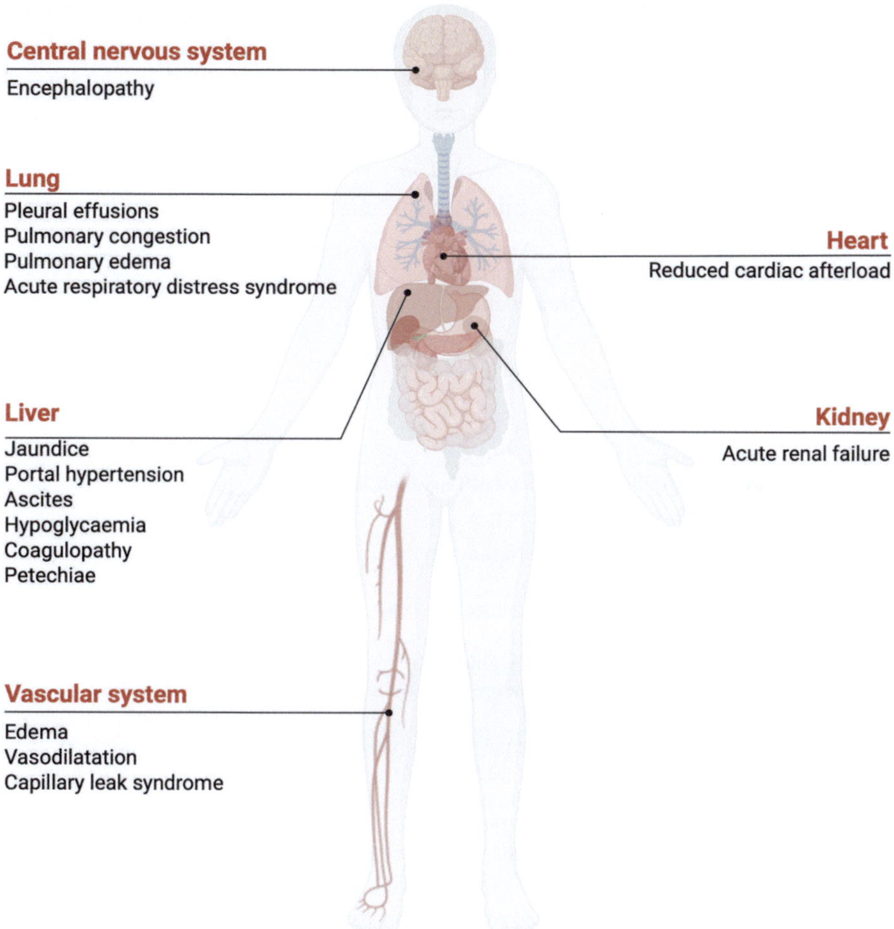

Fig. 5.1 Clinical manifestation of posthepatectomy liver failure. (Created in BioRender. Birgin, E. (2025) https://BioRender.com/vs82cgi)

- *Lung-related symptoms* include pleural effusions, pulmonary congestion, pulmonary edema, and impaired gas exchange leading to acute respiratory distress syndrome.
- *Liver-related symptoms* such as portal hypertension, ascites, coagulopathy, hypoglycemia, and hyperbilirubinemia.
- *Vascular system-related symptoms* can result from systemic inflammation with capillary leak syndrome, causing fluid loss, and vasodilation.
- *Heart-related symptoms* due to reduced cardiac afterload.
- *Kidney-related symptoms* may arise from underlying conditions like chronic kidney disease and cardiovascular diseases, as well as perioperative hypovolemia causing increased retention parameters or reduced urine output.

It is well known that the severity of PHLF and its associated impact on patients' clinical condition can vary significantly. However, prior to the ISGLS definition and grading of PHLF, there had been no severity classification of PHLF. The ISGLS categorizes PHLF into three severity grades based on treatment invasiveness and symptom severity (Table 5.1):

- *Grade A* is associated with biochemical changes without altering clinical management.
- *Grade B* requires noninvasive treatment.
- *Grade C* requires invasive treatment.

Table 5.1 Criteria for grading of posthepatectomy liver failure

	PHLF grade A	PHLF grade B	PHLF grade C
Specific treatment	No	Noninvasive[a]	Invasive[b]
Hepatic function	Adequate coagulation (INR <1.5) No neurological symptoms	Inadequate coagulation (INR ≥1.5/<2.0) Beginning of neurological symptoms	Inadequate coagulation (INR ≥2.0) Severe neurological symptoms/hepatic encephalopathy
Renal function	Adequate urine output (>0.5 ml/kg/h) Blood urea nitrogen <150 mg/dL No symptoms of uremia	Inadequate urine output (≤0.5 ml/kg/h) Blood urine nitrogen <150 mg/dL No symptoms of uremia	Renal dysfunction not manageable with diuretics Blood urine nitrogen ≥150 mg/dL Symptoms of uremia
Pulmonary function	Arterial oxygen saturation > 90%	Arterial oxygen saturation < 90% despite oxygen supply	Severe refractory hypoxemia Arterial oxygen saturation < 85% with high fraction of inspired oxygen
Additional evaluation	Not required	Abdominal ultrasonography/CT Chest radiography Sputum, blood, urine cultures, brain CT	Abdominal ultrasonography/CT Chest radiography/CT Brain CT Sputum, blood, urine cultures Intracranial pressure monitoring device

CT computed tomography, *INR* international normalized ratio, *PHLF* posthepatectomy liver failure
[a] Transfer to intensive care unit, circulatory support (vasoactive drugs), need for glucose infusion, hemodialysis, intubation and mechanical ventilation, extracorporeal liver support, rescue hepatectomy/liver transplantation
[b] Fresh-frozen plasma, albumin, daily diuretics, noninvasive ventilation, transfer to intermediate/intensive care unit

In the ISGLS validation study, 65 out of 576 patients (11%) were diagnosed with PHLF. Grade A was diagnosed in 5 patients (1%), grade B in 47 patients (8%), and grade C in 13 patients (2%), with mortality rates of 0%, 12%, and 54%, respectively.

5.7 Validation of the Definition and Classification of PHLF

The ISGLS aimed to establish a reliable and valid definition and classification of PHLF for practical use in clinical settings. Since its publication in 2010, this definition has been broadly accepted by the scientific community and cited more than 1575 times (source: web of science). Several other studies analyzed the clinical impact of ISGLS definition and grading in external cohorts and validated its applicability [3, 30–32]. Even among patients with preoperative liver damage and jaundice, the definition enables precise diagnosis and distinction between different degrees of PHLF [30]. Furthermore, the ISGLS definition of PHLF is associated with a higher sensitivity in the prediction of postoperative mortality compared of the 50–50 criteria, for which the latter prediction model was designed [1, 10].

A recent systematic review found that the ISGLS definition of PHLF is the most suitable definition for reporting data on *this condition* [33].

5.8 Summary and Outlook

Prevention and—in particular treatment—of PHLF remain clinical challenges. Even though advances in surgical and perioperative care decreased the incidence of PHLF, it still remains associated with significant morbidity and mortality in affected patients. Further improvement of preventive and therapeutic approaches is critically dependent on a definition of this complication, which is accurate, reliable, and applicable in clinical routine. In this regard, it is important to distinguish risk prediction models of postoperative mortality from actual definitions of PHLF, which provide a clinical framework for the diagnosis of this condition. The ISGLS for the first time developed a definition of PHLF diagnosis together with a classification of its severity, which was based on actual patient data and did not include specific cutoff values other than the ones at the local centers. This definition and severity grading were subsequently validated in various cohorts to be accurate and applicable in clinical routine. Future studies need to keep using the ISGLS definition of PHLF in order to facilitate cross-comparisons of results from different studies and further improve perioperative outcome of patients undergoing partial hepatectomy.

References

1. Rahbari NN, et al. The predictive value of postoperative clinical risk scores for outcome after hepatic resection: a validation analysis in 807 patients. Ann Surg Oncol. 2011;18(13):3640–9.

2. Reissfelder C, et al. Postoperative course and clinical significance of biochemical blood tests following hepatic resection. Br J Surg. 2011;98(6):836–44.
3. Sultana A, et al. Prospective evaluation of the International Study Group for liver surgery definition of post hepatectomy liver failure after liver resection: an international multicentre study. HPB (Oxford). 2018;20(5):462–9.
4. Birgin E, et al. Robotic or laparoscopic repeat hepatectomy after open hepatectomy: a cohort study. Surg Endosc. 2024;38(3):1296–305.
5. Birgin E, et al. Minimally invasive mesohepatectomy for centrally located liver lesions-a case series. Surg Endosc. 2022;36(12):8935–42.
6. Birgin E, et al. Robotic versus laparoscopic hepatectomy for liver malignancies (ROC'N'ROLL): a single-centre, randomised, controlled, single-blinded clinical trial. Lancet Reg Health Eur. 2024;43:100972.
7. Rahbari NN, et al. Posthepatectomy liver failure: a definition and grading by the International Study Group of Liver Surgery (ISGLS). Surgery. 2011;149(5):713–24.
8. Balzan S, et al. The "50-50 criteria" on postoperative day 5: an accurate predictor of liver failure and death after hepatectomy. Ann Surg. 2005;242(6):824–8. discussion 828–9
9. Gyoeri GP, et al. The 3-60 criteria challenge established predictors of postoperative mortality and enable timely therapeutic intervention after liver resection. Hepatobiliary Surg Nutr. 2019;8(2):111–24.
10. Mullen JT, et al. Hepatic insufficiency and mortality in 1,059 noncirrhotic patients undergoing major hepatectomy. J Am Coll Surg. 2007;204(5):854–62. discussion 862–4
11. Nagano Y, et al. The impact of advanced age on hepatic resection of colorectal liver metastases. J Am Coll Surg. 2005;201(4):511–6.
12. Azoulay D, et al. Ischemic preconditioning for major liver resection under vascular exclusion of the liver preserving the caval flow: a randomized prospective study. J Am Coll Surg. 2006;202(2):203–11.
13. Hemming AW, et al. Role for extending hepatic resection using an aggressive approach to liver surgery. J Am Coll Surg. 2008;206(5):870–5. discussion 875–8
14. Taura K, et al. Influence of coexisting cirrhosis on outcomes after partial hepatic resection for hepatocellular carcinoma fulfilling the Milan criteria: an analysis of 293 patients. Surgery. 2007;142(5):685–94.
15. Rahman SH, et al. Prognostic utility of postoperative C-reactive protein for posthepatectomy liver failure. Arch Surg. 2008;143(3):247–53. discussion 253
16. Torzilli G, et al. Systematic extended right posterior sectionectomy: a safe and effective alternative to right hepatectomy. Ann Surg. 2008;247(4):603–11.
17. Lodge JP, et al. In-contiguity and non-anatomical extension of right hepatic trisectionectomy for liver metastases. Br J Surg. 2005;92(3):340–7.
18. Rassam F, et al. Current modalities for the assessment of future remnant liver function. Visc Med. 2017;33(6):442–8.
19. Stockmann M, et al. Prediction of postoperative outcome after hepatectomy with a new bedside test for maximal liver function capacity. Ann Surg. 2009;250(1):119–25.
20. Santol J, et al. Comparison of the LiMAx test vs. the APRI+ALBI score for clinical utility in preoperative risk assessment in patients undergoing liver surgery – a European multicenter study. Eur J Surg Oncol. 2024;50(4):108048.
21. Stockmann M, et al. Randomized clinical trial comparing liver resection with and without perioperative assessment of liver function. BJS Open. 2018;2(5):301–9.
22. Wai CT, et al. A simple noninvasive index can predict both significant fibrosis and cirrhosis in patients with chronic hepatitis C. Hepatology. 2003;38(2):518–26.
23. Soubrane O, et al. Predicting high grade lesions of sinusoidal obstruction syndrome related to oxaliplatin-based chemotherapy for colorectal liver metastases: correlation with post-hepatectomy outcome. Ann Surg. 2010;251(3):454–60.
24. Kamiya H, et al. Peak-postoperative serum transaminases correlate with post-hepatectomy liver failure and inflow occlusion after laparoscopic liver resection. Anticancer Res. 2025;45(2):691–700.

25. Boleslawski E, et al. Relevance of postoperative peak transaminase after elective hepatectomy. Ann Surg. 2014;260(5):815–20. discussion 820–1
26. Birgin E, Reissfelder C, Rahbari N. Remote ischemic preconditioning in a cirrhotic patient undergoing major hepatectomy. Cureus. 2020;12(7):e9056.
27. Hardt JLS, et al. Remote ischemic preconditioning for reduction of ischemia-reperfusion injury after hepatectomy: a randomized sham-controlled trial. Surgery. 2024;175(2):424–31.
28. Joliat GR, et al. Postoperative decrease of albumin (ΔAlb) as early predictor of complications after gastrointestinal surgery: a systematic review. Perioper Med (Lond). 2022;11(1):7.
29. Søreide JA, Deshpande R. Post hepatectomy liver failure (PHLF) – recent advances in prevention and clinical management. Eur J Surg Oncol. 2021;47(2):216–24.
30. Birgin E, et al. Evaluation of the new ISGLS definitions of typical posthepatectomy complications. Scand J Surg. 2019;108(2):130–6.
31. Bogner A, et al. Intraoperative increase of portal venous pressure is an immediate predictor of Posthepatectomy liver failure after major hepatectomy: a prospective study. Ann Surg. 2021;274(1):e10–7.
32. Roberts KJ, Bharathy KG, Lodge JP. Kinetics of liver function tests after a hepatectomy for colorectal liver metastases predict post-operative liver failure as defined by the International Study Group for Liver Surgery. HPB (Oxford). 2013;15(5):345–51.
33. Sparrelid E, et al. Current evidence on posthepatectomy liver failure: comprehensive review. BJS Open. 2022;6(6):zrac142.

Part II

Volumetric and Functional Evaluation of Remnant Liver

6 Volumetric Study of the Liver and Cutoffs for a Safe Liver Surgery

Elena Panettieri, Antony Haddad, and Jean-Nicolas Vauthey

6.1 Introduction

Posthepatectomy liver failure (PHLF) has historically represented a threatening complication after major hepatectomy, particularly right or right extended hepatectomy [1]. Improved patient selection and the proper utilization of liver hypertrophy techniques for optimizing the future liver remnant (FLR) are responsible for better postoperative outcomes [2], and are of paramount importance to prevent the occurrence of PHLF in an era where the boundaries of liver surgery for oncologic disease keep being pushed [3, 4]. In this scenario, accurate assessment of preoperative FLR volume and liver hypertrophy is key to performing a safe liver surgery.

6.2 Volumetric Study of the Liver

Liver volumetry is based on the measurement and analysis of the liver's size and structure using imaging techniques, most notably computed tomography (CT) and magnetic resonance imaging (MRI). There are several techniques available to perform liver volumetry: manual, semiautomated, and fully automated [5].

Manual tracing volumetry is the traditional technique to assess liver volumes and is based on two-dimensional (2D) imaging. Typically, the entire perimeter of the liver, liver segments, and tumors is manually outlined on each cross-sectional slice. Subsequently, after the tumor areas are subtracted from the segment areas, the sums of the segment areas are multiplied by the section thickness to obtain the segment volumes [5].

E. Panettieri · A. Haddad · J.-N. Vauthey (✉)
Department of Surgical Oncology, The University of Texas MD Anderson Cancer Center, Houston, TX, USA
e-mail: JVauthey@mdanderson.org

L. Aldrighetti et al. (eds.), *Liver Regeneration Techniques In Hepatic Surgery*,
https://doi.org/10.1007/978-3-032-10997-2_6

Semiautomated volumetry is based on three-dimensional (3D) imaging. First, the software reconstructs liver parenchyma, portal branches, and hepatic veins as 3D structures, allowing for manual corrections as needed. The three components are then combined and, by selecting a branch of interest, the corresponding territory volume is calculated [6, 7]. While there are several software to perform 3D volumetry, semiautomated volumetry overall provides similar measurements as manual volumetry with the advantage of being more reproducible and significantly less time-consuming [5, 7, 8]. Nevertheless, the accuracy of 3D reconstruction in determining individual segment volume remains uncertain [5].

Fully automated liver volumetry has been more recently introduced and does not require any human intervention [9, 10]. While fully automated volumetry overall offers accurate results, it still requires operator intervention to correct any misidentified structures or segments. In addition, the clinical benefit of fully automated liver segmentation over semiautomated volumetry is not pronounced. Thus, its role in planning liver resection still needs to be assessed [5, 11].

6.3 Total Liver Volume and Future Liver Remnant Assessment

The future liver remnant, termed FLR, is obtained with the following formula: FLR = (future liver remnant volume / total liver volume) x 100. Measured FLR (mFLR) is obtained after determining the total liver volume (TLV), tumor volume, and FLR volume from imaging scans using the following formula mFLR (%) = FLR volume / (total liver volume—tumor volume) × 100 [12, 13].

While assessing mFLR is an easily applicable method, it does not take into account patient's body size and physiological needs. The concept of a standardized liver volume was first proposed by transplant surgeons to identify the minimum graft to patient's body weight (BW) ratio required for graft survival [14]. This principle was later adopted to plan liver resection as mFLR does not portray the relationship between liver volume and patient metabolic demands. Notably, of several formulas that have been proposed to correlate BW and body surface area (BSA) to TLV [14–17], two were established at The University of Texas MD Anderson Cancer Center based on liver volume measurements in 292 Western individuals with healthy livers [17]. After calculating BSA utilizing the Mosteller formula [18], a linear regression equation to assess the estimated TLV (eTLV) based on BSA was obtained: eTLV = – 794.41 + (1267.28 × BSA). Additionally, a formula based on patient's BW was also elaborated: eTLV = 191.80 × 18.51 × weight (kilograms). Subsequently, the ability of the formulas to predict PHLF was verified, demonstrating that both methods were appropriate for assessing liver volume in noncirrhotic patients [19]. Further studies comparing different equations reported that the formulas proposed by The University of Texas MD Anderson Cancer Center showed the least bias among all the methods available to assess eTLV [20, 21]. An online calculator accessible through the following website was established for ease of access (LiverVolume.com).

After eTLV is calculated, the ratio of the FLR volume to the baseline eTLV is defined as the standardized FLR (sFLR) and expressed as a percentage, as shown in the following formula: sFLR = (FLR volume / eTLV) × 100 [22]. Ribero et al. [23] aimed at determining which method of liver volumetry was more accurate in predicting a safe resection in 243 noncirrhotic patients undergoing resection of three or more liver segments. Results from their analysis demonstrated that the use of the eTLV, as opposed to a measured TLV, was able to identify a subset of patients (~11%) in whom liver volumetry with the measured TLV underestimated the risk of hepatic insufficiency [23].

6.4 Future Liver Remnant Cutoffs for Safe Hepatectomy

Volumetric evaluation of the liver is pivotal in appropriately planning liver resection and assessing indications to liver hypertrophy techniques since the extent of hepatectomy is inevitably related to the risk of PHLF.

Chun et al. [19] reviewed preoperative FLRs of 68 noncirrhotic patients who underwent major hepatectomy after portal vein embolization (PVE), demonstrating that an FLR/BW ratio of ≤0.4 and an FLR/TLV ratio of ≤20% provided equivalent thresholds to perform safe hepatectomy. While some authors suggested that preoperative PVE is indicated when the sFLR is <30% [24, 25], Kishi et al. [1] reported that rates of PHLF and death from PHLF were similar between patients with an sFLR of 20.1–30% and an sFLR ≥30%, but were higher in patients with an sFLR ≤20% in a cohort of 301 patients who underwent extended right hepatectomy. Additionally, Ribero et al. [26] analyzed outcomes of 112 patients undergoing hepatectomy after PVE, showing that overall, major and liver-related complications, PHLF, hospital stay, and 90-day mortality rate were significantly greater in patients with an sFLR of ≤20%. Based on such evidence, an sFLR >20% is considered the threshold for safe hepatectomy in patients with healthy livers undergoing extended right hepatectomy at The University of Texas MD Anderson Cancer Center [19, 26, 27].

The presence of underlying liver disease should be considered during volumetric evaluation of the liver. In particular, cirrhosis is associated with increased morbidity after major hepatectomy [28] and represents a risk factor for PHLF [29]. For this reason, an sFLR of at least 40% is recommended for safe hepatectomy in cirrhotic patients [30, 31]. A recent report by Reese et al. [32] took into account 1511 major hepatectomies, defining patients as at high-risk for PHLF in the presence of at least one of the following factors: diabetes mellitus, extended right hepatectomy, perihilar cholangiocarcinoma, gallbladder cancer, and cirrhosis. Results from this investigation confirmed that, in patients at high-risk for PHLF, the overall incidence of PHLF was 15% when the sFLR was <30%, increasing to 32% with an FLR of 30–40% [32].

Additionally, the widespread utilization of preoperative chemotherapy may impair liver function. More specifically, chemotherapy-associated liver injury (CALI) appears to be regimen-specific for irinotecan (steatohepatitis) and oxaliplatin (sinusoidal obstruction) [33–35]. This translates into increased overall morbidity, 90-day mortality, and PHLF-related mortality for irinotecan [35], and increased perioperative transfusion rate for oxaliplatin [36]. Shindoh et al. [22] observed that patients undergoing extended right hepatectomy after >12 weeks of chemotherapy for colorectal liver metastases developed PHLF more often than those who received short-course treatment or no chemotherapy (16.3% vs. 3.7%, $p = 0.006$). The best cutoff of FLR for preventing PHLF after long-course chemotherapy was estimated as >30%, with both chemotherapy >12 weeks and FLR $\leq$ 30% being independent predictors of PHLF [22]. Notably, not only is prolonged chemotherapy associated with CALI, but it is not associated with an increase in complete or major pathologic response [37].

6.5 Degree of Hypertrophy and Kinetic Growth Rate

After accurate assessment of preoperative liver volumetry, patients with an insufficient sFLR may be candidate to liver hypertrophy procedures, with PVE being the most widely used technique. Not only is PVE able to increase the sFLR, but it is also a tool to evaluate the regenerative potential of the liver, hence its functional reserve.

The degree of liver hypertrophy (DH), defined as the difference between the sFLR before and after PVE, is a dynamic measure of the liver regeneration capacity. Ribero et al. [26] demonstrated that sFLR increases the most during the first 3 weeks after PVE, reaching a plateau from week 3 to 8. After the eighth week from PVE, another rise in sFLR usually occurs, but it is usually less steep than the first peak. Hence, measuring sFLR during the post-PVE plateau phase provides the most accurate value since it reflects a steady state of liver regeneration [26]. Additionally, a DH < 5% was associated with complications, PHLF, hospital stay, and 90-day mortality after major or extended major hepatectomy [26].

Kinetic growth rate (KGR) is defined as DH at the first volumetric assessment after PVE divided by number of weeks elapsed after PVE. Shindoh et al. [38] demonstrated that KGR is a better predictor of postoperative outcomes after liver resection than sFLR and DH. In particular, in 107 patients undergoing

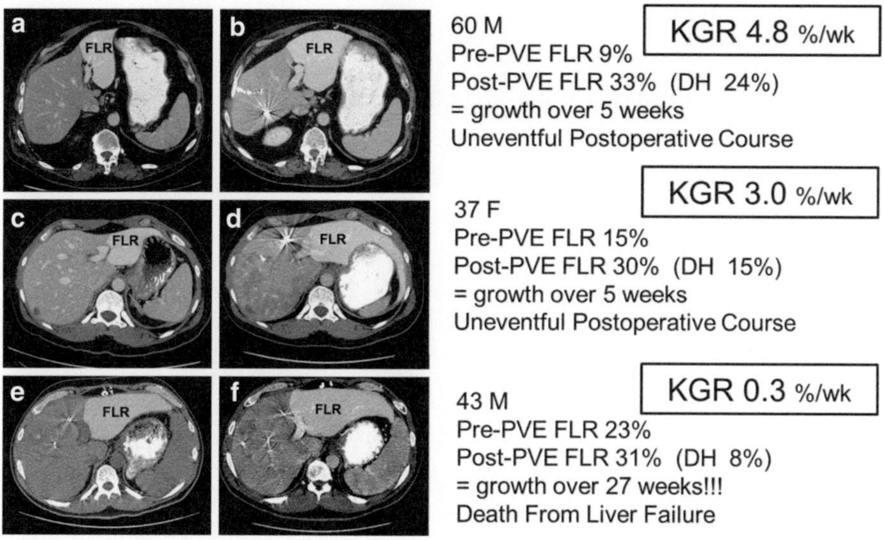

Fig. 6.1 Clinical cases showing how kinetic growth rate correlates with outcomes after hepatectomy following portal vein embolization. Abbreviations: *PVE* portal vein, *FLR* future liver remnant, *DH* degree of hypertrophy, *KGR* kinetic growth rate, *wk*. week

hepatectomy for CLM, a KGR < 2% per week was associated with rates of PHLF and liver-related 90-day mortality [38]. KGR showed to be reliable regardless of sFLR volume or timing of volumetric evaluation, provided that sFLR is assessed within 8 weeks from PVE [38]. Additionally, a KGR ≥ 2% proved to be a safe threshold to prevent PHLF even in patients experiencing significant hepatic atrophy ≥ 10% following preoperative chemotherapy (Fig. 6.1) [39]. Notably, Denbo et al. [40] published that patients with a KGR < 2% have a lower visceral adipose index and were more commonly sarcopenic than patients with a KGR ≥ 4.2%. Similarly, sarcopenic patients showed a lower visceral adipose index, a lesser DH, and lower KGR [39]. An algorithm for safe hepatectomy, including useful formulas, is portrayed in Fig. 6.2.

1) Measure **FLR volume**: manual, semiautomated, or fully automated volumetry

2) Calculate BSA with the **Mosteller formula**: $\sqrt{\frac{\text{weight (kg)} \times \text{height (cm)}}{3600}}$

3) Determine **eTLV**: - 794.41 + (1,267.28 x BSA)

4) Obtain **sFLR**: (FLR / eTLV) x 100

5) Evaluate safe sFLR cutoff based on **underlying liver parenchyma**:

Healthy liver > 20% [1,2]

CALI > 30 % [2]

Cirrhosis > 40% [3]

6) Perform **PVE/LVD** for patients with insufficient sFLR

7) Get new imaging **3-8 weeks** after PVE/LVD

8) Assess **KGR**: $\frac{\text{DH at first post-PVE/LVD volume evaluation (\%)}}{\text{time elapsed since PVE/LVD (weeks)}}$

9) Make sure KGR is **≥ 2% / week**

1. Abdalla EK *Arch Surg* 2002
2. Vauthey JN *Ann Surg* 2004
3. Shindoh J *Annal Surg Oncol* 2013
4. Kubota K *Hematology* 1997

Fig. 6.2 Algorithm for planning safe hepatectomy. Abbreviations: *mFLR* measured future liver remnant, *BSA* body surface area, *kg* kilograms, *cm* centimeters, *eTLV* estimated total liver volume, *sFLR* standardized future liver remnant, *CALI* chemotherapy-associated liver injury, *PVE* portal vein embolization, *LVD* liver KGR, kinetic growth rate, *DH* degree of hypertrophy

6.6 Conclusion

Precise volumetric assessment of the liver is pivotal in planning safe hepatectomy to avoid undesired events such as PHLF and PHLF-related mortality. Liver volume should be evaluated in patients candidate to major or extended hepatectomy to select the best surgical approach and to ascertain the need for liver hypertrophy procedures. At baseline, the presence of underlying liver conditions should be considered and FLR should be standardized based on eTLV accounting for patient's BSA. After performing liver hypertrophy techniques such as PVE, the most reliable metric to confirm appropriate degree of liver regeneration is KGR.

References

1. Kishi Y, Abdalla EK, Chun YS, Zorzi D, Madoff DC, Wallace MJ, et al. Three hundred and one consecutive extended right hepatectomies: evaluation of outcome based on systematic liver volumetry. Ann Surg. 2009 Oct;250(4):540–8. https://doi.org/10.1097/SLA.0b013e3181b674df.
2. Cloyd JM, Mizuno T, Kawaguchi Y, Lillemoe HA, Karagkounis G, Omichi K, et al. Comprehensive complication index validates improved outcomes over time despite increased complexity in 3707 consecutive Hepatectomies. Ann Surg. 2020 Apr;271(4):724–31. https://doi.org/10.1097/SLA.0000000000003043.
3. Torzilli G, Adam R, Viganò L, Imai K, Goransky J, Fontana A, et al. Surgery of colorectal liver metastases: pushing the limits. Liver Cancer. 2016 Nov;6(1):80–9. https://doi.org/10.1159/000449495.
4. Mueller M, Breuer E, Mizuno T, Bartsch F, Ratti F, Benzing C, et al. Perihilar Cholangiocarcinoma – novel benchmark values for surgical and oncological outcomes from 24 expert centers. Ann Surg. 2021;274(5):780–8. https://doi.org/10.1097/SLA.0000000000005103.
5. Haddad A, Lendoire M, Maki H, Kang HC, Habibollahi P, Odisio BC, et al. Liver volumetry and liver-regenerative interventions: history, rationale, and emerging tools. J Gastrointest Surg. 2024 May;28(5):766–75. https://doi.org/10.1016/j.gassur.2024.02.020.
6. Mise Y, Satou S, Shindoh J, Conrad C, Aoki T, Hasegawa K, et al. Three-dimensional volumetry in 107 normal livers reveals clinically relevant inter-segment variation in size. HPB (Oxford). 2014 May;16(5):439–47. https://doi.org/10.1111/hpb.12157.
7. Maki H, Nishioka Y, Haddad A, Lendoire M, Tran Cao HS, Chun YS, et al. Reproducibility and efficiency of liver volumetry using manual method and liver analysis software. HPB (Oxford). 2024 Jul;26(7):911–8. https://doi.org/10.1016/j.hpb.2024.03.1157.
8. Panettieri E, Vega EA, Salirrosas O, Ogiso S, Geller D, Conrad C. Global practice patterns of preoperative image reconstruction for liver surgery. J Gastrointest Surg. 2024 Jan;28(1):26–32. https://doi.org/10.1016/j.gassur.2023.11.014.
9. Koitka S, Gudlin P, Theysohn JM, Oezcelik A, Hoyer DP, Dayangac M, et al. Fully automated preoperative liver volumetry incorporating the anatomical location of the central hepatic vein. Sci Rep. 2022;12(1):16479. https://doi.org/10.1038/s41598-022-20778-4.
10. Lee S, Elton DC, Yang AH, Koh C, Kleiner DE, Lubner MG, et al. Fully automated and explainable liver segmental volume ratio and spleen segmentation at CT for diagnosing cirrhosis. Radiol Artif Intell. 2022;4(5):e210268. https://doi.org/10.1148/ryai.210268.
11. Suzuki K, Epstein ML, Kohlbrenner R, Garg S, Hori M, Oto A, Baron RL. Quantitative radiology: automated CT liver volumetry compared with interactive volumetry and manual volumetry. AJR Am J Roentgenol. 2011;197(4):W706–12. https://doi.org/10.2214/AJR.10.5958. PMID: 21940543; PMCID: PMC4277944
12. Heymsfield SB, Fulenwider T, Nordlinger B, Barlow R, Sones P, Kutner M. Accurate measurement of liver, kidney, and spleen volume and mass by computerized axial tomography. Ann Intern Med. 1979 Feb;90(2):185–7. https://doi.org/10.7326/0003-4819-90-2-185.
13. Kawasaki S, Makuuchi M, Matsunami H, Hashikura Y, Ikegami T, Chisuwa H, et al. Preoperative measurement of segmental liver volume of donors for living related liver transplantation. Hepatology. 1993 Nov;18(5):1115–20.
14. Urata K, Kawasaki S, Matsunami H, Hashikura Y, Ikegami T, Ishizone S, et al. Calculation of child and adult standard liver volume for liver transplantation. Hepatology. 1995 May;21(5):1317–21.

15. DeLand FH, North WA. Relationship between liver size and body size. Radiology. 1968 Dec;91(6):1195–8. https://doi.org/10.1148/91.6.1195.
16. Heinemann A, Wischhusen F, Püschel K, Rogiers X. Standard liver volume in the Caucasian population. Liver Transpl Surg. 1999 Sep;5(5):366–8. https://doi.org/10.1002/lt.500050516.
17. Vauthey JN, Abdalla EK, Doherty DA, Gertsch P, Fenstermacher MJ, Loyer EM, et al. Body surface area and body weight predict total liver volume in Western adults. Liver Transpl. 2002 Mar;8(3):233–40. https://doi.org/10.1053/jlts.2002.31654.
18. Mosteller RD. Simplified calculation of body-surface area. N Engl J Med. 1987;317(17):1098. https://doi.org/10.1056/NEJM198710223171717.
19. Chun YS, Ribero D, Abdalla EK, Madoff DC, Mortenson MM, Wei SH, Vauthey JN. Comparison of two methods of future liver remnant volume measurement. J Gastrointest Surg. 2008 Jan;12(1):123–8. https://doi.org/10.1007/s11605-007-0323-8.
20. Johnson TN, Tucker GT, Tanner MS, Rostami-Hodjegan A. Changes in liver volume from birth to adulthood: a meta-analysis. Liver Transpl. 2005 Dec;11(12):1481–93. https://doi.org/10.1002/lt.20519.
21. Olthof PB, van Dam R, Jovine E, Campos RR, de Santibañes E, Oldhafer K, et al. Accuracy of estimated total liver volume formulas before liver resection. Surgery. 2019;166(3):247–53. https://doi.org/10.1016/j.surg.2019.05.003. Epub 2019 Jun 14
22. Shindoh J, Tzeng CW, Aloia TA, Curley SA, Zimmitti G, Wei SH, et al. Optimal future liver remnant in patients treated with extensive preoperative chemotherapy for colorectal liver metastases. Ann Surg Oncol. 2013 Aug;20(8):2493–500. https://doi.org/10.1245/s10434-012-2864-7.
23. Ribero D, Amisano M, Bertuzzo F, Langella S, Lo Tesoriere R, Ferrero A, et al. Measured versus estimated total liver volume to preoperatively assess the adequacy of the future liver remnant: which method should we use? Ann Surg. 2013;258(5):801–6.; discussion 806-7. https://doi.org/10.1097/SLA.0000000000000213.
24. Clavien PA, Petrowsky H, DeOliveira ML, Graf R. Strategies for safer liver surgery and partial liver transplantation. N Engl J Med. 2007;356(15):1545–59. https://doi.org/10.1056/NEJMra065156.
25. Giraudo G, Greget M, Oussoultzoglou E, Rosso E, Bachellier P, Jaeck D. Preoperative contralateral portal vein embolization before major hepatic resection is a safe and efficient procedure: a large single institution experience. Surgery. 2008 Apr;143(4):476–82. https://doi.org/10.1016/j.surg.2007.12.006.
26. Ribero D, Abdalla EK, Madoff DC, Donadon M, Loyer EM, Vauthey JN. Portal vein embolization before major hepatectomy and its effects on regeneration, resectability and outcome. Br J Surg. 2007 Nov;94(11):1386–94. https://doi.org/10.1002/bjs.5836.
27. Abdalla EK, Barnett CC, Doherty D, Curley SA, Vauthey JN. Extended hepatectomy in patients with hepatobiliary malignancies with and without preoperative portal vein embolization. Arch Surg. 2002;137(6):675–80.; discussion 680–1. https://doi.org/10.1001/archsurg.137.6.675.
28. Cipriani F, Aldrighetti L, Ratti F, Wu AGR, Kabir T, Scatton O, Goh BKP, International Robotic and Laparoscopic Liver Resection Study Group Investigators. Impact of liver cirrhosis, severity of cirrhosis, and portal hypertension on the difficulty and outcomes of laparoscopic and robotic major liver resections for primary liver malignancies. Ann Surg Oncol. 2024;31(1):97–114. https://doi.org/10.1245/s10434-023-14376-5.
29. Baumgartner R, Gilg S, Björnsson B, Hasselgren K, Ghorbani P, Sauter C, et al. Impact of post-hepatectomy liver failure on morbidity and short- and long-term survival after major hepatectomy. BJS Open. 2022;6(4):zrac097. https://doi.org/10.1093/bjsopen/zrac097.
30. Kubota K, Makuuchi M, Kusaka K, Kobayashi T, Miki K, Hasegawa K, et al. Measurement of liver volume and hepatic functional reserve as a guide to decision-making in resectional surgery for hepatic tumors. Hepatology. 1997 Nov;26(5):1176–81. https://doi.org/10.1053/jhep.1997.v26.pm0009362359.
31. Qadan M, Garden OJ, Corvera CU, Visser BC. Management of Postoperative Hepatic Failure. J Am Coll Surg. 2016 Feb;222(2):195–208. https://doi.org/10.1016/j.jamcollsurg.2015.11.007.

32. Reese T, Gilg S, Böcker J, Wagner KC, Vali M, Engstrand J, et al. Impact of the future liver remnant volume before major hepatectomy. Eur J Surg Oncol. 2024 Nov;50(11):108660. https://doi.org/10.1016/j.ejso.2024.108660.
33. Karoui M, Penna C, Amin-Hashem M, et al. Influence of preoperative chemotherapy on the risk of major hepatectomy for colorectal liver metastases. Ann Surg. 2006;243:1–7.
34. Zhao J, van Mierlo KMC, Gómez-Ramírez J, et al. Systematic review of the influence of chemotherapy-associated liver injury on outcome after partial hepatectomy for colorectal liver metastases. Br J Surg. 2017 Jul;104(8):990–1002.
35. Vauthey JN, Pawlik TM, Ribero D, et al. Chemotherapy regimen predicts steatohepatitis and an increase in 90-day mortality after surgery for hepatic colorectal metastases. J Clin Oncol. 2006;24:2065–72.
36. Aloia T, Sebagh M, Plasse M, Karam V, Lévi F, Giacchetti S, et al. Liver histology and surgical outcomes after preoperative chemotherapy with fluorouracil plus oxaliplatin in colorectal cancer liver metastases. J Clin Oncol. 2006;24(31):4983–90. https://doi.org/10.1200/JCO.2006.05.8156.
37. Kishi Y, Zorzi D, Contreras CM, Maru DM, Kopetz S, Ribero D, et al. Extended preoperative chemotherapy does not improve pathologic response and increases postoperative liver insufficiency after hepatic resection for colorectal liver metastases. Ann Surg Oncol. 2010 Nov;17(11):2870–6. https://doi.org/10.1245/s10434-010-1166-1.
38. Shindoh J, Truty MJ, Aloia TA, Curley SA, Zimmitti G, Huang SY, et al. Kinetic growth rate after portal vein embolization predicts posthepatectomy outcomes: toward zero liver-related mortality in patients with colorectal liver metastases and small future liver remnant. J Am Coll Surg. 2013 Feb;216(2):201–9. https://doi.org/10.1016/j.jamcollsurg.2012.10.018.
39. Omichi K, Yamashita S, Cloyd JM, Shindoh J, Mizuno T, Chun YS, et al. Portal vein embolization reduces postoperative hepatic insufficiency associated with Postchemotherapy hepatic atrophy. J Gastrointest Surg. 2018 Jan;22(1):60–7. https://doi.org/10.1007/s11605-017-3467-1.
40. Denbo JW, Kim BJ, Vauthey JN, Tzeng CW, Ma J, Huang SY, et al. Overall body composition and sarcopenia are associated with poor liver hypertrophy following portal vein embolization. J Gastrointest Surg. 2021 Feb;25(2):405–10. https://doi.org/10.1007/s11605-020-04522-9.

7 Functional Study of the Liver: Imaging Tests

Pieter Arntz, Fenna van der Zijden, Thomas Van Gulik, Nienke Wassenaar, Roel Bennink, and Joris Erdmann

Major liver surgery carries significant risks due to the vital role of the liver in metabolic function and its limited regenerative capacity under compromised conditions [1]. Accurate preoperative assessment is essential to predict postoperative functional reserve and evaluate risk of post-hepatectomy liver failure (PHLF) [2–4]. The demand for reliable tools to assess liver function has grown substantially, driven by the increasing complexity of patient profiles, advancements in surgical techniques, and persistent challenges associated with morbidity and mortality [5, 6].

Various modalities have been developed to help clinicians tailor surgical and perioperative strategies, optimizing patient outcomes by balancing the need for radical resection with the preservation of sufficient functional reserve [7]. Initially developed to stratify patients for transplant eligibility, clinical grading systems such as the Child–Turcotte–Pugh score or model for end-stage liver disease have been adopted for risk prediction in liver surgery [8]. However, their utility is limited by their focus on advanced or end-stage liver disease and their inability to provide quantitative or regional assessments of liver function [9, 10]. This has driven the development of quantitative tools to better predict PHLF risk, guide preoperative

P. Arntz · F. van der Zijden · T. Van Gulik · J. Erdmann (✉)
Cancer Center, Amsterdam, The Netherlands

Department of Surgery, Amsterdam UMC, University of Amsterdam, Amsterdam, The Netherlands
e-mail: t.m.vangulik@amsterdamumc.nl; j.i.erdmann@amsterdamumc.nl

N. Wassenaar
Department of Radiology and Nuclear Medicine, Amsterdam UMC, Vrije Universiteit Amsterdam, Amsterdam, The Netherlands

Imaging and Biomarkers, Cancer Center Amsterdam, Amsterdam, The Netherlands

R. Bennink
Department of Radiology and Nuclear Medicine, Amsterdam UMC, Vrije Universiteit Amsterdam, Amsterdam, The Netherlands

L. Aldrighetti et al. (eds.), *Liver Regeneration Techniques In Hepatic Surgery*,
https://doi.org/10.1007/978-3-032-10997-2_7

liver conditioning strategies, and assess whether a liver resection should be avoided in cases of insufficient liver function [11, 12].

7.1 Quantitative Nonimaging Tests

Whole liver function tests such as the indocyanine green (ICG) clearance and methacetin breath test (LiMAx®, Humedics GmbH, Berlin, Germany) provide quantitative measurement of global liver function and are applicable in patients suspected of having underlying liver disease [13, 14]. While both tests effectively reflect liver functionality, their inability to assess regional variations limits their applicability in complex liver surgery planning.

7.2 Imaging Tests

Imaging modalities are integral to the assessment of the future liver remnant (FLR), including both volumetric and function-based measurements [3, 15]. Liver volumetry is used to quantify total and segmental liver volume, providing an estimate of the FLR to guide surgical planning (Fig. 1a1, a2). A cutoff of at least 30% for healthy livers and 40% for livers with parenchymal disease or perihilar cholangiocarcinoma is considered sufficient for safe resection. In patients with healthy liver parenchyma, volumetry serves as a reliable surrogate marker for hepatic functional reserve, assuming a homogeneous distribution of liver function. However, in patients with parenchymal disease or other underlying liver pathologies, such as fibrosis, cholestatic liver damage, or chemotherapy-induced liver injury, additional functional testing of remnant liver function is recommended [3, 16].

7.3 Hepatobiliary Scintigraphy

Hepatobiliary scintigraphy (HBS) has been developed as a practical tool for quantitative preoperative assessment of liver function and provides insights into global and regional liver function. This offers the ability to use the technique both as a screening method for patients with suspected underlying liver disease and as a targeted measure in high-risk patients [17–19]. These include patients undergoing liver augmentation procedures or extended resections, those with biliary tumors or underlying liver disease, and patients exposed to extensive chemotherapy regimens [20, 21].

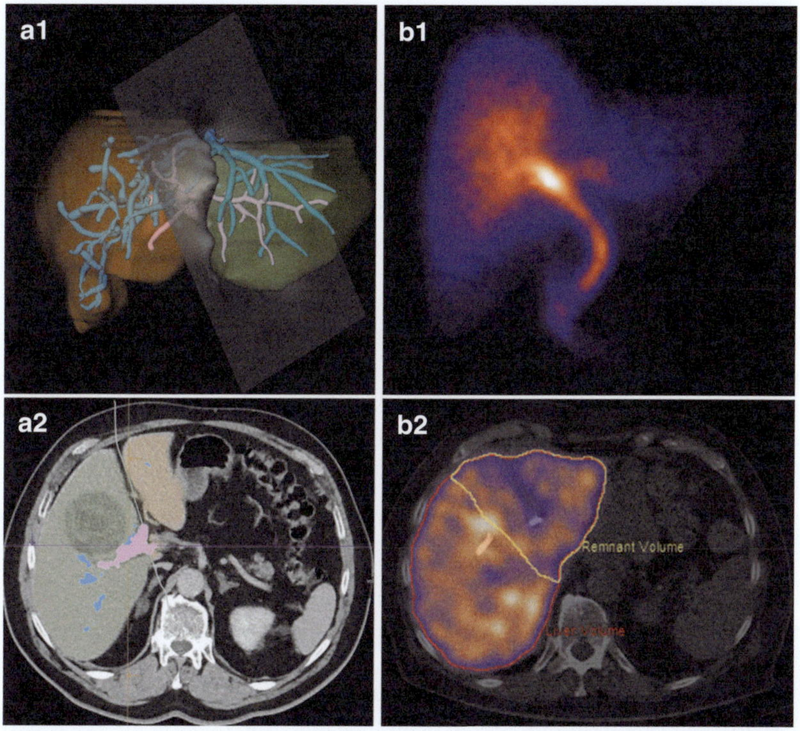

Fig. 1 (**a1**) 3D volumetric reconstruction for hepatic resection planning. The portal and hepatic veins are segmented to facilitate liver segmentation according to Couinaud segments. (**a2**) Axial CT volumetry segmentation (FLR S2–3) in a patient scheduled for an extended right hemihepatectomy. (**b1**) Hepatobiliary scintigraphy 3D heat map showing hepatic uptake and early biliary excretion after administration of 99mTc-mebrofenin. (**b2**) Axial view of hepatobiliary scintigraphy postprocessing and segmentation (FLR S1–4) in a patient scheduled for a right hemihepatectomy

7.4 Radiopharmaceutical

HBS combines dynamic liver uptake scintigraphy with single photon emission computed tomography and computed tomography (SPECT-CT), providing noninvasive quantitative measurement of total and regional liver function [22, 23]. The most commonly used radiopharmaceutical tracer in Western countries is technetium-99 m (^{99m}Tc)-mebrofenin (2,4,6 trimethyl-3-bromoiminodiacetic acid) [24]. The properties of this type of iminodiacetic acid ensure nearly exclusive hepatocyte uptake, along with rapid blood clearance and minimal renal excretion. Alternatively, ^{99m}Tc-galactosyl human serum albumin (Tc-GSA) receptor-mediated hepatic uptake followed by endocytosis and lysosomal degradation enables exclusive uptake within the liver without biliary excretion [25]. The limited availability of ^{99m}Tc-GSA restricted to Japan makes it unsuitable for global application.

7.5 Uptake Mechanism

Hepatic uptake of ^{99m}Tc-mebrofenin is almost exclusively mediated by the organic anion transporting polypeptides 1B1 and 1B3, exhibiting negligible renal excretion [24]. Biliary excretion of ^{99m}Tc-mebrofenin is facilitated by the multidrug resistance protein 2. In the presence of elevated serum bilirubin levels (>50 µmol/L), which in this patient group is likely due to primary (hepatic comorbidity, chemotherapy) or secondary (biliary obstruction) hepatocyte dysfunction, uptake of 99mTc-mebrofenin is impaired due to receptor competition, however, reflecting true impaired hepatocyte function [26]. The uptake mechanism of ^{99m}Tc-GSA differs from that of ^{99m}Tc-mebrofenin. After binding to asialoglycoprotein receptors on hepatocytes, ^{99m}Tc-GSA undergoes receptor-mediated endocytosis followed by lysosomal degradation [27]. This receptor-specific uptake mechanism ensures that elevated bilirubin levels do not interfere with ^{99m}Tc-GSA uptake, making it particularly suitable for use in cholestatic conditions.

7.6 Protocol: ^{99m}Tc-mebrofenin

HBS with ^{99m}Tc-mebrofenin acquisition involves a gamma camera and includes two dynamic planar scans with an interspersed three-dimensional SPECT-CT. Following an intravenous bolus injection of the radiopharmaceutical (200 MBq), the first dynamic planar scan measures the hepatic uptake rate of the liver. This is followed by a three-dimensional SPECT scan during peak uptake to map variation in functional distribution. Finally, a second dynamic planar acquisition measures biliary excretion to assess potential biliary obstruction. The low-dose CT for anatomical mapping is obtained at the end of the SPECT acquisition. Differences in regional liver measured activity on planar dynamic scans (due to the difference in depth of right and left liver lobes and distance-based signal body attenuation) are corrected by calculating the pixel-based geometric mean of the anterior and posterior datasets [28]. Post-processing is required to determine both total liver function and FLR function. Three regions of interest are defined within the image matrix to determine time–activity curves across the total field of view, the liver, and the left ventricle. The region of interest in the left ventricle represents blood pool activity, which serves as a reference for correcting the liver time–activity curve for nonspecific (vascular) uptake to calculate the hepatic mebrofenin uptake rate (%/min) with the Ekman formula [29]. To account for individual metabolic differences, the mebrofenin uptake rate is divided by the patient body surface area, calculated with the Mosteller formula [30]. This results in the corrected mebrofenin uptake rate, expressed as %/min/m^2, which denotes total liver function.

7.7 Protocol: ^{99m}Tc-GSA

The acquisition for ^{99m}Tc-GSA involves a dual or triple-head gamma camera and includes a single series of dynamic 3D SPECT imaging, 1 min post bolus injection of the radiopharmaceutical (185 MBq), The regional hepatic clearance of ^{99m}Tc-GSA is determined for each voxel using a Patlak plot [31]. The sum of hepatic clearance across all voxels yields the total hepatic clearance, expressed in mL/min. Clearance normalized by functional liver volume provides an index of hepatic function expressed in mL/min/mL.

The planned resection margins are delineated on the fused SPECT and low-dose CT images, providing anatomical detail and enabling the calculation of the functional share of the FLR. By aligning the functional distribution with the resection boundaries, the proportion of functional capacity within the FLR relative to the total liver function is determined (Fig. 1b1, b2).

7.8 Volume versus Function

Whether the practical determination of remnant liver function with HBS offers better prediction of PHLF than volumetry remains debated. The incidence of PHLF varies widely and is primarily dependent on the patient population undergoing liver surgery, the extent of resection, and the specific criteria used for defining and scoring PHLF [32–34]. In a recent large cohort study in 547 patients, both methods could predict liver failure in univariate analysis and demonstrate excellent negative predictive value [17–19, 35]. Interestingly, only liver function remained a significant predictor of liver failure in multivariate analysis [20]. HBS incorporates not only volumetry but also harbors information of known and unknown risk factors, making it a good screening tool for unexpected poor remnant liver function.

7.9 Evaluation of Preoperative Augmentation Procedures

The evaluation of preoperative augmentation procedures such as portal vein embolization (PVE), associating liver partition and portal vein ligation for staged hepatectomy (ALPPS), and liver venous deprivation (LVD) is complemented by HBS, portraying the strong redistribution of liver function to the contralateral liver [36]. In these patients, the volumetric kinetic growth rate may be employed, which is used to assess the rate of hypertrophy over time and predict overall and liver-specific postoperative morbidity and mortality [37]. Kinetic growth rate is calculated as the degree of hypertrophy observed during the initial volume assessment divided by the number of weeks elapsed since the procedure. Discrepancies between volumetric and functional assessment across interventions become more pronounced, as either volume or function may be overestimated or underestimated [38–40]. This mismatch increases the risk of misinterpreting remnant liver function, potentially leading to unsafe resections or deeming resection futile despite sufficient functional capacity.

7.10 Magnetic Resonance Imaging

Magnetic resonance imaging (MRI) presents a promising alternative in the preoperative assessment of liver function and evaluation of underlying liver disease. Gadolinium ethoxybenzyl diethylenetriamine pentaacetic acid (Gd-EOB-DTPA, Primovist®), a liver-specific contrast agent routinely used in clinical MRI lesion characterization, demonstrates specific accumulation in liver parenchyma with normal hepatocyte function [41, 42]. By shortening relaxation times in tissues, Gd-EOB-DTPA induces quantifiable alterations in signal intensity on MRI, which correlate with its uptake and excretion by hepatocytes. The mechanism of uptake of Gd-EOB-DTPA is similar to that of [99mTc]Tc-mebrofenin, relying on largely overlapping hepatocytes uptake receptors. This makes it a surrogate for liver function and a potential alternative for HBS [43].

7.11 Semi-quantitative

Semi-quantitative MRI techniques to estimate liver function include signal intensity (SI)-based indices such as relative liver enhancement, liver-to-spleen ratio, and liver-to-muscle ratio. These methods compare the pre- and post-contrast difference in SI, measured on T1-weighted MRI of the liver [44]. Ratio variants normalize hepatic SI changes to a reference organ, reducing variability caused by patient or scanner-related factors. SI-based indices are straightforward and clinically feasible but are significantly influenced by technical factors such as field strength and scanner variability, limiting their reliability for consistent comparisons over time, between patients, and across centers [45]. Combined with clinically validated techniques for quantitative measurement for whole liver function, SI may be valuable in the evaluation of regional distribution [46].

7.12 Relaxometry

T1 relaxometry is a quantitative measurement of longitudinal relaxation times in tissues. Unlike semi-quantitative methods, which rely on relative SI-based metrics such as peak enhancement, relaxometry relies on multiple acquisitions at different inversion or saturation times to provide a more absolute measurement [47]. In patients with liver cirrhosis, T1 relaxometry has been shown valuable in assessing parenchymal status and to differentiate between Child–Pugh score, separating mild to moderate from severe disease [48]. Additionally, T1 relaxation times have been correlated to markers of liver synthesis, such as albumin levels, in both cirrhotic and noncirrhotic patients [49].

7.13 Contrast-Enhanced

Contrast-enhanced T1 relaxometry further improves the evaluation by measurement of changes in T1 relaxation after the administration of contrast agents. These changes give static information in key physiological processes as hepatocyte uptake and biliary excretion. Evaluation of hepatic uptake with Gd-EOB-DTPA is therefore a promising modality for estimation of liver function. By using T1 mapping, a parametric image is generated where each pixel represents a T1 value, making it more intuitive and useful for visual assessment in clinical application as well as resection planning on a segmental level [50]. Its reliability can be affected by variability in imaging timing during the hepatobiliary phase, as well as physiological or pathological conditions such as altered perfusion or biliary dynamics. To maximize the clinical utility of T1 relaxometry, standardized imaging protocols and careful interpretation are essential.

7.14 Dynamic Contrast-Enhanced

Dynamic contrast-enhanced (DCE)-MRI potentially provides a novel quantitative method for the assessment of liver function [51, 52], enables imaging across multiple time points, and has the ability to capture contrast uptake and washout kinetics over time. DCE-MRI scans are analyzed by fitting a pharmacokinetic model with physiological parameters to quantify hepatocyte uptake kinetics. This approach also accounts for effect of hepatic blood flow [53]. This approach is designed to be more physiologically accurate compared to other MRI techniques. The extraction of these parameters requires precise timing of the contrast bolus, conversion of signal intensity into contrast agent concentration, and the fitting of pharmacokinetic models. A limitation of DCE is the complex and intricate evaluation of the process, combined with the lack of standardization across protocols and models, posing challenges for implementation in routine clinical application despite its potential to provide detailed liver function assessments.

Several qMRI techniques beyond T1-based methods have been developed to assess parenchymal status and estimate liver function based on underlying pathology. Intravoxel incoherent motion (IVIM) and diffusion-weighted imaging (DWI) evaluate tissue microperfusion and water diffusion, providing insights into fibrosis and cellular density [54, 55]. Magnetic resonance elastography (MRE) quantifies liver stiffness with high diagnostic accuracy for staging fibrosis and predicting liver-related complications [56]. Proton density fat fraction (PDFF) accurately quantifies hepatic steatosis, while T2 relaxometry measures iron overload, both of which can significantly impact liver function [57–59]. Iron-corrected T1 (cT1) relaxometry serves as a metric for liver fibrosis and inflammation, correlating well with functional impairment [60]. Multiple qMRI techniques can be integrated into multiparametric MRI (mpMRI), offering a comprehensive assessment of liver composition and functionality.

A critical limitation of mpMRI is that, while several commercially available protocols integrate qMRI methods into an mpMRI workflow to support volumetry, their utility for direct liver function assessment remains underdeveloped. These protocols can differentiate between healthy and diseased liver parenchyma by incorporating data on parenchymal status and vascular characteristics. However, they lack clinical applicability for precise liver function assessment, particularly in borderline cases where subtle functional impairments must be considered. Moreover, liver disease does not always correlate directly with decreased liver function. The absence of validated cutoff values to distinguish borderline insufficient livers limits their ability to provide actionable insights for clinical decision-making. Without robust validation and standardization, mpMRI remains a supplementary tool rather than a definitive method for liver function evaluation.

7.15 Summary

Volumetry is the gold standard for predicting and preventing PHLF as it is inexpensive and widely available. However, the addition of functional tests is recommended. HBS provides spatial information on the distribution of liver function, complementing volumetry and enhancing the detection of (unexpected) poor remnant liver function. Following augmentative procedures, volume and function do not correlate in a 1:1 manner. While HBS allows direct measurement of absolute remnant function, volumetry alone requires KGR to assess liver regenerative capacity. Evaluation of liver function with MRI is complex, prone to inter-observer variability, and lacks clinically validated cutoff values for predicting the risk of PHLF.

References

1. Friedman LS. The risk of surgery in patients with liver disease. Hepatology. 1999;29(6):1617–23.
2. Sparrelid E, Olthof PB, Dasari BV, Erdmann JI, Santol J, Starlinger P, Gilg S. Current evidence on posthepatectomy liver failure: comprehensive review. BJS Open. 2022;6(6):zrac142.
3. Primavesi F, Maglione M, Cipriani F, Denecke T, Oberkofler CE, Starlinger P, et al. E-AHPBA–ESSO–ESSR Innsbruck consensus guidelines for preoperative liver function assessment before hepatectomy. Br J Surg. 2023;110(10):1331–47.
4. Arntz P, Olthof PB. Assessment of liver function before major hepatectomy. Br J Surg. 2023;110(12):1588–9.
5. Madoff DC, Odisio BC, Schadde E, Gaba RC, Bennink RJ, van Gulik TM, Guiu B. Improving the safety of major resection for hepatobiliary malignancy: portal vein embolization and recent innovations in liver regeneration strategies. Curr Oncol Rep. 2020;22:1–20.
6. Baumgartner R, Gilg S, Björnsson B, Hasselgren K, Ghorbani P, Sauter C, et al. Impact of post-hepatectomy liver failure on morbidity and short-and long-term survival after major hepatectomy. BJS Open. 2022;6(4):zrac097.
7. Guglielmi A, Ruzzenente A, Conci S, Valdegamberi A, Iacono C. How much remnant is enough in liver resection? Dig Surg. 2012;29(1):6–17.
8. Farnsworth N, Fagan SP, Berger DH, Awad SS. Child-Turcotte-Pugh versus MELD score as a predictor of outcome after elective and emergent surgery in cirrhotic patients. Am J Surg. 2004;188(5):580–3.

9. Morandi A, Risaliti M, Montori M, Buccianti S, Bartolini I, Moraldi L. Predicting post-hepatectomy liver failure in HCC patients: a review of liver function assessment based on laboratory tests scores. Medicina. 2023;59(6):1099.
10. Teh SH, Sheppard BC, Schwartz J, Orloff SL. Model for end-stage liver disease score fails to predict perioperative outcome after hepatic resection for hepatocellular carcinoma in patients without cirrhosis. Am J Surg. 2008;195(5):697–701.
11. Morris-Stiff G, Gomez D, Prasad R. Quantitative assessment of hepatic function and its relevance to the liver surgeon. J Gastrointest Surg. 2009;13(2):374–85.
12. Rassam F, Olthof PB, Bennink RJ, van Gulik TM. Current modalities for the assessment of future remnant liver function. Visceral Med. 2017;33(6):442–8.
13. Lau H, Man K, Fan ST, Yu WC, Lo CM, Wong J. Evaluation of preoperative hepatic function in patients with hepatocellular carcinoma undergoing hepatectomy. Br J Surg. 1997;84(9):1255–9.
14. Stockmann M, Lock JF, Riecke B, Heyne K, Martus P, Fricke M, et al. Prediction of postoperative outcome after hepatectomy with a new bedside test for maximal liver function capacity. Ann Surg. 2009;250(1):119–25.
15. Reese T, Gilg S, Böcker J, Wagner KC, Vali M, Engstrand J, et al. Impact of the future liver remnant volume before major hepatectomy. Eur J Surg Oncol. 2024;50(11):108660.
16. Rio Bartulos C, Senk K, Schumacher M, Plath J, Kaiser N, Bade R, et al. Assessment of liver function with MRI: where do we stand? Front Med. 2022;9:839919.
17. Bennink RJ, Dinant S, Erdogan D, Heijnen BH, Straatsburg IH, van Vliet AK, van Gulik TM. Preoperative assessment of postoperative remnant liver function using hepatobiliary scintigraphy. J Nucl Med. 2004;45(6):965–71.
18. Dinant S, de Graaf W, Verwer BJ, Bennink RJ, van Lienden KP, Gouma DJ, et al. Risk assessment of posthepatectomy liver failure using hepatobiliary scintigraphy and CT volumetry. J Nucl Med. 2007;48(5):685–92.
19. Cieslak KP, Bennink RJ, de Graaf W, van Lienden KP, Besselink MG, Busch OR, et al. Measurement of liver function using hepatobiliary scintigraphy improves risk assessment in patients undergoing major liver resection. HPB. 2016;18(9):773–80.
20. Olthof PB, Arntz P, Truant S, El Amrani M, Dasari BV, Tomassini F, et al. Hepatobiliary scintigraphy to predict postoperative liver failure after major liver resection; a multicenter cohort study in 547 patients. HPB. 2023;25(4):417–24.
21. Olthof PB, Coelen RJ, Bennink RJ, Heger M, Lam MF, Besselink MG, et al. 99mTc-mebrofenin hepatobiliary scintigraphy predicts liver failure following major liver resection for perihilar cholangiocarcinoma. HPB. 2017;19(10):850–8.
22. Arntz PJ, Deroose CM, Marcus C, Sturesson C, Panaro F, Erdmann J, et al. Joint EANM/SNMMI/IHPBA procedure guideline for [99mTc] Tc-mebrofenin hepatobiliary scintigraphy SPECT/CT in the quantitative assessment of the future liver remnant function. HPB. 2023;25(10):1131–44.
23. Rassam F, Olthof PB, Richardson H, van Gulik TM, Bennink RJ. Practical guidelines for the use of technetium-99m mebrofenin hepatobiliary scintigraphy in the quantitative assessment of liver function. Nucl Med Commun. 2019;40(4):297–307.
24. Krishnamurthy S, Krishnamurthy GT. Technetium-99m-iminodiacetic acid organic anions: review of biokinetics and clinical application in hepatology. Hepatology. 1989;9(1):139–53.
25. Kudo M, Todo A, Ikekubo K, Hino M. Receptor index via hepatic asialoglycoprotein receptor imaging: correlation with chronic hepatocellular damage. Am J Gastroenterol (Springer Nature). 1992;87(7):865–70.
26. Slijepcevic D, Roscam Abbing RL, Fuchs CD, Haazen LC, Beuers U, Trauner M, et al. Na+-taurocholate cotransporting polypeptide inhibition has hepatoprotective effects in cholestasis in mice. Hepatology. 2018;68(3):1057–69.
27. Ha-Kawa SK, Tanaka Y. A quantitative model of technetium-99m-DTPA-galactosyl-HSA for the assessment of hepatic blood flow and hepatic binding receptor. J Nucl Med. 1991;32(12):2233–40.
28. de Graaf W, van Lienden KP, van Gulik TM, Bennink RJ. 99mTc-mebrofenin hepatobiliary scintigraphy with SPECT for the assessment of hepatic function and liver functional volume before partial hepatectomy. J Nucl Med. 2010;51(2):229–36.

29. Ekman M, Fjälling M, Holmberg S, Person H. IODIDA clearance rate: a method for measuring hepatocyte uptake function. In: Transplantation proceedings; 1992.
30. Mosteller RD. Simplified calculation of body surface area. N Engl J Med. 1987;317:1098.
31. Hwang E-H, Taki J, Shuke N, Nakajima K, Kinuya S, Konishi S, et al. Preoperative assessment of residual hepatic functional reserve using 99mTc-DTPA-galactosyl-human serum albumin dynamic SPECT. J Nucl Med. 1999;40(10):1644–51.
32. Rahbari NN, Garden OJ, Padbury R, Brooke-Smith M, Crawford M, Adam R, et al. Posthepatectomy liver failure: a definition and grading by the International Study Group of Liver Surgery (ISGLS). Surgery. 2011;149(5):713–24.
33. Ray S, Mehta N, Golhar A, Nundy S. Post hepatectomy liver failure–a comprehensive review of current concepts and controversies. Ann Med Surg. 2018;34:4–10.
34. Schreckenbach T, Liese J, Bechstein WO, Moench C. Posthepatectomy liver failure. Dig Surg. 2012;29(1):79–85.
35. Serenari M, Bonatti C, Zanoni L, Peta G, Tabacchi E, Cucchetti A, et al. The role of hepatobiliary scintigraphy combined with spect/ct in predicting severity of liver failure before major hepatectomy: a single-center pilot study. Updat Surg. 2021;73:197–208.
36. Franken L, Rassam F, Van Lienden K, Bennink R, Besselink M, Busch O, et al. Effect of structured use of preoperative portal vein embolization on outcomes after liver resection of perihilar cholangiocarcinoma. BJS Open. 2020;4(3):449–55.
37. Shindoh J, Truty MJ, Aloia TA, Curley SA, Zimmitti G, Huang SY, et al. Kinetic growth rate after portal vein embolization predicts posthepatectomy outcomes: toward zero liver-related mortality in patients with colorectal liver metastases and small future liver remnant. J Am Coll Surg. 2013;216(2):201–9.
38. Rassam F, Olthof PB, van Lienden KP, Bennink RJ, Besselink MG, Busch OR, van Gulik TM. Functional and volumetric assessment of liver segments after portal vein embolization: differences in hypertrophy response. Surgery. 2019;165(4):686–95.
39. Rassam F, Olthof PB, van Lienden KP, Bennink RJ, Erdmann JI, Swijnenburg R-J, et al. Comparison of functional and volumetric increase of the future remnant liver and postoperative outcomes after portal vein embolization and complete or partial associating liver partition and portal vein ligation for staged hepatectomy (ALPPS). Ann Transl Med. 2020;8(7):436.
40. Rassam F, Van Lienden K, Olthof P, Bennink R, Busch O, Erdmann J, et al. Hypertrophy responses after portal vein embolization, complete and partial ALPPS in patients undergoing major liver resection. HPB. 2020;22:S373.
41. Baleato-González S, Vilanova JC, Luna A, Menéndez de Llano R, Laguna-Reyes JP, Machado-Pereira DM, et al. Current and advanced applications of Gadoxetic acid–enhanced MRI in hepatobiliary disorders. Radiographics. 2023;43(4):e220087.
42. Reimer P, Schneider G, Schima W. Hepatobiliary contrast agents for contrast-enhanced MRI of the liver: properties, clinical development and applications. Eur Radiol. 2004;14:559–78.
43. Leonhardt M, Keiser M, Oswald S, Kühn J, Jia J, Grube M, et al. Hepatic uptake of the magnetic resonance imaging contrast agent Gd-EOB-DTPA: role of human organic anion transporters. Drug Metab Dispos. 2010;38(7):1024–8.
44. Kukuk GM, Schaefer SG, Fimmers R, Hadizadeh DR, Ezziddin S, Spengler U, et al. Hepatobiliary magnetic resonance imaging in patients with liver disease: correlation of liver enhancement with biochemical liver function tests. Eur Radiol. 2014;24:2482–90.
45. Mazzola M, Cannella R, Pilato G, Blandino AA, Milazzo M, Matteini F, et al. Quantitative liver MRI biomarkers: what the radiologist should know. J Med Imaging Interv Radiol. 2024;11(1):13.
46. Nilsson H, Karlgren S, Blomqvist L, Jonas E. The inhomogeneous distribution of liver function: possible impact on the prediction of post-operative remnant liver function. HPB. 2015;17(3):272–7.
47. Haimerl M, Verloh N, Zeman F, Fellner C, Nickel D, Lang SA, et al. Gd-EOB-DTPA-enhanced MRI for evaluation of liver function: comparison between signal-intensity-based indices and T1 relaxometry. Sci Rep. 2017;7(1):43347.

48. Heye T, Yang S-R, Bock M, Brost S, Weigand K, Longerich T, et al. MR relaxometry of the liver: significant elevation of T1 relaxation time in patients with liver cirrhosis. Eur Radiol. 2012;22:1224–32.
49. Fahlenkamp UL, Kunkel J, Ziegeler K, Neumann K, Adams LC, Engel G, et al. Correlation of native liver parenchyma T1 and T2 relaxation times and liver synthetic function tests: a pilot study. Diagnostics. 2021;11(6):1125.
50. Zhou Z-P, Long L-L, Qiu W-J, Cheng G, Huang L-J, Yang T-F, Huang Z-K. Evaluating segmental liver function using T1 mapping on Gd-EOB-DTPA-enhanced MRI with a 3.0 Tesla. BMC Med Imaging. 2017;17:1–7.
51. Nilsson H, Blomqvist L, Douglas L, Nordell A, Jonas E. Assessment of liver function in primary biliary cirrhosis using Gd-EOB-DTPA-enhanced liver MRI. HPB. 2010;12(8):567–76.
52. Rassam F, Zhang T, Cieslak K, Lavini C, Stoker J, Bennink R, et al. Comparison between dynamic gadoxetate-enhanced MRI and 99m Tc-mebrofenin hepatobiliary scintigraphy with SPECT for quantitative assessment of liver function. Eur Radiol. 2019;29:5063–72.
53. Materne R, Smith A, Peeters F, Dehoux J-P, Keyeux A, Horsmans Y, Van Beers B. Assessment of hepatic perfusion parameters with dynamic MRI. Magn Reson Med. 2002;47(1):135–42.
54. Chow AM, Gao DS, Fan SJ, Qiao Z, Lee FY, Yang J, et al. Liver fibrosis: an intravoxel incoherent motion (IVIM) study. J Magn Reson Imaging. 2012;36(1):159–67.
55. Tao Y-Y, Zhou Y, Wang R, Gong X-Q, Zheng J, Yang C, et al. Progress of intravoxel incoherent motion diffusion-weighted imaging in liver diseases. World J Clin Cases. 2020;8(15):3164.
56. Berzigotti A, Tsochatzis E, Boursier J, Castera L, Cazzagon N, Friedrich-Rust M, et al. EASL clinical practice guidelines on non-invasive tests for evaluation of liver disease severity and prognosis–2021 update. J Hepatol. 2021;75(3):659–89.
57. Caussy C, Reeder SB, Sirlin CB, Loomba R. Noninvasive, quantitative assessment of liver fat by MRI-PDFF as an endpoint in NASH trials. Hepatology. 2018;68(2):763–72.
58. Horng DE, Hernando D, Reeder SB. Quantification of liver fat in the presence of iron overload. J Magn Reson Imaging. 2017;45(2):428–39.
59. St. Pierre TG, Clark PR, Chua-anusorn W, Fleming AJ, Jeffrey GP, Olynyk JK, et al. Noninvasive measurement and imaging of liver iron concentrations using proton magnetic resonance. Blood. 2005;105(2):855–61.
60. Dillman JR, Serai SD, Miethke AG, Singh R, Tkach JA, Trout AT. Comparison of liver T1 relaxation times without and with iron correction in pediatric autoimmune liver disease. Pediatr Radiol. 2020;50:935–42.

Functional Study of the Liver: Nonimaging Tests

8

Takashi Kokudo and Norihiro Kokudo

8.1 Introduction

Most patients with hepatocellular carcinoma (HCC) exhibit underlying liver disease [1]. HCC has many therapeutic options, including transplantation, ablation, transarterial chemoembolization, and systemic therapy. Liver resection is predominantly accepted as an effective curative treatment for HCC, and the capacity of the liver to regenerate and restore its volume and function enables lesion removal in the hepatic parenchyma [2]. However, excessive diseased liver volume resection causes insufficient functional reserve of the remnant liver, resulting in posthepatectomy liver failure (PHLF). The mortality rate after liver resection in patients with HCC reaches up to 5.0% [3–5]. Furthermore, PHLF significantly influences the long-term survival of patients with HCC [6, 7]. Therefore, PHLF remains a leading cause of hepatectomy-related mortality and has hindered expanding the surgical indications for HCC, despite advances in surgical techniques and perioperative management. Preventing PHLF occurrence by accurately estimating the liver functional reserve and identifying the permissive future remnant volume during preoperative planning is crucial. Several studies attempted to develop criteria for liver function for safe liver resection [8–11]. However, accurate PHLF predictors based on preoperative liver function evaluation remain controversial [2]. Portal hypertension is considered a contraindication for liver resection in Western countries, and the indocyanine green (ICG) test is predominantly used in East Asian countries to decide surgery in patients with HCC [12–20].

This review aimed to summarize the utility of the current options for the preoperative nonimaging assessment of liver function.

T. Kokudo · N. Kokudo (✉)
National Center for Global Health and Medicine, Tokyo, Japan
e-mail: nkokudo@hosp.ncgm.go.jp

L. Aldrighetti et al. (eds.), *Liver Regeneration Techniques In Hepatic Surgery*,
https://doi.org/10.1007/978-3-032-10997-2_8

8.2 Routine Blood Biochemical Tests and Clinical Scoring Systems

The Child–Pugh score is a classical and popular scoring system for stratifying the prognosis of patients with HCC and as a general guide for surgical resection indication [21, 22]. This score is based on five simple parameters, including encephalopathy, ascites, serum total bilirubin level, serum albumin level, and prothrombin time [23]. Additionally, the model for end-stage liver disease (MELD) score is a widely utilized liver function scoring system that is useful for the prognostication of patients with HCC. The MELD score, which incorporates renal function and general liver functional indicators, was originally designed to predict survival in patients with cirrhosis after a transjugular intrahepatic portosystemic shunt insertion [24]. The MELD score has been employed to prioritize candidates for liver transplantation [25]. Further, the MELD score has been applied for the early prediction of postoperative morbidity and mortality in patients undergoing liver resection [26], but its predictive performance in patients without advanced cirrhosis remains controversial [27, 28].

The Child–Pugh score has conventionally been utilized for the risk assessment of surgical treatment for patients with HCC, but it has limitations, such as subjective parameters and arbitrary cutoff points. The albumin–bilirubin (ALBI) score has emerged as an evidence-based scoring system to evaluate liver function in patients with HCC. This score involves only the albumin and bilirubin values and is, therefore, more objective [29]. The ALBI score has been predominantly accepted as a prognostic tool and has a good correlation with survival, time to recurrence, and tolerability of surgical, locoregional, and systemic therapies for HCC [30, 31]. Additionally, the ALBI score is more capable of predicting postoperative outcomes and major complications, including PHLF, than the Child–Pugh and MELD scores [32–37]. However, retrospective studies mainly demonstrated the use of the preoperative ALBI grade for estimating the risk for PHLF, and further investigations with high-quality designs to assess its predictive accuracy are warranted [38].

The ALBI score has gained popularity because of its simple and objective parameters for predicting prognosis in patients with HCC, but attempts have been performed to identify more accurate predictive models for PHLF using routine blood tests, including prothrombin time, aminotransferase, and platelet count, as well as specific indicators such as the ICG test [5]. Importantly, the platelet count, which is a conventional item not included in the ALBI score, generally affects the postoperative outcome for HCC, as it reflects clinically significant portal hypertension [39]. Additionally, a scoring system adds the platelet count to the ALBI grade, also known as the PALBI grade [40].

8.3 Dynamic Liver Function Tests

8.3.1 ICG Test

The clearance of intravenously administered exogenous substances that are metabolized or excreted via liver perfusion has been performed to quantitatively assess liver function [41]. The ICG retention test is routinely conducted to preoperatively assess the liver functional reserve in Japan and other Asian countries [42]. It is a dynamic method that measures the hepatic clearance of ICG 15 min following its intravenous injection (ICG-R15). ICG clearance is often delayed in patients with liver damage, and an increase in ICG-R15 indicates the degree of liver dysfunction. The Makuuchi criteria, a decisional algorithm for the extent of hepatectomy based on the ICG-R15, have reduced the mortality after hepatectomy and developed safe liver surgery in Japan [43].

The ICG test has gained popularity as a preoperative liver functional test, especially in Japan, and the plasma disappearance rate of ICG (KICG) is reported as useful for liver function quantification in combination with the estimated future liver remnant volume, correlating with PHLF occurrence [44]. Some studies have utilized predictive models incorporating the ICG-R15 [45–48], including the albumin–indocyanine green evaluation model [49]. The ICG clearance test is limited, with its results being affected by biliary obstruction and hemodynamic alterations, including intrahepatic shunt, portal hypertension, and thrombosis.

8.3.2 Liver Maximum Capacity (LiMAx)

The LiMAx test assesses hepatic metabolism by measuring the 13CO2:12CO2 ratio in the exhaled breath, which is derived from the metabolism rate of intravenously injected 13C-methacetin [2]. The LiMAx test result strongly correlates with liver function reserve, and a preoperative volume/function analysis combining future liver remnant and LiMAx enables an accurate remnant liver function estimation preoperatively [50, 51]. The LiMAx test has gained acceptance mostly in Western countries, and the LiMAx decision tree algorithm has improved preoperative PHLF and postoperative outcome assessments [52, 53].

8.4 Serum Markers of Liver Fibrosis

8.4.1 Aspartate Transaminase to Platelet Ratio Index (APRI) and the Fibrosis-4 (FIB-4) Index

Liver fibrosis is a prevalent consequence of chronic liver injury, and the extent of fibrosis is highly correlated with liver functional reserve and prognosis in patients with HCC. Liver biopsy is the standard option for assessing liver fibrosis, but it is an invasive procedure and has several limitations, including complications, sampling errors, intra- and interobserver variability, and expense [54]. Hence, noninvasive liver fibrosis markers suitable for routine use have been developed to address these limitations [2]. The APRI (aspartate aminotransferase/[upper limit of normal] × 100/platelet count [10^9/L]) [55] and the FIB-4 index ([age (in years) × aspartate aminotransferase (U/L)]/[platelet count (10^9/L) × alanine aminotransferase $(U/L)^{1/2}$]) [56] are predominantly assessed using simple and conventional parameters. These liver fibrosis indices demonstrate excellent accuracy in predicting significant fibrosis and cirrhosis, and they have recently gained attention as noninvasive tools for nonalcoholic steatohepatitis (NASH) diagnosis and prognostication. This is important as NASH incidence is rapidly increasing globally, and it is becoming a major etiology of chronic liver disease [57–60]. Additionally, the APRI and FIB-4 index are useful for estimating liver functional reserve as they correlate with the risk of perioperative mortality [61].

8.4.2 Specific Liver Fibrosis Markers

Hyaluronic acid, type IV collagen 7S, and M2BPGi are other specific markers for liver fibrosis investigated by blood tests. Serum hyaluronic acid, which reflects sinusoidal endothelial cell function correlated with hepatic fibrosis, is a reliable liver functional reserve indicator and a useful postoperative complication predictor [62–66]. Type IV collagen 7S is a liver fibrogenesis biomarker, and its serum concentration correlates with hepatic dysfunction after liver resection [67, 68]. More recently, M2BPGi, which is a unique fibrosis-related glycol-alteration detected by a glycan sugar chain-based immunoassay, has been considered a novel marker for liver fibrosis [69]. Further, M2BPGi predicts PHLF better than other preoperative parameters, including KICG, especially in patients with HCV-related HCC [70]. Altogether, the results of these studies indicate that serum markers for liver fibrosis are useful for preoperative liver functional reserve assessment. However, these results are mostly based on a retrospective analysis in a limited number of centers, and further well-designed prospective studies are warranted to identify the markers with the best accuracy.

8.5 Extent of Liver Resection

The extent of liver resection certainly affects the risk of PHLF during liver resection for patients with HCC. The relatively well-known Makuuchi criteria identified the extent of liver resection according to ICG values (Fig. 8.1) [71]. Kokudo et al. developed criteria based on ICG and albumin, the so-called albumin–indocyanine green evaluation (ALICE) grade (Fig. 8.2). The ALICE grade was calculated as follows: linear predictor = 0.663 × $\log_{10}$ICG R15 (%) − 0.0718 × albumin (g/L) (cut-off value: −2.20 and −1.39) [49].

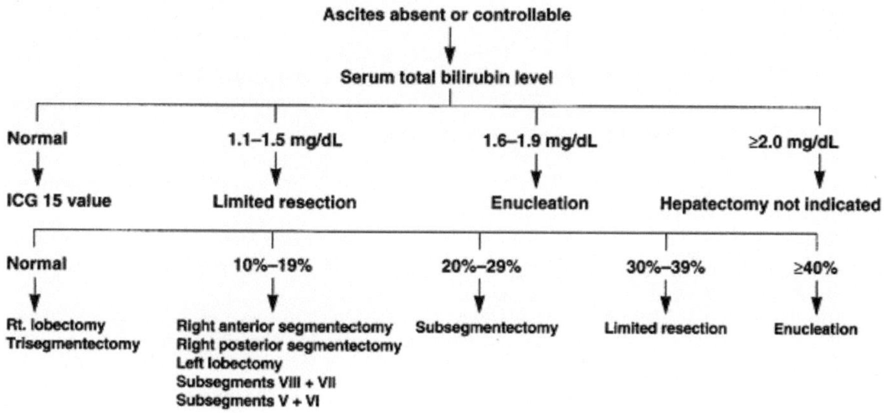

Fig. 8.1 Makuuchi criteria based on the indocyanine green retention rate at 15 min (ICG 15) [71]

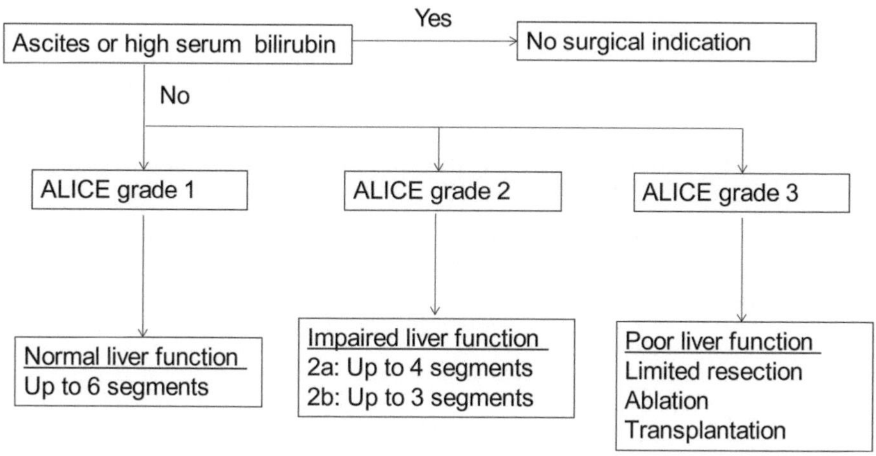

Fig. 8.2 Proposed surgical strategy based on albumin–indocyanine green evaluation (ALICE) grade [49]

8.6 Conclusion

Several nonimaging tests were conducted to examine preoperative liver function to avoid PHLF. However, a universally used test to determine the extent of liver resection remains unavailable. Hopefully, in the coming years, comprehensive prospective clinical trials will be conducted to help develop the best test to predict PHLF.

References

1. Forner A, Llovet JM, Bruix J. Hepatocellular carcinoma. Lancet. 2012;379:1245–55.
2. Nishio T, Taura K, Koyama Y, Ishii T, Hatano E. Current status of preoperative risk assessment for posthepatectomy liver failure in patients with hepatocellular carcinoma. Ann Gastroenterol Surg. 2023;7(6):871–86.
3. Vibert E, Schwartz M, Olthoff KM. Advances in resection and transplantation for hepatocellular carcinoma. J Hepatol. 2020;72(2):262–76.
4. Prodeau M, Drumez E, Duhamel A, Vibert E, Farges O, Lassailly G, et al. An ordinal model to predict the risk of symptomatic liver failure in patients with cirrhosis undergoing hepatectomy. J Hepatol. 2019;71(5):920–9.
5. Yoshino K, Yoh T, Taura K, Seo S, Ciria R, Briceño-Delgado J. A systematic review of prediction models for post-hepatectomy liver failure in patients undergoing liver surgery. HPB (Oxford). 2021;23(9):1311–20.
6. Iguchi K, Hatano E, Yamanaka K, Tanaka S, Taura K, Uemoto S. The impact of posthepatectomy liver failure on the recurrence of hepatocellular carcinoma. World J Surg. 2014;38(1):150–8.
7. Fukushima K, Fukumoto T, Kuramitsu K, Kido M, Takebe A, Tanaka M, et al. Assessment of ISGLS definition of posthepatectomy liver failure and its effect on outcome in patients with hepatocellular carcinoma. J Gastrointest Surg. 2014;18(4):729–36.
8. Donadon M, Costa G, Cimino M, Procopio F, Fabbro DD, Palmisano A, et al. Safe hepatectomy selection criteria for hepatocellular carcinoma patients: a validation of 336 consecutive hepatectomies. The BILCHE score. World J Surg. 2015;39:237–43.
9. Ichikawa T, Uenishi T, Takemura S, Oba K, Ogawa M, Kodai S, et al. A simple, noninvasively determined index predicting hepatic failure following liver resection for hepatocellular carcinoma. J Hepato-Biliary-Pancreat Surg. 2009;16:42–8.
10. Malinchoc M, Kamath PS, Gordon FD, Peine CJ, Rank J, ter Borg PC. A model to predict poor survival in patients undergoing transjugular intrahepatic portosystemic shunts. Hepatology. 2000;31:864–71.
11. Pugh RN, Murray-Lyon IM, Dawson JL, Pietroni MC, Williams R. Transection of the oesophagus for bleeding oesophageal varices. Br J Surg. 1973;60:646–9.
12. Bruix J, Castells A, Bosch J, Feu F, Fuster J, Garcia-Pagan JC, et al. Surgical resection of hepatocellular carcinoma in cirrhotic patients: prognostic value of preoperative portal pressure. Gastroenterology. 1996;111:1018–22.
13. Santambrogio R, Kluger MD, Costa M, Belli A, Barabino M, Laurent A, et al. Hepatic resection for hepatocellular carcinoma in patients with child-Pugh's A cirrhosis: is clinical evidence of portal hypertension a contraindication? HPB. 2013;15:78–84.
14. Ishizawa T, Hasegawa K, Aoki T, Takahashi M, Inoue Y, Sano K, et al. Neither multiple tumors nor portal hypertension are surgical contraindications for hepatocellular carcinoma. Gastroenterology. 2008;134:1908–16.
15. Berzigotti A, Reig M, Abraldes JG, Bosch J, Bruix J. Portal hypertension and the outcome of surgery for hepatocellular carcinoma in compensated cirrhosis: a systematic review and meta-analysis. Hepatology. 2015;61:526–36.
16. Cucchetti A, Cescon M, Golfieri R, Piscaglia F, Renzulli M, Neri F, et al. Hepatic venous pressure gradient in the preoperative assessment of patients with resectable hepatocellular carcinoma. J Hepatol. 2016;64:79–86.
17. Kokudo N, Hasegawa K, Akahane M, Igaki H, Izumi N, Ichida T, et al. Evidence-based clinical practice guidelines for hepatocellular carcinoma: the Japan Society of Hepatology 2013 update (3rd JSHHCC guidelines). Hepatol Res. 2015;45(2) https://doi.org/10.1111/hepr.12464.
18. Seyama Y, Kokudo N. Assessment of liver function for safe hepatic resection. Hepatol Res. 2009;39:107–16.
19. Makuuchi M, Hasegawa H, Yamazaki S. Indication of hepatectomy in patients with hepatocellular carcinoma and cirrhosis (in Japanese). Shindan Chiryo. 1986;74:1225–30.

20. Kokudo T, Hasegawa K, Amikura K, Uldry E, Shirata C, Yamaguchi T, Arita J, Kaneko J, Akamatsu N, Sakamoto Y, Takahashi A, Sakamoto H, Makuuchi M, Matsuyama Y, Demartines N, Malagó M, Kokudo N, Halkic N. Assessment of preoperative liver function in patients with hepatocellular carcinoma—the albumin-indocyanine green evaluation (ALICE) grade. PLoS One. 2016;11:e0159530.
21. Galle PR, Forner A, Llovet JM, Mazzaferro V, Piscaglia F, Raoul J-L, et al. EASL clinical practice guidelines: management of hepatocellular carcinoma. J Hepatol. 2018;69(1):182–236.
22. Marrero JA, Kulik LM, Sirlin CB, Zhu AX, Finn RS, Abecassis MM, et al. Diagnosis, staging, and management of hepatocellular carcinoma: 2018 practice guidance by the American Association for the Study of Liver Diseases. Hepatology. 2018;68(2):723–50.
23. Pugh RN, Murray-Lyon IM, Dawson JL, Pietroni MC, Williams R. Transection of the oesophagus for bleeding oesophageal varices. Br J Surg. 1973;60(8):646–9.
24. Malinchoc M, Kamath PS, Gordon FD, Peine CJ, Rank J, ter-Borg PL. A model to predict poor survival in patients undergoingtransjugular intrahepatic portosystemic shunts. Hepatology. 2000;31:864–71.
25. Wiesner R, Edwards E, Freeman R, Harper A, Kim R, Kamath P, Kremers W, Lake J, Howard T, Merion RM, Wolfe RA, Krom R, United Network for Organ Sharing Liver Disease Severity Score Committee. Model for end-stage liver disease (MELD) and allocation of donor livers. Gastroenterology. 2003;124:91–6.
26. Rahbari NN, Reissfelder C, Koch M, Elbers H, Striebel F, Büchler MW, et al. The predictive value of postoperative clinical risk scores for outcome after hepatic resection: a validation analysis in 807 patients. Ann Surg Oncol. 2011;18(13):3640–9.
27. Schroeder RA, Marroquin CE, Bute BP, Khuri S, Henderson WG, Kuo PC. Predictive indices of morbidity and mortality after liver resection. Ann Surg. 2006;243(3):373–9.
28. Cholongitas E, Papatheodoridis GV, Vangeli M, Terreni N, Patch D, Burroughs AK. Systematic review: the model for end-stage liver disease—should it replace child-Pugh's classification for assessing prognosis in cirrhosis? Aliment Pharmacol Ther. 2005;22(11–12):1079–89.
29. Johnson PJ, Berhane S, Kagebayashi C, Satomura S, Teng M, Reeves HL, et al. Assessment of liver function in patients with hepatocellular carcinoma: a new evidence-based approach—the ALBI grade. J Clin Oncol. 2015;33(6):550–8.
30. Demirtas CO, D'Alessio A, Rimassa L, Sharma R, Pinato DJ. ALBI grade: evidence for an improved model for liver functional estimation in patients with hepatocellular carcinoma. JHEP Rep. 2021;3(5):100347.
31. Pinato DJ, Sharma R, Allara E, Yen C, Arizumi T, Kubota K, et al. The ALBI grade provides objective hepatic reserve estimation across each BCLC stage of hepatocellular carcinoma. J Hepatol. 2017;66(2):338–46.
32. Wang YY, Zhong JH, Su ZY, Huang JF, Lu SD, Xiang BD, et al. Albumin–bilirubin versus child–Pugh score as a predictor of outcome after liver resection for hepatocellular carcinoma. Br J Surg. 2016;103(6):725–34.
33. Fagenson AM, Gleeson EM, Pitt HA, Lau KN. Albumin-bilirubin score vs model for end-stage liver disease in predicting post-hepatectomy outcomes. J Am Coll Surg. 2020;230(4):637–45.
34. Taylor GA, Fagenson AM, Kuo LE, Pitt HA, Lau KN. Predicting operative outcomes in patients with liver disease: albumin-bilirubin score vs model for end-stage liver disease-sodium score. J Am Coll Surg. 2021;232(4):470–80.e2.
35. Shi J-Y, Sun L-Y, Quan B, Xing H, Li C, Liang L, et al. A novel online calculator based on non-invasive markers (ALBI and APRI) for predicting post-hepatectomy liver failure in patients with hepatocellular carcinoma. Clin Res Hepatol Gastroenterol. 2021;45(4):101534.
36. Takahashi K, Gosho M, Kim J, Shimomura O, Miyazaki Y, Furuya K, et al. Prediction of posthepatectomy liver failure with a combination of albumin-bilirubin score and liver resection percentage. J Am Coll Surg. 2022;234(2):155–65.
37. Zou H, Wen Y, Yuan K, Miao X-Y, Xiong L, Liu K-J. Combining albumin-bilirubin score with future liver remnant predicts post-hepatectomy liver failure in HBV-associated HCC patients. Liver Int. 2018;38(3):494–502.

38. Marasco G, Alemanni LV, Colecchia A, Festi D, Bazzoli F, Mazzella G, et al. Prognostic value of the albumin-bilirubin grade for the prediction of post-hepatectomy liver failure: a systematic review and meta-analysis. J Clin Med. 2021;10(9):2011.
39. Berzigotti A, Reig M, Abraldes JG, Bosch J, Bruix J. Portal hypertension and the outcome of surgery for hepatocellular carcinoma in compensated cirrhosis: a systematic review and meta-analysis. Hepatology. 2015;61(2):526–36.
40. Liu PH, Hsu CY, Hsia CY, Lee YH, Chiou YY, Huang YH, Lee FY, Lin HC, Hou MC, Huo TI. ALBI and PALBI grade predict survival for HCC across treatment modalities and BCLC stages in the MELD era. J Gastroenterol Hepatol. 2017 Apr;32(4):879–86.
41. Seyama Y, Kokudo N. Assessment of liver function for safe hepatic resection. Hepatol Res. 2009;39(2):107–16.
42. Kokudo T, Hasegawa K, Shirata C, Tanimoto M, Ishizawa T, Kaneko J, et al. Assessment of preoperative liver function for surgical decision making in patients with hepatocellular carcinoma. Liver Cancer. 2019;8(6):447–56.
43. Makuuchi M, Kosuge T, Takayama T, Yamazaki S, Kakazu T, Miyagawa S, et al. Surgery for small liver cancers. Semin Surg Oncol. 1993;9(4):298–304.
44. Nagino M, Kamiya J, Nishio H, Ebata T, Arai T, Nimura Y. Two hundred forty consecutive portal vein embolizations before extended hepatectomy for biliary cancer: surgical outcome and long-term follow-up. Ann Surg. 2006;243(3):364–72.
45. Honmyo N, Kobayashi T, Kuroda S, Oshita A, Onoe T, Kohashi T, et al. A novel model for predicting posthepatectomy liver failure based on liver function and degree of liver resection in patients with hepatocellular carcinoma. HPB (Oxford). 2021;23(1):134–43.
46. Tomassini F, Giglio MC, De Simone G, Montalti R, Troisi RI. Hepatic function assessment to predict post-hepatectomy liver failure: what can we trust? A systematic review. Updates Surg. 2020;72(4):925–38.
47. Li J, Lei B, Nie X, Lin L, Tahir SA, Shi W, et al. A comprehensive method for predicting fatal liver failure of patients with liver cancer resection. Medicine (Baltimore). 2015;94(17):e784.
48. Kim HJ, Kim CY, Park EK, Hur YH, Koh YS, Kim HJ, et al. Volumetric analysis and indocyanine green retention rate at 15 min as predictors of post-hepatectomy liver failure. HPB (Oxford). 2015;17(2):159–67.
49. Kokudo T, Hasegawa K, Amikura K, Uldry E, Shirata C, Yamaguchi T, et al. Assessment of preoperative liver function in patients with hepatocellular carcinoma—the albumin-indocyanine green evaluation (ALICE) grade. PLoS One. 2016;11(7):e0159530.
50. Stockmann M, Lock JF, Riecke B, Heyne K, Martus P, Fricke M, et al. Prediction of postoperative outcome after hepatectomy with a new bedside test for maximal liver function capacity. Ann Surg. 2009;250(1):119–25.
51. Blüthner E, Jara M, Shrestha R, Faber W, Pratschke J, Stockmann M, et al. The predictive value of future liver remnant function after liver resection for HCC in noncirrhotic and cirrhotic patients. HPB (Oxford). 2019;21(7):912–22.
52. Stockmann M, Lock JF, Malinowski M, Niehues SM, Seehofer D, Neuhaus P. The LiMAx test: a new liver function test for predicting postoperative outcome in liver surgery. HPB (Oxford). 2010;12(2):139–46.
53. Jara M, Reese T, Malinowski M, Valle E, Seehofer D, Puhl G, et al. Reductions in post-hepatectomy liver failure and related mortality after implementation of the LiMAx algorithm in preoperative work-up: a single-Centre analysis of 1170 hepatectomies of one or more segments. HPB (Oxford). 2015;17(7):651–8.
54. Bedossa P, Dargère D, Paradis V. Sampling variability of liver fibrosis in chronic hepatitis C. Hepatology. 2003;38(6):1449–57.
55. Wai CT, Greenson JK, Fontana RJ, Kalbfleisch JD, Marrero JA, Conjeevaram HS, et al. A simple noninvasive index can predict both significant fibrosis and cirrhosis in patients with chronic hepatitis C. Hepatology. 2003;38(2):518–26.
56. Sterling RK, Lissen E, Clumeck N, Sola R, Correa MC, Montaner J, et al. Development of a simple noninvasive index to predict significant fibrosis in patients with HIV/HCV coinfection. Hepatology. 2006;43(6):1317–25.

57. Nielsen MJ, Leeming DJ, Goodman Z, Friedman S, Frederiksen P, Rasmussen DGK, et al. Comparison of ADAPT, FIB-4 and APRI as non-invasive predictors of liver fibrosis and NASH within the CENTAUR screening population. J Hepatol. 2021;75(6):1292–300.
58. Younossi ZM, Loomba R, Anstee QM, Rinella ME, Bugianesi E, Marchesini G, et al. Diagnostic modalities for nonalcoholic fatty liver disease, nonalcoholic steatohepatitis, and associated fibrosis. Hepatology. 2018;68(1):349–60.
59. Younossi ZM, Anstee QM, Wai-Sun Wong V, Trauner M, Lawitz EJ, Harrison SA, et al. The association of histologic and noninvasive tests with adverse clinical and patient-reported outcomes in patients with advanced fibrosis due to nonalcoholic steatohepatitis. Gastroenterology. 2021;160(5):1608–19.e13.
60. Younes R, Caviglia GP, Govaere O, Rosso C, Armandi A, Sanavia T, et al. Long-term outcomes and predictive ability of non-invasive scoring systems in patients with non-alcoholic fatty liver disease. J Hepatol. 2021;75(4):786–94.
61. Maegawa FB, Shehorn L, Aziz H, Kettelle J, Jie T, Riall TS. Association between noninvasive fibrosis markers and postoperative mortality after hepatectomy for hepatocellular carcinoma. JAMA Netw Open. 2019;2(1):e187142.
62. Nanashima A, Yamaguchi H, Tanaka K, Shibasaki S, Tsuji T, Ide N, et al. Preoperative serum hyaluronic acid level as a good predictor of posthepatectomy complications. Surg Today. 2004;34(11):913–9.
63. Ueno M, Uchiyama K, Ozawa S, Hayami S, Kiriyama S, Yamaue H. A new prediction model of postoperative complications after major hepatectomy for hepatocellular carcinoma. Dig Surg. 2009;26(5):392–9.
64. Mizuguchi T, Katsuramaki T, Nobuoka T, Kawamoto M, Oshima H, Kawasaki H, et al. Serum hyaluronate level for predicting subclinical liver dysfunction after hepatectomy. World J Surg. 2004;28(10):971–6.
65. Yachida S, Wakabayashi H, Okano K, Suzuki Y. Prediction of posthepatectomy hepatic functional reserve by serum hyaluronate. Br J Surg. 2009;96(5):501–8.
66. Murtha-Lemekhova A, Fuchs J, Ghamarnejad O, Nikdad M, Probst P, Hoffmann K. Influence of cytokines, circulating markers and growth factors on liver regeneration and post-hepatectomy liver failure: a systematic review and meta-analysis. Sci Rep. 2021;11(1):13739.
67. Kubo S, Tsukamoto T, Hirohashi K, Tanaka H, Shuto T, Takemura S, et al. Correlation between preoperative serum concentration of type IV collagen 7s domain and hepatic failure following resection of hepatocellular carcinoma. Ann Surg. 2004;239(2):186–93.
68. Ishii M, Itano O, Shinoda M, Kitago M, Abe Y, Hibi T, et al. Pre-hepatectomy type IV collagen 7S predicts post-hepatectomy liver failure and recovery. World J Gastroenterol. 2020;26(7):725–39.
69. Kuno A, Ikehara Y, Tanaka Y, Ito K, Matsuda A, Sekiya S, et al. A serum "sweet-doughnut" protein facilitates fibrosis evaluation and therapy assessment in patients with viral hepatitis. Sci Rep. 2013;3(1):1065.
70. Okuda Y, Taura K, Yoshino K, Ikeno Y, Nishio T, Yamamoto G, et al. Usefulness of mac-2 binding protein glycosylation isomer for prediction of posthepatectomy liver failure in patients with hepatocellular carcinoma. Ann Surg. 2017;265(6):1201–8.
71. Miyagawa S, Makuuchi M, Kawasaki S, Kakazu T. Criteria for safe hepatic resection. Am J Surg. 1995;169(6):589–94.

9 Portal Flow and Pressure Modulation in Major Hepatectomies

Goudarz T. Passand and Nicolas Golse

Abbreviations

ALPPS	Associating liver partition and portal vein ligation for staged hepatectomy
FLR	Future liver remnant
HCC	Hepatocellular carcinoma
HVPG	Hepatic vein pressure gradient
PCS	Porto-caval shunt
PHLF	Posthepatectomy liver failure
PHT	Portal hypertension
PVF	Portal vein flow
PVP	Portal vein pressure
SAE	Splenic artery embolization
SAL	Splenic artery ligation
SFSS	Small for size syndrome
TLV	Total liver volume

9.1 Introduction

Posthepatectomy liver failure (PHLF) is recognized as the leading cause of mortality after major hepatectomy [1]. Despite recent advances to improve outcomes, the incidence of PHLF can reach 30% [2] and its severity can range from a simple disorder in biological liver function to a state of multiorgan failure with refractory ascites, jaundice, renal and respiratory failure, hemodynamic instability, and encephalopathy. In major hepatectomies, PHLF accounts for approximately 40% of

G. T. Passand · N. Golse (✉)
Paul Brousse University Hospital, Centre Hépato-Biliaire, Villejuif, France

L. Aldrighetti et al. (eds.), *Liver Regeneration Techniques In Hepatic Surgery*,
https://doi.org/10.1007/978-3-032-10997-2_9

the 90-day postoperative mortality [3]. Liver transplantation, which is rarely available in this setting, remains the only definitive treatment for patients with persistent PHLF.

While multifactorial, the main risk factor for PHLF is an insufficient volume of the future liver remnant (FLR). It is generally admitted that FLR/total liver volume >20% (or FLR/body weight ratio >0.5) [4] in healthy livers and >40% in cirrhotic livers is required, but the cutoff is less consensual in this pathological setting. Moreover, any underlying liver hepatopathy (steatosis, cholestasis, chemotherapy, radiotherapy…) must be considered even if the theoretical minimum required FLR volume is reached.

Means to increase the FLR such as portal vein embolization (possibly associated with hepatic vein—liver venous deprivation), two-staged hepatectomy and associating liver partition and portal vein ligation for staged hepatectomy (ALPPS) are discussed in Part III.

A maintained high portal venous flow into a small remnant volume induces a small for size syndrome (SFSS) [5]. This situation occurs after major hepatectomies or even after minor resections in cirrhotic livers, notably due to reduced regenerative capacities [6]. High venous pressure causes mechanical damage to the sinusoidal endothelial cells, leading to capillary leakage. Histologically, this is associated with sinusoidal dilatation and hepatocyte swelling. It also increases the risk of bacterial translocation. High portal flow also has the effect of reducing hepatic artery perfusion through the hepatic artery buffer, possibly responsible for ischemic cholangitis [7]. These changes are rapidly irreversible and liver parenchyma loses its ability to regenerate.

Therefore, monitoring portal flow and pressure at the end of high-risk surgery is mandatory to prevent the onset of SFSS.

9.2 Portal Flow

9.2.1 Methods for Measuring Portal Venous Pressure

- Preoperative assessment

Portal venous pressure (PVP) is defined as the product of portal blood flow and vascular resistance; a rise in either increases portal pressure. Portal hypertension (PHT) can be related to prehepatic, intrahepatic or posthepatic obstruction, it may pre-exist preoperatively or occur after resection.

Assessment of PVP can be performed according to noninvasive methods corresponding to clinical–biological consequences of PHT (e.g., gastro-esophageal varices, ascites, splenomegaly, thrombopenia) or invasive methods that are currently recommended because they are more accurate. Direct measurement of PVP by laparotomy or percutaneous transhepatic puncture is gradually being abandoned in favor of indirect measurement: it consists of inserting a balloon catheter into the hepatic vein through a transjugular approach to measure occluded and free hepatic venous pressures. The hepatic venous pressure gradient (HVPG), which is an estimate of portocaval gradient, is calculated as the difference between these two pressures; PHT is defined as HVPG ≥5 mmHg.

- Intraoperative assessment

Gradient measurement can be performed during hepatectomy by direct puncture of the portal vein as well as the retro- (or ideally supra-) hepatic inferior vena cava. However, this method is not routinely feasible by a minimally invasive approach.

9.2.2 Methods for Measuring Portal Venous Flow

Preoperative assessment of the portal vein flow (PVF) is performed with a percutaneous pulsed-wave Doppler ultrasound, which highlights a hepatopetal monophasic flow varying with respiration. The flow rate can be deduced from the velocity and diameter of the vessel; a normal portal flow velocity should be >25 cm/s. This device can also be used intraoperatively.

A more precise assessment of the portal flow can also be made with a flow meter after dissection of the portal pedicle during open hepatectomy.

9.2.3 Hemodynamic Consequences of Hepatectomy in Noncirrhotic Livers

The deleterious effect of elevated posthepatectomy PVP on liver function in humans was first studied in the context of living donor liver transplantation (LDLT). Yagi et al. analyzed 32 patients during the first 3 days after LDLT and concluded that a postoperative PVP greater than 20 mmHg was associated with higher incidence of graft dysfunction characterized by hyper-bilirubinemia, coagulopathy, and development of severe ascites [8]. Similarly, Shimamura et al. demonstrated that the postoperative peak level of total bilirubin was significantly higher in patients with portal flow exceeding 260 mL/min/100 g graft [9]. These results were confirmed by other studies retaining that a postperfusion PVP above 15 mmHg was associated with increased graft dysfunction and mortality [10–12]. Troisi et al. further reported in a cohort of 24 LDLT that a portal flow exceeding 250 mL/min/100 g of graft was associated with an increased risk of SFSS and mortality [13].

These findings were later extrapolated to the field of extended resections in noncirrhotic livers:

1. Bucur et al. demonstrated the negative effect of a high portal flow on postoperative liver function in an experimental study [14]. They performed a 75% hepatectomy in 17 noncirrhotic pigs and allocated them into two groups: a group with portal flow modulation using a constrictive ring around the portal vein and a control group. The authors found a significantly lower postoperative bilirubinemia level and a higher Ki67 rate in the group with the portal modulation. After

sacrifice on postoperative day 7, the microarchitecture of liver specimens in the ring group was significantly richer in bile canaliculi.

2. In a clinical study including 277 major hepatectomies, Allard et al. demonstrated that a posthepatectomy PVP greater than 20 mmHg was an independent predictor for PHLF and 90-day mortality [15]. Therefore, intraoperative modulation of PVP would be advisable when PVP exceeds this threshold, although no other large-scale study has yet confirmed these results. To date, in contrast to LDLT, there are no studies recommending specific management based on the portal flow rate in major hepatectomies.

9.2.4 Impact of Pre-existing Portal Hypertension on Outcomes

In cirrhotic liver, normal parenchyma is replaced by fibrotic scar tissue and regenerative nodules responsible for higher resistance to intrahepatic blood flow; cirrhosis is considered the main cause of PHT, accounting for approximately 90% of cases.

The European Association for the Study of the Liver (EASL) guidelines considers preoperative PHT as a contraindication for surgical resection due to the high risk of postoperative liver decompensation. Therefore, measurement of the HVPG is the gold standard for risk stratification of PHLF in cirrhotic livers. In two prospective studies, the Barcelona Clinic Liver Cancer (BCLC) group showed that a preoperative HVPG >10 mmHg in hepatocellular carcinoma (HCC) patients was associated with increased postoperative morbimortality. Bruix et al. analyzed 29 patients and found that all patients with unresolved postoperative decompensation after 3 months had a preoperative HVPG >10 mmHg [16]. Llovet et al. confirmed these findings, reporting an odds ratio of 13 for postoperative decompensation among patients with HVPG >10 mmHg [17].

A systematic review of 1124 hepatectomies in HCC patients found that indirect signs of PHT were not significantly associated with postoperative complications or mortality, highlighting the need for invasive assessment of preoperative HVPG. Liver resection in patients with HVPG ≥10 mmHg significantly increased the risk of overall complications, PHLF, and refractory decompensation. Interestingly, PHT was not associated to postoperative complications in mini-invasive approach [18]. Cucchetti et al. prospectively included 70 patients who underwent resection of HCC and assessed the severity of PHLF according to preoperative HVPG. They found that the cutoff of 10 mmHg excluded approximately one-quarter of the patients who would benefit from surgery without short- to mid-term postoperative sequelae, illustrating that this threshold may not be optimal [19].

To date, no post-resection threshold for PVP or PVF to predict PHLF in cirrhotic livers is available in the literature.

9.3 Means of Portal Modulation

9.3.1 Pharmacological

Somatostatin is a peptide hormone secreted by the hypothalamus and by delta cells located in the stomach, the duodenum, and the pancreas. Its main function is the inhibition of the growth factor and thyroid hormones. In the gastrointestinal tract, among others, somatostatin blocks the SSTR2 receptors on the endothelial cells of splanchnic vasculature. Thus, the vasoconstriction of the splanchnic flow decreases the PVP.

Experimental works on pigs proved the benefit of somatostatin in modulating the portal flow. Mohkam et al. administered intraoperative somatostatin during extended hepatectomy in pigs, leading to a decrease of PVF in both the 70% and 90% hepatectomy groups. Somatostatin restored a normal HVPG in the 90% hepatectomy group [20].

The administration of somatostatin for portal flow modulation in humans was first published in LDLT. Troisi et al. analyzed 29 patients undergoing LDLT who were randomized to receive either somatostatin or placebo. The study drug was administered intraoperatively as bolus (somatostatin: 500 μg), followed by a continuous 250 μg/h infusion for 5 days. At graft reperfusion, HVPG was significantly lower in patients receiving somatostatin [21]. Rhaiem et al. used an intraoperative bolus of somatostatin (250 μg) followed by a continuous 250 μg/h infusion for 5 days in 10 noncirrhotic patients who underwent a major hepatectomy. All patients had a PVP above 20 mmHg after the end of hepatectomy and somatostatin perfusion permitted a median PVP decrease of 3.5 mmHg [22].

Terlipressin, an analog of vasopressin, exerts a vasoconstrictive effect in the splanchnic system. It is commonly used to treat complications of PHT in cirrhotic patients such as gastro-esophageal varices bleeding or hepato-renal syndrome.

Jo et al. evaluated 20 pigs undergoing 90% hepatectomy, divided into a terlipressin and a control group. Terlipressin 0.5 mg was injected subcutaneously three times a day, starting immediately before hepatectomy to 7 days after surgery. Postoperative endothelin-1 level, reflecting liver injury, was lower in the terlipressin group, as was PVP at 1 and 6 hours post-hepatectomy. The 7-day survival rate was also significantly higher in the terlipressin group [23].

However, these experimental results were not confirmed in humans. In a randomized double-blind placebo-controlled trial including 150 cirrhotic and non-cirrhotic patients undergoing major hepatectomy, terlipressin administration did not reduce the incidence of PHLF or postoperative mortality [24].

9.3.2 Splenectomy

The spleen is an abdominal organ connected to the portal vein system through the splenic vein, contributing about one-third of the total portal blood flow. HCC most commonly develops in cirrhotic livers, where congestion of the portal vein causes splenomegaly. Therefore, performing a splenectomy significantly reduces the input into portal flow.

Yao et al. analyzed 319 LDLT in a retrospective study evaluating the benefits of PVP modulation through systematic splenectomy when postimplantation PVP exceeded 15 mmHg ($n = 130$ patients). When successful, defined as achieving a postmodulation PVP below 15 mmHg, splenectomy improved prognosis to a level comparable with that of patients who did not require modulation. However, about 30% of modulations failed, essentially in patients with extended portal thrombosis or very small grafts (graft-to-recipient weight ratio <0.8%). Importantly, splenectomy did not increase the rate of readmission for bacterial infection [25]. Yoshizumi et al. analyzed 320 LDLT in a retrospective study. Among them, 232 patients had a simultaneous splenectomy for graft-to-standard liver weight ratio <35% or clinical signs of PHT while 26 patients underwent a post-unclamping splenectomy due to post-implantation PVP higher than 20 mmHg. After propensity score matching, patients undergoing splenectomy had a lower frequency of early graft dysfunction and significantly lower postoperative bilirubinemia and international normalized ratio levels. Univariate analysis revealed a hazard ratio of 3 for graft loss in patients who did not undergo splenectomy [26].

The role of splenectomy in modulating blood flow and preventing SFSS is well established in LDLT. However, its impact in major hepatectomies has only been explored in experimental studies. Arakawa et al. [27] and Ren et al. [28] compared groups of major hepatectomies with and without splenectomy in remnant models. They found that the association of hepatectomy + splenectomy improved postoperative liver functions and increased survival rate. Arakawa et al. notably found that this association favorized liver regeneration through upregulation of hemeoxygenase-1 and downregulation of tumor necrosis factor-α.

9.3.3 Splenic Artery Ligation/Embolization

Reduction of PHT by splenic artery ligation (SAL) has historically been performed for the management of recurrent gastroesophageal variceal bleeding.

In the setting of LDLT, maintaining sufficient hepatic arterial flow is necessary in order to prevent graft loss due to biliary ischemia or hepatic artery thrombosis. Troisi et al. measured the flow in seven LDLT patients and found that SAL decreased portal vein flow and increased hepatic artery flow into the graft [29]. In an animal model, Carrapita et al. studied 48 rats divided into two groups: 85% hepatectomy alone or 85% hepatectomy with SAL. SAL induced a portal flow modulation, promoting an increase in hepatocellular viability and regeneration, with a less marked elevation of oxidative stress during the first 48 hours [30]. In humans, Sato et al. compared 6 major hepatectomies associated to SAL to 15 major hepatectomies without modulation all operated for HCC. They found a reduction in PVP and improved postoperative liver function in the modulated group [31].

Splenic artery embolization (SAE) is a less invasive alternative to surgical ligation. Umeda et al. compared 30 patients undergoing SAE prior an LDLT to 30 other LDLT without SAE. SAE was associated with improved outcomes, characterized by major hepatic artery flow and decreased PVF [32].

9.3.4 Porto-Caval Shunt

Animal experimental studies have shown that the creation of a meso- or porto-caval shunt (PCS) to partially divert the portal flow into the systemic circulation in LDLT improved the graft function [33, 34]. It is explained by a more limited PHT, thus inducing less microvascular injury after reperfusion. Golriz et al. applied these findings by performing PCS during major hepatectomies in 40 pigs. The diversion of the portal flow permitted to decrease and correct the elevated PVP and PVF to pre-resection levels. Also, the lowered hepatic artery flow in the remnant liver is increased and corrected through PCS [35]. These results were later confirmed on histopathology. Wang et al. performed a major hepatectomy in 14 pigs, seven of which underwent a PCS. Post-hepatectomy PVP was significantly lower in the shunt group and survival time was prolonged. In the non-shunt group, significant damage to the sinusoidal lining and edema of the portal triad were observed 1 hour after hepatectomy. In contrast, these changes were not seen in the shunt group [36].

Troisi et al. analyzed 13 patients who underwent LDLT with a low graft-to-recipient weight ratio. Eight of them underwent a PCS. PVF was significantly reduced in the shunt group, improving graft function and patient survival by preventing SFSS. Notably, no postoperative encephalopathy occurred in the shunt group [37].

To date, no published study has reported the use of PCS performed to modulate the PVP in major hepatectomy in humans.

9.4 Portal Modulation Thresholds and Timing

9.4.1 Thresholds in Healthy Livers

Pre-hepatectomy measurement of HVPG or portal flow is not recommended and probably unnecessary in healthy livers as values are usually normal. Indications of pre-resection liver hypertrophy procedures are only based on volumetric measurements.

Given the paucity of studies in the area of post-major hepatectomy pressure modulation, analogies can be made with LDLT. An international consensus published by Hakeem et al. recommended the realization of a portal modulation in LDLT if the PVF is exceeds 250 mL/min/100 g or if the PVP is greater than15 mmHg [38].

Moreover, Sainz-Barriga et al. explored PHT during liver transplantations and concluded that there is no direct correlation between PVF and PVP; thus, these two data should not be used individually to assess the severity of PHT [39]. Contrary to the PVP, there is currently no clear indication for routine assessment of the PVF.

Allard et al. demonstrated that a posthepatectomy PVP greater than 20 mmHg in non-cirrhotic was an independent predictor of PHLF and 90-day mortality. Thus, intraoperative modulation of PVP would be advisable when PVP exceeds this threshold [15]. To date, there is no available data regarding the optimal sequence of the mean of modulation in the setting of an elevated PVP after major hepatectomy but it seems reasonable to escalate progressively from somatostatin administration to more invasive procedures. Splenectomy and splenic artery ligation showed benefits in animal experimentations and LDLT cases. However, their impact in the setting of major hepatectomy should be further explored, especially in cases of postoperative PHT without splenomegaly, where their benefit is expected to be limited. Finally, the creation of a PCS, due to its invasive character, and the potential risk of post-procedural encephalopathy, should be retained as the last option.

9.4.2 Thresholds in Cirrhotic Livers

Aliseda et al. demonstrated that indirect signs of PHT were not significantly associated to postoperative complications nor mortality, recalling the importance of pre-hepatectomy measurements of HVPG [18]. The Barcelona Clinic Liver Cancer (BCLC) group reported that a preoperative HVPG greater than 10 mmHg in HCC patients was associated with increased morbidity and unresolved postoperative decompensation. Thus, a preoperative HVPG higher than 10 mmHg should contraindicate any major hepatectomy, or, at the very least, strongly rediscuss the indication.

As for healthy livers, no data is available on the optimal sequence of the mean of modulation, and it seems reasonable to upgrade progressively from somatostatin to more invasive procedures. The clinical efficacy of somatostatin, evaluated by the reduction of postoperative ascites, after partial hepatectomy in HCC patients is currently being analyzed by a French prospective double-blind multicentric trial [40].

As mentioned previously, splenomegaly is an indirect sign of PHT and is often present in cirrhotic patients. In contrast to noncirrhotic patients, almost half of the portal flow in patients with splenomegaly comes from the splenic vein, making splenectomy an interesting option. By the way, perioperative elevated PVP can lead to immediate modulation by means previously described, but this could also be done later. Takamatsu et al. reported the case of a right hepatectomy performed by laparotomy for an HCC in a 58-year-old woman with chronic hepatitis C. She had also a portal thrombosis and a splenomegaly. Postoperative period was marked by refractory ascites and the development of gastric varices bleeding, secondary to the PHT. The authors performed a splenectomy on postoperative day 41 to reduce PVP from 32 to 23 mmHg. Thereafter, she had a complete recovery from PHLF [41]. This case report suggests the possibility of delayed procedure of PVP modulation for treating PHLF, although irreversible histological damage may already be present by that stage.

Further studies are needed to determine the optimal timing for PVP modulation after major hepatectomy in cirrhotic livers.

9.5 Conclusion

Posthepatectomy liver failure occurs essentially after major resection. It is mainly explained by the maintained high portal venous flow into a small remnant volume, thus inducing irreversible damage on hepatocytes.

Little data is currently available in the field of portal modulation in major hepatectomies. Portal modulation by pharmacological (somatostatin) or invasive (splenectomy, splenic artery ligation, portocaval shunt) means has shown a clear benefit in LDLT, less obviously after partial hepatectomy.

The HVPG, measured preoperatively by trans-jugular approach, contraindicates resection if higher than 10 mmHg in cirrhotic patients. Perioperative measurement of the portal pressure highlights an increase after major hepatectomy. If postresection pressure is higher than 20 mmHg, portal modulation is indicated in healthy livers but no data is currently available in cirrhotic livers.

However, as there is no direct correlation between PVF and PVP, thresholds for modulation in LDLT are based on both portal pressure (>15 mmHg) and flow (>250 mL/min/100 g). No study clearly explored the PVF modulation thresholds after major hepatectomy.

The optimal timing of portal modulation has yet to be determined.

References

1. Rahnemai-Azar AA, Cloyd JM, Weber SM, Dillhoff M, Schmidt C, Winslow ER, Pawlik TM. Update on liver failure following hepatic resection: strategies for prediction and avoidance of post-operative liver insufficiency. J Clin Transl Hepatol. 2018;6(1):97–104.
2. Baumgartner R, Gilg S, Björnsson B, Hasselgren K, Ghorbani P, Sauter C, Stål P, Sandstöm P, Sparrelid E, Engstrand J. Impact of post-hepatectomy liver failure on morbidity and short- and long-term survival after major hepatectomy. BJS Open. 2022;6(4):zrac097.
3. Gilg S, Sandström P, Rizell M, Lindell G, Ardnor B, Strömberg C, Isaksson B. The impact of post-hepatectomy liver failure on mortality: a population-based study. Scand J Gastroenterol. 2018;53(10-11):1335–9.
4. Truant S, Oberlin O, Sergent G, Lebuffe G, Gambiez L, Ernst O, Pruvot FR. Remnant liver volume to body weight ratio > or =0.5%: a new cut-off to estimate postoperative risks after extended resection in noncirrhotic liver. J Am Coll Surg. 2007;204(1):22–33.
5. Dahm F, Georgiev P, Clavien PA. Small-for-size syndrome after partial liver transplantation: definition, mechanisms of disease and clinical implications. Am J Transplant. 2005;5(11):2605–10.
6. Golse N, Bucur PO, Adam R, Castaing D, Sa Cunha A, Vibert E. New paradigms in post-hepatectomy liver failure. J Gastrointest Surg. 2013;17(3):593–605.
7. Demetris AJ, Kelly DM, Eghtesad B, Fontes P, Wallis Marsh J, Tom K, Tan HP, Shaw-Stiffel T, Boig L, Novelli P, Planinsic R, Fung JJ, Marcos A. Pathophysiologic observations and histopathologic recognition of the portal hyperperfusion or small-for-size syndrome. Am J Surg Pathol. 2006;30(8):986–93.
8. Yagi S, Iida T, Taniguchi K, Hori T, Hamada T, Fujii K, Mizuno S, Uemoto S. Impact of portal venous pressure on regeneration and graft damage after living-donor liver transplantation. Liver Transpl. 2005;11(1):68–75.
9. Shimamura T, Taniguchi M, Jin MB, Suzuki T, Matsushita M, Furukawa H, Todo S. Excessive portal venous inflow as a cause of allograft dysfunction in small-for-size living donor liver transplantation. Transplant Proc. 2001;33(1-2):1331.
10. Salman A, El-Garem N, Sholkamy A, Hosny K, Abdelaziz O. Exploring portal vein hemodynamic velocities as a promising, attractive horizon for small-for-size syndrome prediction after living-donor liver transplantation: an Egyptian center study. Transplant Proc. 2016;48:2135–9.

11. Osman AMA, Hosny AA, El-Shazli MA, Uemoto S, Abdelaziz O, Helmy AS. A portal pressure cut-off of 15 versus a cut-off of 20 for prevention of small-for-size syndrome in liver transplantation: a comparative study. Hepatol Res. 2017;47:293–302.
12. Ito T, Kiuchi T, Yamamoto H, et al. Changes in portal venous pressure in the early phase after living donor liver transplantation: pathogenesis and clinical implications. Transplantation. 2003;75:1313–7.
13. Troisi R, de Hemptinne B. Clinical relevance of adapting portal vein flow in living donor liver transplantation in adult patients. Liver Transpl. 2003;9(9):S36–41.
14. Bucur PO, Bekheit M, Audebert C, Othman A, Hammad S, Sebagh M, Allard MA, Decante B, Friebel A, Miquelestorena-Standley E, Drasdo D, Hengstler JG, Vignon-Clementel IE, Vibert E. Modulating portal hemodynamics with vascular ring allows efficient regeneration after partial hepatectomy in a porcine model. Ann Surg. 2018;268(1):134–42.
15. Allard MA, Adam R, Bucur PO, Termos S, Cunha AS, Bismuth H, Castaing D, Vibert E. Posthepatectomy portal vein pressure predicts liver failure and mortality after major liver resection on noncirrhotic liver. Ann Surg. 2013;258(5):822–9. discussion 829–30.
16. Bruix J, Castells A, Bosch J, Feu F, Fuster J, Garcia-Pagan JC, Visa J, Bru C, Rodés J. Surgical resection of hepatocellular carcinoma in cirrhotic patients: prognostic value of preoperative portal pressure. Gastroenterology. 1996;111(4):1018–22.
17. Llovet JM, Fuster J, Bruix J. Intention-to-treat analysis of surgical treatment for early hepatocellular carcinoma: resection versus transplantation. Hepatology. 1999;30(6):1434–40.
18. Aliseda D, Zozaya G, Martí-Cruchaga P, Herrero I, Iñarrairaegui M, Argemí J, Martínez De La Cuesta A, Blanco N, Sabatella L, Sangro B, Rotellar F. The impact of portal hypertension assessment method on the outcomes of hepatocellular carcinoma resection: a meta-analysis of matched cohort and prospective studies. Ann Surg. 2024;280(1):46–55.
19. Cucchetti A, Cescon M, Golfieri R, Piscaglia F, Renzulli M, Neri F, Cappelli A, Mazzotti F, Mosconi C, Colecchia A, Ercolani G, Pinna AD. Hepatic venous pressure gradient in the preoperative assessment of patients with resectable hepatocellular carcinoma. J Hepatol. 2016;64(1):79–86.
20. Mohkam K, Darnis B, Schmitt Z, Duperret S, Ducerf C, Mabrut JY. Successful modulation of portal inflow by somatostatin in a porcine model of small-for-size syndrome. Am J Surg. 2016;212(2):321–6.
21. Troisi RI, Vanlander A, Giglio MC, Van Limmen J, Scudeller L, Heyse B, De Baerdemaeker L, Croo A, Voet D, Praet M, Hoorens A, Antoniali G, Codarin E, Tell G, Reynaert H, Colle I, Sainz-Barriga M. Somatostatin as inflow modulator in liver-transplant recipients with severe portal hypertension: a randomized trial. Ann Surg. 2019;269(6):1025–33.
22. Rhaiem R, Piardi T, Chetboun M, Pessaux P, Lestra T, Memeo R, Kianmanesh R, Sommacale D. Portal inflow modulation by somatostatin after major liver resection: a pilot study. Ann Surg. 2018;267(6):e101–3.
23. Jo HS, Park HJ, Choi YY, Seok JI, Han JH, Yoon YI, Kim DS. Portal modulation effects of terlipressin on liver regeneration and survival in a porcine model subjected to 90% hepatectomy. Am J Transl Res. 2021;13(6):5880–91.
24. Kohler A, Perrodin S, De Gottardi A, Candinas D, Beldi G. Effectiveness of terlipressin for prevention of complications after major liver resection—a randomized placebo-controlled trial. HPB (Oxford). 2020;22(6):884–91.
25. Yao S, Kaido T, Uozumi R, Yagi S, Miyachi Y, Fukumitsu K, Anazawa T, Kamo N, Taura K, Okajima H, Uemoto S. Is portal venous pressure modulation still indicated for all recipients in living donor liver transplantation? Liver Transpl. 2018;24(11):1578–88.
26. Yoshizumi T, Itoh S, Shimokawa M, Inokuchi S, Harada N, Takeishi K, Mano Y, Yoshiya S, Kurihara T, Nagao Y, Ikegami T, Soejima Y, Mori M. Simultaneous splenectomy improves outcomes after adult living donor liver transplantation. J Hepatol. 2021;74(2):372–9.
27. Arakawa Y, Shimada M, Uchiyama H, Ikegami T, Yoshizumi T, Imura S, Morine Y, Kanemura H. Beneficial effects of splenectomy on massive hepatectomy model in rats. Hepatol Res. 2009;39(4):391–7.

28. Ren YS, Qian NS, Tang Y, Liao YH, Liu WH, Raut V, Tao KS, Dou KF. Beneficial effects of splenectomy on liver regeneration in a rat model of massive hepatectomy. Hepatobiliary Pancreat Dis Int. 2012;11(1):60–5.
29. Troisi R, Hoste E, Van Langenhove P, Decruyenaere J, Voet D, Hesse UJ, Cuomo O, de Hemptinne B. Modulation of liver graft hemodynamics by partial ablation of the splenic circuit: a way to increase hepatic artery flow? Transplant Proc. 2001;33(1-2):1445–6.
30. Carrapita J, Abrantes AM, Campelos S, Gonçalves AC, Cardoso D, Sarmento-Ribeiro AB, Rocha C, Santos JN, Botelho MF, Tralhão JG, Farges O, Barbosa JM. Impact of splenic artery ligation after major hepatectomy on liver function, regeneration and viability. Sci Rep. 2016;6:34731.
31. Sato Y, Kobayashi T, Nakatsuka H, Yamamoto S, Oya H, Watanabe T, Hatakeyama K. Splenic arterial ligation prevents liver injury after a major hepatectomy by a reduction of surplus portal hypertension in hepatocellular carcinoma patients with cirrhosis. Hepato-Gastroenterology. 2001;48(39):831–5.
32. Umeda Y, Yagi T, Sadamori H, Matsukawa H, Matsuda H, Shinoura S, Mizuno K, Yoshida R, Iwamoto T, Satoh D, Tanaka N. Effects of prophylactic splenic artery modulation on portal overperfusion and liver regeneration in small-for-size graft. Transplantation. 2008;86(5):673–80.
33. Ku Y, Fukumoto T, Nishida T, Tominaga M, Maeda I, Kitagawa T, Takao S, Shiotani M, Tseng A, Kuroda Y, et al. Evidence that portal vein decompression improves survival of canine quarter orthotopic liver transplantation. Transplantation. 1995;59(10):1388–92.
34. Smyrniotis VE, Kostopanagiotou G, Theodoraki K, Gamaletsos E, Kondi-Pafiti A, Mystakidou K, Arkadopoulos N. Effect of mesocaval shunt on survival of small-for-size liver grafts: experimental study in pigs. Transplantation. 2003;75(10):1737–40.
35. Golriz M, Majlesara A, Khajeh E, Rezaei N, Saffari A, Arwin J, Hafezi M, El Sakka S, Abbasi S, Emami G, Ramouz A, Mehrabi A. Portocaval shunt can optimize transhepatic flow following extended hepatectomy: a short-term study in a porcine model. Sci Rep. 2022;12(1):1668.
36. Wang H, Ohkohchi N, Enomoto Y, Usuda M, Miyagi S, Masuoka H, Sekiguchi S, Kawagishi N, Fujimori K, Sato A, Satomi S. Effect of portocaval shunt on residual extreme small liver after extended hepatectomy in porcine. World J Surg. 2006;30(11):2014–22. discussion 2023–4.
37. Troisi R, Ricciardi S, Smeets P, Petrovic M, Van Maele G, Colle I, Van Vlierberghe H, de Hemptinne B. Effects of hemi-portocaval shunts for inflow modulation on the outcome of small-for-size grafts in living donor liver transplantation. Am J Transplant. 2005;5(6):1397–404.
38. Hakeem AR, Mathew JS, Aunés CV, Mazzola A, Alconchel F, Yoon YI, Testa G, Selzner N, Sarin SK, Lee KW, Soin A, Pomposelli J, Menon K, Goyal N, Kota V, Abu-Gazala S, Rodriguez-Davalos M, Rajalingam R, Kapoor D, Durand F, Kamath P, Jothimani D, Sudhindran S, Vij V, Yoshizumi T, Egawa H, Lerut J, Broering D, Berenguer M, Cattral M, Clavien PA, Chen CL, Shah S, Zhu ZJ, Ascher N, Bhangui P, Rammohan A, Emond J, Rela M. Preventing small-for-size syndrome in living donor liver transplantation: guidelines from the ILTS-iLDLT-LTSI consensus conference. Transplantation. 2023;107(10):2203–15.
39. Sainz-Barriga M, Scudeller L, Costa MG, de Hemptinne B, Troisi RI. Lack of a correlation between portal vein flow and pressure: toward a shared interpretation of hemodynamic stress governing inflow modulation in liver transplantation. Liver Transpl. 2011;17(7):836–48.
40. Mohkam K, Rayar M, Adam JP, Muscari F, Rode A, Merle P, Pradat P, Bauler S, Delfour I, Chiche L, Ducerf C, Boudjema K, Lesurtel M, Laurent C, Mabrut JY. Evaluation of postoperative ascites after somatostatin infusion following hepatectomy for hepatocellular carcinoma by laparotomy: a multicenter randomized double-blind controlled trial (SOMAPROTECT). BMC Cancer. 2018;18(1):844.
41. Takamatsu Y, Hori T, Machimoto T, Hata T, Kadokawa Y, Ito T, Kato S, Yasukawa D, Aisu Y, Kimura Y, Kitano T, Yoshimura T. Intentional modulation of portal venous pressure by splenectomy saves the patient with liver failure and portal hypertension after major hepatectomy: is delayed splenectomy an acceptable therapeutic option for secondary portal hypertension? Am J Case Rep. 2018;19:137–44.

Part III

Techniques to Induce Liver Hypertrophy

Portal Vein Embolization

10

Yujiro Nishioka and Kiyoshi Hasegawa

Abbreviations

DH	Degree of liver hypertrophy
FLR	Future liver remnant
ICG-R15	Indocyanine green retention rate at 15 min
KGR	Kinetic growth ratio
NBCA	N-butyl-cyanoacrylate
POHF	Postoperative hepatic failure
PTPE	Percutaneous transhepatic portal vein embolization
PVA	Polyvinyl alcohol
PVE	Portal vein embolization
RLV-BWR	Remnant liver volume to body weight ratio
SLV	Standardized liver volume
TIPE	Trans-ileocolic portal vein embolization
TLV	Total liver volume

10.1 Introduction

Liver resection is the only curative treatment for patients with liver malignancy, including hepatocellular carcinoma, colorectal liver metastases, intrahepatic cholangiocarcinoma, and hilar cholangiocarcinoma. However, in patients with advanced liver tumors, aggressive liver resection such as extended hemihepatectomy and

Y. Nishioka · K. Hasegawa (✉)
Hepato-Biliary-Pancreatic Surgery Division, Department of Surgery, Graduate School of Medicine, The University of Tokyo, Tokyo, Japan
e-mail: hasegawa-2su@h.u-tokyo.ac.jp

L. Aldrighetti et al. (eds.), *Liver Regeneration Techniques In Hepatic Surgery*,
https://doi.org/10.1007/978-3-032-10997-2_10

trisectionectomy may be required, which leads to the increased risk of postoperative mortality mainly due to postoperative hepatic failure (POHF) followed by the insufficient functional liver remnant (FLR) volume. Due to the difficulty of screening and diagnosis for patients with liver malignancy, less than 25% of patients are reportedly to be initially surgical candidates and it is a crucial issue for surgeons to expand the indication of hepatectomy safely.

Preoperative portal vein embolization (PVE) is a strategy for producing hypertrophy of the future liver remnant, which improves the safety of extended hepatectomy. PVE was first introduced by Makuuchi in 1984 [1, 2] and now has become an established technique performed globally. However, with recent advancements in the 3D simulation software and the perioperative management, including chemotherapy, surgeons are required to plan more complexed hepatectomy and assess the future liver remnant volume and the background liver function precisely before surgery. During this process, the indication of PVE needs to be carefully considered and it is also essential to evaluate whether the liver hypertrophy after PVE is enough for achieving the scheduled hepatectomy safely.

Furthermore, the combination of PVE with other modalities is recently being developed to enhance its trophic effects and expand the resectability of initially unresectable tumors. These approaches include associating liver partition and PVE for staged hepatectomy (ALPPS) [3], hepatic vein deprivation (HVD) [4], and radioembolization [5]. This chapter aims to provide an overview of the current evidence of the indication, the efficacy evaluation, the safety and approach variation, and the combined use of PVE during two-stage hepatectomy [6].

10.2 Indication of PVE

As mentioned above, the purpose of PVE is to provide a "sufficient" FLR preoperatively for patients with an "insufficient" FLR. Defining what constitutes a "sufficient" FLR is crucial in determining the indication for PVE in patients with liver malignancies. Currently, there is no definitive consensus on the indication of PVE, as FLR status depends not only on its volume but also on the background liver function. Therefore, surgeons need to follow three key steps when deciding to perform PVE: measuring the FLR volume accurately, evaluating the background liver function, and determining the minimal FLR for preventing POHF.

10.2.1 Accurate Measurement of the FLR Volume: 3D Simulation and Virtual Hepatectomy

In the 1990s, the quantitative assessment of FLR from preoperative imaging was performed by the manual tracing of computed tomography (CT) images for each slice, followed by the integration of planar dimensions. This process was labor-intensive and time-consuming, and it could only delineate segment boundaries based on anatomical landmarks, resulting in discrepancies with the true FLR as defined by portal territory.

The emergence of 3D simulation software in the 2000s enabled the extraction of vascular structures from preoperative images and the calculation of their governing regions [7, 8]. This technique revealed the fact that intrahepatic vascular anatomy has a variety of branching pattern [9] and the plains between each segment/sector are not so simple [10]. "Virtual hepatectomy" using 3D simulation software provided surgeons a more accurate evaluation of portal territory and the more detailed imagination of cut surface after hepatectomy [11]. Also, this technique was reported to be reproducible, quick, and friendly for even inexperienced physicians [12]. Recent dramatic advance in artificial intelligence accelerated the shortening of liver volumetry process and simple liver volumetry such as hemihepatectomy could be obtained within a couple of minutes [13].

An additional advantage of 3D simulation is its ability to calculate venous perfusion territories. Liver function can be impaired by approximately 70% in the congestion area caused by concomitant sacrifice of hepatic veins due to tumor invasion [14]. Therefore, it is crucial to accurately calculate the noncongested remnant liver volume in the expected FLR.

10.2.2 Evaluation of the Background Liver Function

Not only viral hepatitis, the recent increase of metabolic dysfunction-associated steatotic liver disease and chemotherapy-associated liver injury has led to the increased risk of incidental liver damage and made liver function assessment increasingly important. In Asia, including Japan, the indocyanine green retention rate at 15 min (ICG-R15) has long been used as the gold standard for assessing background liver function [15, 16]. Its use has recently expanded to Western countries, and it has been reported to correlate with portal pressure [17, 18].

As a quantitative assessment of liver functional reserve, the ALBI grade, which combines serum albumin and bilirubin levels, has been proposed [19]. However, serum bilirubin levels are often within the normal range in candidates for hepatic resection, and the utility of ALBI grade is limited. To address this limitation, the ALICE score, which is calculated using serum albumin levels and ICG-R15, has been introduced [20].

10.2.3 Determining the Minimal FLR for Preventing POHF

Makuuchi proposed to determine the minimal FLR based on serum bilirubin levels and ICG-R15, that is, "Makuuchi Criteria" [15]. Subsequently, Kubota et al. reported that PVE in cases with expected FLR <40% allows for safe liver resection [21]. Since these criteria aimed for "zero mortality" and were considered too strict, expanded criteria were proposed in European countries, setting the minimal FLR at 30% for patients with normal liver and 50% for those with impaired liver (ICG-R15 <20%) [22, 23].

In the United States, the ratio of FLR to standardized liver volume (SLV), calculated based on height and weight, is commonly used. The proposed minimal FLR thresholds are 20% of SLV for patients with normal liver, 30% for those who underwent preoperative chemotherapy, and 40% for those with hepatic fibrosis or cirrhosis [24–27]. Additionally, Truant et al. introduced the remnant liver volume to body weight ratio (RLV-BWR) and reported that an RLV-BWR of 0.5% is the lower limit to avoid POHF in patients with normal liver [28].

Regarding the degree of liver hypertrophy (DH), namely the percentage point difference between the liver volume before and after PVE, Shindoh et al. reported a median value of 10.9% based on the data from 358 patients [29], Alvarez et al. reported 11.1% based on 431 patients [30], and Yamashita et al. reported 9.6%–10% based on 319 patients [31]. Yamashita also noted that DH did not differ by the underlying disease, whether hepatocellular carcinoma, metastatic liver cancer, or cholangiocarcinoma.

Given these reports, a threshold of 25%–30% is currently considered safe for patients with a normal liver, while those with an injured or cirrhotic liver require additional 10% or more FLR for safe surgery [32]. PVE typically results in about 10% of DH, although it remains debatable to choose TLV or SLV as the standard. Therefore, if the expected FLR does not reach 15% below the safety limit, proceeding with resection after PVE is unlikely to be feasible and PVE should not be indicated.

10.3 Evaluation of the Effect of PVE

10.3.1 Timing for the Evaluation of DH

Nagasue et al. evaluated the remnant liver volume over time in 28 patients after hepatectomy and reported that the remnant liver volume reaches a plateau within 2 months after hepatectomy in both patients with normal liver and impaired liver [33]. Ribero et al. assessed DH in 112 patients who underwent PVE and found that 75% of the growth in the FLR within the first 2 months after PVE occurs in the first 3 weeks [26]. Based on these findings, it is generally accepted to evaluate DH 2–4 weeks after PVE to determine whether to proceed with resection.

10.3.2 Continuous Evaluation of Liver Hypertrophy Considering Background Liver Function

The minimal FLR criteria for safe hepatectomy based on ICG-R15 had some limitations. First, they did not integrate background liver function and FLR in a continuous manner. To address this issue, Nagino et al. analyzed 193 patients with cholangiocarcinoma who underwent PVE followed by hepatectomy and proposed the Krem-ICG defined by the formula: kICG (the elimination rate constant) × FLR [ml]/TLV [ml]. They reported that Krem-ICG ≥0.05 is necessary for safe liver resection [34].

However, this method still did not account for the second limitation: the dynamic changes in FLR over time. Shindoh et al. introduced the kinetic growth rate (KGR), defined as DH at initial volume assessment divided by number of weeks elapsed after PVE. Analyzing data from 107 patients who underwent liver resection after PVE, they found that KGR <2.0% predicted POHF rather than static parameters like FLR/SLV or DH [35]. Furthermore, it was also reported that chemotherapy-associated liver injury and diabetes are predictors of low KGR, supporting the use of PVE for selecting suitable surgical candidates [36].

Another limitation of ICG clearance testing is that it cannot assess functional heterogeneity in the liver, particularly in the embolized area scheduled for resection, which is expected to exhibit functional decline after PVE. To overcome this problem, efforts have been made to quantitatively evaluate functional FLR using: Scintigraphy (e.g., 99mTc-labeled mebrofenin hepatobiliary scintigraphy, 99mTc-labeled GSA hepatobiliary scintigraphy) [37–39], and EOB-MRI assessing the hepatocellular uptake index in FLR [40, 41] (Table 10.1). However, the evidence is

Table 10.1 Evaluation for liver hypertrophy after PVE and proposed minimal limit for safety

Author	Published year	Modality	Evaluation	Definition	Minimal limit for safety
Kubota [21]	1997	CT	FLR volume	Post-PVE FLR/TLV	40%[a]; 50%[b]
Clavien [22]	2007	CT	FLR volume	Post-PVE FLR/TLV	30%[a]; 50%[b]
Ribero [26]	2007	CT	Standardized FLR Degree of hypertrophy	FLR/SLV (Post-PVE FLR − pre-PVE FLR)/SLV	20%[a]; 30%[b] 5%
Nagino [34]	2006	CT	Krem-ICG	kICG (the elimination rate constant) × FLR [ml]/TLV [ml]	0.05
Shindoh [35]	2013	CT	Kinetic growth rate	Degree of hypertrophy (%)/number of weeks after PVE	2.0%
Tomita [38]	2021	^{99m}Tc GSA scintigraphy	FLR-LU15	Liver uptake 15 min after injection	16.7
de Graaf [39]	2010	^{99m}Tc mebrofenin scintigraphy	Uptake in the FLR		2.69%/min/m^2
Kim [40]	2018	EOB-MRI	Hepatocyte uptake index (BW adjusted)	FLR × [(liver EOB uptake/spleen EOB uptake) − 1]/BW	12.38
Akabane [41]	2023	EOB-MRI	Hepatocyte uptake index	FLR × [(liver EOB uptake/spleen EOB uptake) − 1]	927.1

FLR future liver remnant, *TLV* total liver volume, *SLV* standardized liver volume, *EOB-MRI* gadolinium ethoxybenzyl diethylenetriamine pentaacetic acid-enhanced magnetic resonance imaging, *BW* body weight

[a]Patients with normal liver

[b]Patients with injured or cirrhotic liver

scarce and these functional assessments still cannot be integrated with precise FLR calculations sufficiently.

Therefore, there is no gold standard for the indication and evaluation of liver hypertrophy after PVE. To improve predictive accuracy, recent research suggests that radiomics and laboratory tests combined with artificial intelligence could effectively predict FLR, KGR, and TLV after PVE [42]. This advanced approach may enhance decision-making for patients with marginal FLR, potentially refining PVE indications and improving surgical outcomes.

10.4 Safety and Approach of PVE

10.4.1 Complication Related to PVE

Alvarez reported that 72 of 431 patients (16.7%) experienced complications after PVE, and the most frequent complication was accidental embolization of part of the FLR, occurring in 7.4% of patients. The rate of severe complications (Clavien–Dindo grade > IIIa) was 2.5%, and one patient (0.2%) died [30]. Similarly, Yamashita et al. reported that 34 of 338 patients (10.0%) experienced PVE-related complications [31]. One cause of erratic embolization is the enlargement of a thrombus formed in the embolized right portal vein branch, which can extend into the main portal vein. Therefore, it is crucial to embolize the anterior and posterior branches of the portal vein separately (Fig. 10.1).

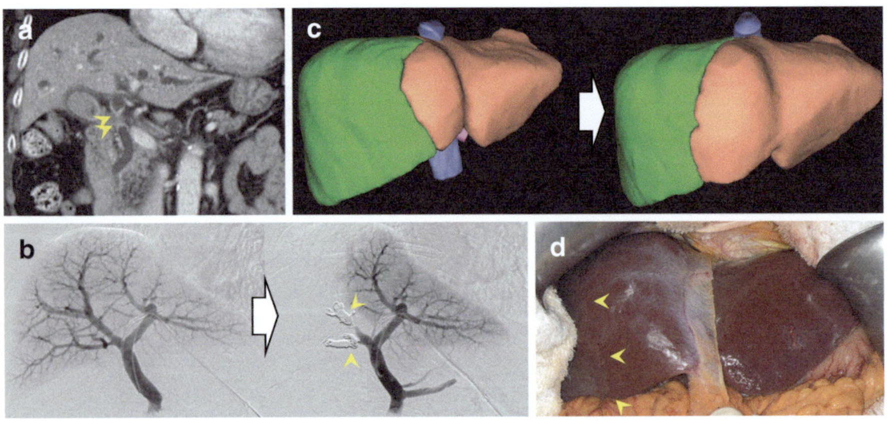

Fig. 10.1 A case who underwent conventional PVE followed by right hemihepatectomy with bile duct resection. (**a**) Preoperative CT image showing widespread hilar cholangiocarcinoma (arrowhead in yellow). (**b**) Portography before and after PVE using absolute alcohol with coils. Anterior and posterior portal vein branch was embolized separately (arrowhead in yellow). (**c**) 3D CT simulation showing liver hypertrophy (FLR/TLV 33.9% → 45.9%, KGR 6.0%). (**d**) Intraoperative view showing the atrophy of right liver along Rex–Cantlie line (arrowhead in yellow)

10.4.2 Percutaneous Transhepatic Approach Versus Trans-ileocolic Approach

For accessing portal vein, two major methods are available: percutaneous transhepatic portal vein embolization (PTPE), trans-ileocolic portal vein embolization (TIPE). A meta-analysis by Abulkhir et al. reported significantly greater FLR hypertrophy after PTPE than after TIPE (11.9% vs. 9.7%), with no significant difference in major complications [43]. Additionally, PTPE offers several advantages over TIPE: it eliminates the need for general anesthesia, is less invasive with lower costs and a shorter recovery time, and avoids the risk of adhesions around the hepatic hilum, which could complicate subsequent surgery. As a result, TIPE is no longer recommended as a first-line option.

10.4.3 Ipsilateral Approach Versus Contralateral Approach

PTPE can be performed using two access routes to the portal vein: the ipsilateral approach and the contralateral approach. The ipsilateral approach accesses the portal vein through the liver to be resected (usually anterior segment of the right portal vein), while the contralateral approach accesses the portal vein in the FLR (usually segment 3). The primary advantage of the ipsilateral approach is that it avoids trauma to the FLR and provides easier access to segment 4 if needed. In contrast, the contralateral approach allows for easier catheter manipulation by radiologists and reduces the risk of tumor dissemination in patients with high tumor burden. Alvarez et al. reported that the ipsilateral approach was associated with significantly fewer complications than the contralateral approach (10.3% vs 19.4%), particularly a lower risk of erratic embolization (6.9% vs. 11.1%) [30]. However, the choice of approach should be decided considering, based on tumor burden, the extent of the embolization and the local expertise.

10.4.4 Embolic Materials for PVE

Several embolic agents have been studied for embolizing the portal vein. Operators need to choose materials considering the expected speed and extent of liver hypertrophy, complications, and ease of handling [44].

Gelatin foam is one of the oldest materials. It is very inexpensive and has a temporary occlusion nature, but that leads to recanalization and limits its effectiveness in PVE compared to other nontemporary embolic material [45].

Polyvinyl alcohol (PVA) particles also belong to the oldest materials, but the combination of PVA particles and coils or vascular plugs is currently a widely used approach in Western countries. Studies report significantly improved liver regeneration using these materials, with the increase of FLR/TLV reaching 7.7%–8.5%. However, complications like portal vein thrombosis have been observed in 8% [46, 47].

N-butyl-cyanoacrylate (NBCA) is a liquid embolic agent that polymerizes upon contact with ionic fluids, forming a strong bond. It is mixed with lipiodol for visibility and controlled polymerization. A recent systematic review including 2896 patients by Ali et al. reported its superiority compared to microparticles including PVA in terms of %FLR (the increased ratio of FLR/TLV increase after to before PVE, 49.1% vs. 42.2%), shorter procedure time (215 min vs. 348 min), and less radiation dose, with no difference of major complication (4% vs. 5%) [48].

At last, absolute alcohol, primarily used in Japan, is a highly aggressive liquid embolic material applied with anti-reflux techniques. It denatures proteins and induces immediate thrombosis. Although no large cohort studies have evaluated the use of absolute alcohol for PVE, several Japanese retrospective studies have demonstrated strong hypertrophy outcomes, with an FLR/TLV increase of 10.8%–13.0%, which was comparable to or superior to PVE using other embolic materials, including NBCA [49–51]. The reported complication rate of PVE with ethanol ranged from 3.7% to 6.0%, similar to that of other embolic materials. However, absolute alcohol has significant drawbacks, including severe pain, rapid vascular dilution, and high toxicity, often leading to elevated liver enzyme levels post-procedure. Recently, Shibata et al. reported that the combination of ethanol and coils resulted in lower recanalization rates and reduced liver damage compared with ethanol alone [52].

10.5 Extended PVE and Combined Use of PVE in Two-Stage Hepatectomy

In addition to conventional PVE (i.e., embolization of the right lobe portal branch), several variations have been reported. This section reviews extended PVE and the combined use of PVE with two-stage hepatectomy. ALPPS, HVD, and radioembolization will be discussed in detail in subsequent chapters.

10.5.1 Efficacy of PVE Extended to Segment 4

For patients requiring a right-sided trisectionectomy for curative resection, PVE extended to segment 4 can be considered. Kishi et al. analyzed data from 73 patients and reported that PVE extended to segment 4 portal vein resulted in a significantly higher hypertrophy rate in segments 2 + 3 compared to conventional PVE (54% vs. 26%), with a comparable complication rate [53]. However, controversy remains regarding the hypertrophy rate and the risk of erratic embolization in the left portal venous system [54–57].

Segment 4 has typically 2–4 portal vein branches, making complete embolization technically challenging (Fig. 10.2). Furthermore, candidates for anatomical right-sided trisectionectomy should be highly selected, including cases of advanced

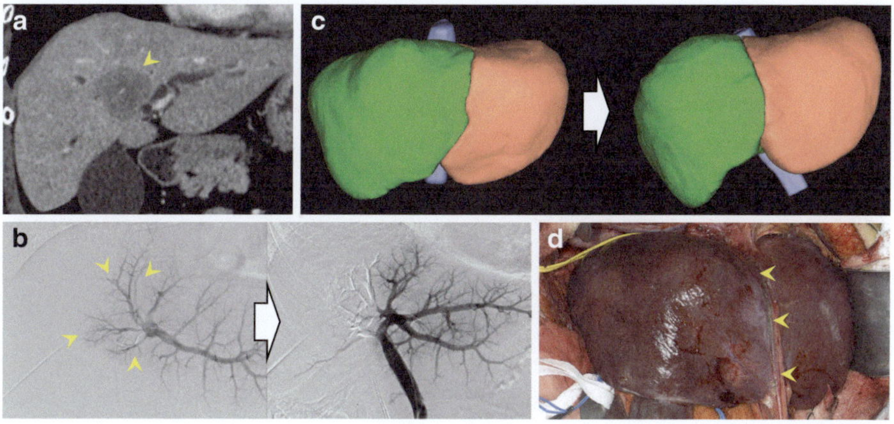

Fig. 10.2 A case who underwent extended PVE to segment 4 followed by right trisectorectomy. (**a**) Preoperative CT image showing intrahepatic cholangiocarcinoma infiltrating to hilar plate and segment 4 bile duct branch (arrowhead in yellow). (**b**) Portography before and after PVE using absolute alcohol with coils. Four branches of segment 4 portal vein branches were completely embolized (arrowhead in yellow) *Segment 4 branches were too thin for using absolute alcohol or coils, then NBCA was injected in them. (**c**) 3D CT simulation showing liver hypertrophy (FLR/TLV 30.3% → 36.0%, KGR 2.9%). (**d**) Intraoperative view showing the atrophy of right liver along falciform ligament (arrowhead in yellow)

biliary tract cancer, because liver parenchyma-preserving hepatectomy is currently recommended for patients with colorectal liver metastases.

10.5.2 Two-Stage Hepatectomy

For patients with multiple bilateral colorectal liver metastases, two-stage hepatectomy combined with PVE has been established as a safe and effective treatment strategy. Adam et al. first reported this approach in 2000 based on data from 16 patients, showing a completion rate of 81% and a postoperative mortality rate of 15% [6]. In 2016, Passot et al. analyzed 109 patients planned for two-stage hepatectomy, reporting a completion rate of 82% and a postoperative mortality rate of 7% [58]. Patients who completed two-stage hepatectomy had significantly better survival (5-year overall survival 49% vs. 0%). However, despite recent advancements in colorectal cancer chemotherapy, the completion rate has remained at 70%–80% [59–64] (Table 10.2).

The primary cause of the 20%–30% drop-out rate is tumor progression during the interval between the first and second hepatectomy [58]. To shorten this interval, "fast-track" two-stage hepatectomy has been proposed, in which first-stage hepatectomy is performed concurrently with PTPE in a hybrid intervention/operating room suite [65]. Although the reported completion rate was 59%, the pilot study included patients who had a very high tumor burden and poor tumor biology. Similarly, in the

Table 10.2 Outcomes of two-stage hepatectomy combined with PVE for bilateral colorectal liver metastases

Author	Published year	Number of patients	PVE (%)	Interval of hepatectomy	Completion rate (%)	Postoperative morbidity (%)	Postoperative mortality (%)	3y-OS (%)
Adam	2000	16	44	4 months	81	38	15	35
Tanaka	2007	21	100	NA	100	23	0	33
Wicherts	2008	59	78	3.3 months	69	59	7	60
Tsim	2011	38	95	NA	87	33	0	50
Narita	2011	80	86	3 months	76	54	0	59
Turini	2012	48	100	2.4 months	71	20	6	59
Passot	2016	109	73	NA	82	27	6	68
Chavez	2021	196	65.3	4 months	100	47	5	64
Nishioka	2021	19	89	1.5 months[a]	59	10	0	NA

OS overall survival
[a] Fast-track two-stage hepatectomy

context of ALPPS, a first-stage hepatectomy with concurrent TIPE has been proposed [66]. Its efficacy requires further validation in larger cohorts.

10.6 Conclusion

Preoperative PVE plays a crucial role in enhancing liver regeneration and expanding the eligibility for extended hepatectomy in patients with liver malignancies. Recent advancements in 3D simulation, liver function assessment, and embolic materials have improved the precision and effectiveness of PVE; however, there does not yet exist a gold standard for the evaluation of liver hypertrophy after PVE. The optimal PVE approach, timing of evaluation, and combination with other treatments must be carefully tailored to each patient to maximize safety and surgical success. While PVE remains a standard technique, other emerging strategies offer additional options for patients with initially unresectable tumors.

References

1. Makuuchi M, Takayasu K, Takuma T, et al. Preoperative transcatheter embolization of the portal venous branch for patients receiving extended lobectomy due to the bile duct carcinoma. J Jpn Pract Surg Soc. 1984;45(12):1558–64.
2. Makuuchi M, Thai BL, Takayasu K, et al. Preoperative portal embolization to increase safety of major hepatectomy for hilar bile duct carcinoma: a preliminary report. Surgery. 1990;107(5):521–7.
3. Schnitzbauer AA, Lang SA, Goessmann H, et al. Right portal vein ligation combined with in situ splitting induces rapid left lateral liver lobe hypertrophy enabling 2-staged extended right hepatic resection in small-for-size settings. Ann Surg. 2012;255(3):405–14.
4. Kobayashi K, Yamaguchi T, Denys A, et al. Liver venous deprivation compared to portal vein embolization to induce hypertrophy of the future liver remnant before major hepatectomy: a single center experience. Surgery. 2020;167(6):917–23.
5. Addeo P, de Mathelin P, De Marini P, et al. Sequential Y(90) liver radioembolization and portal vein embolization: an additional strategy to downstage liver tumors and to enhance liver hypertrophy before major hepatectomies. Langenbeck's Arch Surg. 2023;408(1):339.
6. Adam R, Laurent A, Azoulay D, et al. Two-stage hepatectomy: a planned strategy to treat irresectable liver tumors. Ann Surg. 2000;232(6):777–85.
7. Lamadé W, Glombitza G, Fischer L, et al. The impact of 3-dimensional reconstructions on operation planning in liver surgery. Arch Surg. 2000;135(11):1256–61.
8. Saito S, Yamanaka J, Miura K, et al. A novel 3D hepatectomy simulation based on liver circulation: application to liver resection and transplantation. Hepatology. 2005;41(6):1297–304.
9. Mise Y, Satou S, Shindoh J, et al. Three-dimensional volumetry in 107 normal livers reveals clinically relevant inter-segment variation in size. HPB (Oxford). 2014;16(5):439–47.
10. Shindoh J, Mise Y, Satou S, et al. The intersegmental plane of the liver is not always flat--tricks for anatomical liver resection. Ann Surg. 2010;251(5):917–22.
11. Takamoto T, Hashimoto T, Ogata S, et al. Planning of anatomical liver segmentectomy and subsegmentectomy with 3-dimensional simulation software. Am J Surg. 2013;206(4):530–8.
12. Maki H, Nishioka Y, Haddad A, et al. Reproducibility and efficiency of liver volumetry using manual method and liver analysis software. HPB (Oxford). 2024;26(7):911–8.

13. Kazami Y, Kaneko J, Keshwani D, et al. Two-step artificial intelligence algorithm for liver segmentation automates anatomic virtual hepatectomy. J Hepatobiliary Pancreat Sci. 2023;30(11):1205–17.
14. Kawaguchi Y, Ishizawa T, Miyata Y, et al. Portal uptake function in veno-occlusive regions evaluated by real-time fluorescent imaging using indocyanine green. J Hepatol. 2013;58(2):247–53.
15. Imamura H, Seyama Y, Kokudo N, et al. One thousand fifty-six hepatectomies without mortality in 8 years. Arch Surg. 2003;138(11):1198–206. discussion 1206.
16. Hwang S, Ha TY, Song GW, et al. Quantified risk assessment for major hepatectomy via the indocyanine green clearance rate and liver volumetry combined with standard liver volume. J Gastrointest Surg. 2015;19(7):1305–14.
17. Le Roy B, Gregoire E, Cosse C, et al. Indocyanine green retention rates at 15 min predicted hepatic decompensation in a Western population. World J Surg. 2018;42(8):2570–8.
18. Kobayashi K, Uldry E, Kokudo T, et al. Correlation between portal pressure and indocyanine green retention rate is unaffected by the cause of cirrhosis: a prospective study. World J Surg. 2021;45(8):2546–55.
19. Johnson PJ, Berhane S, Kagebayashi C, et al. Assessment of liver function in patients with hepatocellular carcinoma: a new evidence-based approach-the ALBI grade. J Clin Oncol. 2015;33(6):550–8.
20. Kokudo T, Hasegawa K, Amikura K, et al. Assessment of preoperative liver function in patients with hepatocellular carcinoma—the albumin-indocyanine green evaluation (ALICE) grade. PLoS One. 2016;11(7):e0159530.
21. Kubota K, Makuuchi M, Kusaka K, et al. Measurement of liver volume and hepatic functional reserve as a guide to decision-making in resectional surgery for hepatic tumors. Hepatology. 1997;26(5):1176–81.
22. Clavien PA, Petrowsky H, DeOliveira ML, et al. Strategies for safer liver surgery and partial liver transplantation. N Engl J Med. 2007;356(15):1545–59.
23. Seyama Y, Kokudo N. Assessment of liver function for safe hepatic resection. Hepatol Res. 2009;39(2):107–16.
24. Vauthey JN, Chaoui A, Do KA, et al. Standardized measurement of the future liver remnant prior to extended liver resection: methodology and clinical associations. Surgery. 2000;127(5):512–9.
25. Abdalla EK, Adam R, Bilchik AJ, et al. Improving resectability of hepatic colorectal metastases: expert consensus statement. Ann Surg Oncol. 2006;13(10):1271–80.
26. Ribero D, Abdalla EK, Madoff DC, et al. Portal vein embolization before major hepatectomy and its effects on regeneration, resectability and outcome. Br J Surg. 2007;94(11):1386–94.
27. Kishi Y, Abdalla EK, Chun YS, et al. Three hundred and one consecutive extended right hepatectomies: evaluation of outcome based on systematic liver volumetry. Ann Surg. 2009;250(4):540–8.
28. Truant S, Oberlin O, Sergent G, et al. Remnant liver volume to body weight ratio > or =0.5%: a new cut-off to estimate postoperative risks after extended resection in noncirrhotic liver. J Am Coll Surg. 2007;204(1):22–33.
29. Shindoh J, Tzeng CW, Aloia TA, et al. Safety and efficacy of portal vein embolization before planned major or extended hepatectomy: an institutional experience of 358 patients. J Gastrointest Surg. 2014;18(1):45–51.
30. Alvarez FA, Castaing D, Figueroa R, et al. Natural history of portal vein embolization before liver resection: a 23-year analysis of intention-to-treat results. Surgery. 2018;163(6):1257–63.
31. Yamashita S, Sakamoto Y, Yamamoto S, et al. Efficacy of preoperative portal vein embolization among patients with hepatocellular carcinoma, biliary tract cancer, and colorectal liver metastases: a comparative study based on single-center experience of 319 cases. Ann Surg Oncol. 2017;24(6):1557–68.
32. Kishi Y, Vauthey JN. Issues to be considered to address the future liver remnant prior to major hepatectomy. Surg Today. 2021;51(4):472–84.

33. Nagasue N, Yukaya H, Ogawa Y, et al. Human liver regeneration after major hepatic resection. A study of normal liver and livers with chronic hepatitis and cirrhosis. Ann Surg. 1987;206(1):30–9.
34. Nagino M, Kamiya J, Nishio H, et al. Two hundred forty consecutive portal vein embolizations before extended hepatectomy for biliary cancer: surgical outcome and long-term follow-up. Ann Surg. 2006;243(3):364–72.
35. Shindoh J, Truty MJ, Aloia TA, et al. Kinetic growth rate after portal vein embolization predicts posthepatectomy outcomes: toward zero liver-related mortality in patients with colorectal liver metastases and small future liver remnant. J Am Coll Surg. 2013;216(2):201–9.
36. Omichi K, Yamashita S, Cloyd JM, et al. Portal vein embolization reduces postoperative hepatic insufficiency associated with postchemotherapy hepatic atrophy. J Gastrointest Surg. 2018;22(1):60–7.
37. Iimuro Y, Kashiwagi T, Yamanaka J, et al. Preoperative estimation of asialoglycoprotein receptor expression in the remnant liver from CT/99mTc-GSA SPECT fusion images correlates well with postoperative liver function parameters. J Hepatobiliary Pancreat Sci. 2010;17(5):673–81.
38. Tomita K, Chiba N, Ochiai S, et al. Prognostic value of future liver remnant LU15 index of 99mTc-galactosyl serum albumin scintigraphy for predicting posthepatectomy liver failure. PLoS One. 2021;16(2):e0247675.
39. de Graaf W, van Lienden KP, Dinant S, et al. Assessment of future remnant liver function using hepatobiliary scintigraphy in patients undergoing major liver resection. J Gastrointest Surg. 2010;14(2):369–78.
40. Kim DK, Choi JI, Choi MH, et al. Prediction of posthepatectomy liver failure: MRI with hepatocyte-specific contrast agent versus indocyanine green clearance test. AJR Am J Roentgenol. 2018;211(3):580–7.
41. Akabane M, Shindoh J, Kobayashi Y, et al. Risk stratification of patients with marginal hepatic functional reserve using the remnant hepatocyte uptake index in gadoxetic acid-enhanced magnetic resonance imaging for safe liver surgery. World J Surg. 2023;47(4):1042–8.
42. Kuhn TN, Engelhardt WD, Kahl VH, et al. Artificial intelligence-driven patient selection for preoperative portal vein embolization for patients with colorectal cancer liver metastases. J Vasc Interv Radiol. 2025;36(3):477–88.
43. Abulkhir A, Limongelli P, Healey AJ, et al. Preoperative portal vein embolization for major liver resection: a meta-analysis. Ann Surg. 2008;247(1):49–57.
44. Luz JHM, Gomes FV, Coimbra E, et al. Preoperative portal vein embolization in hepatic surgery: a review about the embolic materials and their effects on liver regeneration and outcome. Radiol Res Pract. 2020;2020:9295852.
45. de Baere T, Roche A, Elias D, et al. Preoperative portal vein embolization for extension of hepatectomy indications. Hepatology. 1996;24(6):1386–91.
46. Madoff DC, Hicks ME, Abdalla EK, et al. Portal vein embolization with polyvinyl alcohol particles and coils in preparation for major liver resection for hepatobiliary malignancy: safety and effectiveness—study in 26 patients. Radiology. 2003;227(1):251–60.
47. Geisel D, Malinowski M, Powerski MJ, et al. Improved hypertrophy of future remnant liver after portal vein embolization with plugs, coils and particles. Cardiovasc Intervent Radiol. 2014;37(5):1251–8.
48. Ali A, Ahle M, Björnsson B, et al. Portal vein embolization with N-butyl cyanoacrylate glue is superior to other materials: a systematic review and meta-analysis. Eur Radiol. 2021;31(8):5464–78.
49. Sakuhara Y, Abo D, Hasegawa Y, et al. Preoperative percutaneous transhepatic portal vein embolization with ethanol injection. AJR Am J Roentgenol. 2012;198(4):914–22.
50. Sofue K, Arai Y, Shimada K, et al. Right portal vein embolization with absolute ethanol in major hepatic resection for hepatobiliary malignancy. Br J Surg. 2014;101(9):1122–8.
51. Sugawara S, Arai Y, Sone M, et al. Retrospective comparative study of absolute ethanol with N-butyl-2-cyanoacrylate in percutaneous portal vein embolization. J Vasc Interv Radiol. 2019;30(8):1215–22.

52. Shibata E, Takao H, Kaiume M, et al. Preoperative portal vein embolization: a comparison of ethanol and coils versus ethanol alone. Minim Invasive Ther Allied Technol. 2022;31(6):939–47.
53. Kishi Y, Madoff DC, Abdalla EK, et al. Is embolization of segment 4 portal veins before extended right hepatectomy justified? Surgery. 2008;144(5):744–51.
54. Hammond CJ, Ali S, Haq H, et al. Segment 2/3 hypertrophy is greater when right portal vein embolisation is extended to segment 4 in patients with colorectal liver metastases: a retrospective cohort study. Cardiovasc Intervent Radiol. 2019;42(4):552–9.
55. Björnsson B, Hasselgren K, Røsok B, et al. Segment 4 occlusion in portal vein embolization increase future liver remnant hypertrophy—a Scandinavian cohort study. Int J Surg. 2020;75:60–5.
56. van Gulik TM, van den Esschert JW, de Graaf W, et al. Controversies in the use of portal vein embolization. Dig Surg. 2008;25(6):436–44.
57. Massimino KP, Kolbeck KJ, Enestvedt CK, et al. Safety and efficacy of preoperative right portal vein embolization in patients at risk for postoperative liver failure following major right hepatectomy. HPB (Oxford). 2012;14(1):14–9.
58. Passot G, Chun YS, Kopetz SE, et al. Predictors of safety and efficacy of 2-stage hepatectomy for bilateral colorectal liver metastases. J Am Coll Surg. 2016;223(1):99–108.
59. Tanaka K, Shimada H, Matsuo K, et al. Remnant liver regeneration after two-stage hepatectomy for multiple bilobar colorectal metastases. Eur J Surg Oncol. 2007;33(3):329–35.
60. Wicherts DA, Miller R, de Haas RJ, et al. Long-term results of two-stage hepatectomy for irresectable colorectal cancer liver metastases. Ann Surg. 2008;248(6):994–1005.
61. Tsim N, Healey AJ, Frampton AE, et al. Two-stage resection for bilobar colorectal liver metastases: R0 resection is the key. Ann Surg Oncol. 2011;18(7):1939–46.
62. Narita M, Oussoultzoglou E, Jaeck D, et al. Two-stage hepatectomy for multiple bilobar colorectal liver metastases. Br J Surg. 2011;98(10):1463–75.
63. Turrini O, Ewald J, Viret F, et al. Two-stage hepatectomy: who will not jump over the second hurdle? Eur J Surg Oncol. 2012;38(3):266–73.
64. Chavez MI, Gholami S, Kim BJ, et al. Two-stage hepatectomy for bilateral colorectal liver metastases: a multi-institutional analysis. Ann Surg Oncol. 2021;28(3):1457–65.
65. Nishioka Y, Odisio BC, Velasco JD, et al. Fast-track two-stage hepatectomy by concurrent portal vein embolization at first-stage hepatectomy in hybrid interventional radiology/operating suite. Surg Oncol. 2021;39:101648.
66. Sakamoto Y, Inagaki F, Omichi K, et al. Associating liver partial partition and transileocecal portal vein embolization for staged hepatectomy. Ann Surg. 2016;264(6):e21–2.

Portal Vein Ligation

11

Francesco Ardito and Felice Giuliante

The use of portal vein occlusion to induce the hypertrophy of the future liver remnant volume (FLRV) has represented one of the most relevant advancement in liver surgery by allowing to expand the number of patients with resectable disease [1]. Portal vein occlusion can be performed by percutaneous portal vein embolization (PVE) or by intraoperative portal vein ligation (PVL). The efficacy of PVE in stimulating the hypertrophy of FLRV and in improving the safety of extended hepatectomy has been widely published in the literature [2, 3] since the first report by Makuuchi et al. in 1990 [4]. In 2003 a new strategy design, defined as two-stage hepatectomy (TSH), was described to treat patients with multiple and bilateral colorectal liver metastases (CRLM) who were classified as primarily unresectable due to insufficient FLRV [5]. The two surgical steps of this strategy are combined with PVE, which is performed 2–5 weeks after the first-stage hepatectomy [6].

TSH is often planned in patients with synchronous CRLM with primary tumor in site. Such patients may be considered as ideal candidates for the intraoperative PVL, which can be performed during the first stage, instead of the postoperative PVE [7]. Indeed, during the first step, the primary tumor and all left-sided CRLM are resected. Simultaneously, right PVL may be performed to induce hypertrophy in the left lobe. The advantage associated with PVL could be that the portal vein occlusion is obtained during the same intervention, avoiding further percutaneous procedures after surgery.

In the literature, several papers compared the efficacy between PVE and PVL in inducing liver hypertrophy with controversial results [8–10]. The study by Broering

F. Ardito · F. Giuliante (✉)
Hepatobiliary Surgery Unit, Fondazione Policlinico Universitario Agostino Gemelli, IRCCS, Rome, Italy

Department of Translational Medicine and Surgery, Università Cattolica del Sacro Cuore, Rome, Italy
e-mail: felice.giuliante@unicatt.it

L. Aldrighetti et al. (eds.), *Liver Regeneration Techniques In Hepatic Surgery*, https://doi.org/10.1007/978-3-032-10997-2_11

et al. [8] showed that PVE resulted in a significantly more efficient increase in liver volume and a shorter hospital stay. On the other hand, the French results by Belghiti [9] and the study by Capussotti et al. [10] showed that the PVL was as effective as PVE in inducing hypertrophy of the FLRV. A recent meta-analysis [11] did not reveal significant differences in future liver remnant hypertrophy rates between PVE and PVL, nor in post-procedure morbidity.

Possible explanations of these controversial results may be the limited number of PVL patients and the limited quality of the PVL studies. Another possible bias may be the surgical technique of PVL, which is not always similarly described in most centers. One critical issue is the association, or not, of absolute alcohol injection into the right portal vein after its proximal ligation. It has been demonstrated that the only proximal occlusion of the right portal vein by coil embolization or by surgical ligation may be not sufficient in inducing the hypertrophy of the future remnant liver. Indeed, the venous intrahepatic system is naturally anastomosed by porto-portal collaterals between portal branches of segment 4 and the branches of the adjacent right segments 5 and 8. The development and the hypertrophy of such veins have been described in patients with portal vein thrombosis [12]. The hypertrophy of these collateral veins after the proximal portal vein occlusion may limit the benefits of portal flow redistribution and may have a negative impact on the degree of hypertrophy of the future liver remnant [12].

Since its introduction in 1986, PVE has evolved technically and various embolic agents have been used and tested to date [13]. This long experience has demonstrated that a permanent proximal and distal embolization is the key to induce a greater hypertrophy of the future liver remnant. The level of embolization has an impact on the efficacy of the procedure in inducing the hypertrophy. After the only proximal PVL, a hepatopetal flow in the occluded lobe due to intrahepatic porto-portal neocollaterals can be documented. This phenomenon is less frequent after a distal percutaneous PVE with embolic materials and it may explain why the hypertrophy achieved with PVE seems greater than that achieved with only proximal PVL [14].

The same effect of distal embolization by embolic agents used during PVE can be obtained by the injection of absolute alcohol (ethanol) into the right portal vein after its proximal ligation (Figs. 11.1, 11.2, and 11.3). The injection of alcohol is associated with a sclerosing effect into the peripheral portal branches with a consequent peripheral vessel occlusion. This phenomenon prevent the development of collateral vessels and the recanalization of the occluded portal branch. A recent study by Russolillo et al. [15] showed that PVL associated with alcohol injection significantly increased the liver regeneration rate when compared with PVL alone in patients with CRLM [14]. Indeed, in such patients the FLRV after PVL was significantly higher in the group of patients with alcohol injection than that observed in patients with only PVL. Moreover, in CT scan, both the recanalization rate of the occluded portal vein and the rate of cavernous transformation of the portal vein were higher in patients with only proximal PVL [15].

Given the comparable results of efficacy in inducing hypertrophy of the future liver remnant, PVL has been used in many centers as a surgical step during the first

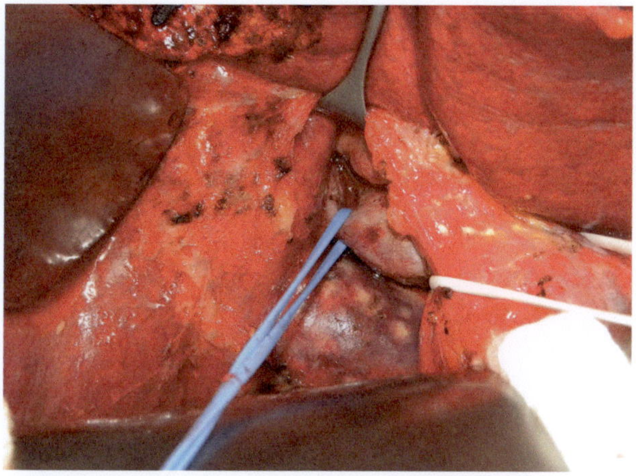

Fig. 11.1 Isolation of the right portal vein (blue tape) during a TSH for bilateral CRLM

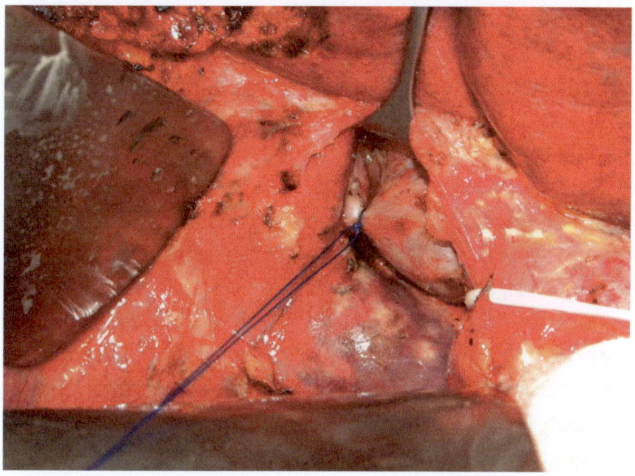

Fig. 11.2 Ligation of the right portal vein

stage of TSH in the treatment of bilateral CRLM. In a multicenter Italian study on 130 TSH performed between 2002 and 2011, PVL was performed in 51.8% of patients at the time of the first stage [16]. PVE was used in the remaining 48.2% of patients after the first hepatectomy [16]. In a more recent French series, out of 85 patients resected between 2010 and 2020 after portal vein occlusion [17], 33% underwent PVL. In this study, the authors confirmed that PVL and PVE were both effective to provide FRLV hypertrophy before right hepatectomy. This study highlights that PVL may be still relevant for the left hemi-liver hypertrophy, suggesting that it should be considered for the simultaneous treatment of CRLM and the primary tumor [17].

The possible technical disadvantages of the intraoperative PVL may be represented by the consequences of surgical dissection of the portal bifurcation and of the right portal vein. In fact, after PVL with alcohol injection, heavy inflammation of the hepatic hilum may occur and may be responsible for intraoperative difficulties

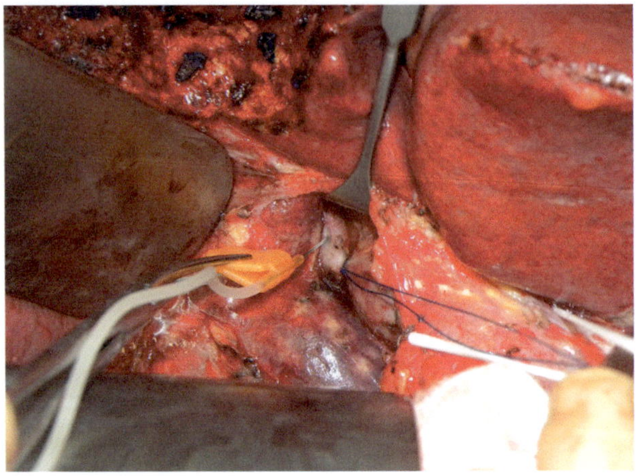

Fig. 11.3 Ethanol injection (10 mL) into the right portal vein

during the second step. In order to facilitate the dissection of the right pedicle during the second stage, it should be recommended to preserve the gallbladder intact during the first stage. However, some centers prefer postoperative PVE to PVL, arguing that the first surgery step could negatively interfere with the subsequent major hepatectomy.

In the era of the minimally invasive liver surgery (MILS), several centers reported their first series of laparoscopic TSH, showing that laparoscopic TSH was associated with less postoperative complications and a lesser hospital stay, compared to open TSH [18–20].

On the other hand, if during open TSH some authors showed that PVL was not responsible for intraoperative difficulties during the second step [17], during laparoscopic right hepatectomy the right portal vein dissection after PVL may be more difficult because of the periportal fibrosis [19]. To facilitate the laparoscopic vascular control during the second stage, some authors avoid PVL and systematically perform percutaneous PVE [18]. In this setting, in case of metastases, experienced interventional radiologists during the procedure should leave at least 1 cm of the right portal vein in order to avoid heavy inflammation and keep the vessels soft [18].

It seems that in the laparoscopic series of TSH, the surgical intraoperative PVL was less frequently performed than the PVE, but of course it is technically possible.

The choice to perform a PVL instead of a subsequent PVE ca be preferred also in cases where the metastases for dimensions or relationship with portal pedicle do not allow a safe percutaneous puncture of portal veins.

In conclusion, given the minimal invasive nature of the PVE procedure that could also be associated with the hepatic vein embolization (liver venous deprivation) to increase the future liver remnant hypertrophy, percutaneous PVE should be considered as the preferred strategy in case of planned minimally invasive TSH with an inadequate FLRV. In this way, by leaving free the first part of the right portal vein, periportal fibrosis could be limited and technical difficulties of laparoscopic portal vein dissection during the second stage may be reduced. Moreover, we think that cases of portal trifurcation or cases with short right portal vein could be better managed by percutaneous distal PVE, avoiding intrahepatic hilar surgical dissection that could injury the left portal vein and may increase the intraoperative difficulties during the second stage. Possible current indications to laparoscopic intraoperative PVL during the first stage of TSH could be an easy access to the right portal vein, which does not present any anatomical variants and can be easily ligated at a distance of at least 1 cm from the portal bifurcation.

References

1. Minagawa M, Makuuchi M, Torzilli G, et al. Extension of the frontiers of surgical indications in the treatment of liver metastases from colorectal cancer: longterm results. Ann Surg. 2000;231(4):487–99.
2. Ebata T, Yokoyama Y, Igami T, et al. Portal vein embolization before extended hepatectomy for biliary cancer: current technique and review of 494 consecutive embolizations. Dig Surg. 2012;29(1):23–9.
3. Shindoh J, Tzeng CW, Aloia TA, et al. Safety and efficacy of portal vein embolization before planned major or extended hepatectomy: an institutional experience of 358 patients. J Gastrointest Surg. 2014;18(1):45–51.
4. Makuuchi M, Thai BL, Takayasu K, et al. Preoperative portal embolization to increase safety of major hepatectomy for hilar bile duct carcinoma: a preliminary report. Surgery. 1990;107:521–7.
5. Jaeck D, Bachellier P, Nakano H, et al. One or two-stage hepatectomy combined with portal vein embolization for initially nonresectable colorectal liver metastases. Am J Surg. 2003;185(3):221–9.
6. Jaeck D, Oussoultzoglou E, Rosso E, et al. A two-stage hepatectomy procedure combined with portal vein embolization to achieve curative resection for initially unresectable multiple and bilobar colorectal liver metastases. Ann Surg. 2004;240(6):1037–49.
7. Kianmanesh R, Farges O, Abdalla EK, et al. Right portal vein ligation: a new planned two-step all-surgical approach for complete resection of primary gastrointestinal tumors with multiple bilateral liver metastases. J Am Coll Surg. 2003;197(1):164–70.
8. Broering DC, Hillert C, Krupski G, et al. Portal vein embolization vs. portal vein ligation for induction of hypertrophy of the future liver remnant. J Gastrointest Surg. 2002;6(6):905–13.
9. Aussilhou B, Lesurtel M, Sauvanet A, et al. Right portal vein ligation is as efficient as portal vein embolization to induce hypertrophy of the left liver remnant. J Gastrointest Surg. 2008;12(2):297–303.
10. Capussotti L, Muratore A, Baracchi F, et al. Portal vein ligation as an efficient method of increasing the future liver remnant volume in the surgical treatment of colorectal metastases. Arch Surg. 2008;143(10):978–82.
11. Isfordink CJ, Samim M, Braat MNGJA, et al. Portal vein ligation versus portal vein embolization for induction of hypertrophy of the future liver remnant: a systematic review and meta-analysis. Surg Oncol. 2017;26(3):257–67.
12. Denys AL, Abehsera M, Sauvanet A, et al. Failure of right portal vein ligation to induce left lobe hypertrophy due to intrahepatic portoportal collaterals: successful treatment with portal vein embolization. AJR Am J Roentgenol. 1999;173(3):633–5.
13. Ali A, Ahle M, Björnsson B, et al. Portal vein embolization with N-butyl cyanoacrylate glue is superior to other materials: a systematic review and meta-analysis. Eur Radiol. 2021;31(8):5464–78.

14. Robles R, Marín C, Lopez-Conesa A, et al. Comparative study of right portal vein ligation versus embolisation for induction of hypertrophy in two-stage hepatectomy for multiple bilateral colorectal liver metastases. Eur J Surg Oncol. 2012;38(7):586–93.
15. Russolillo N, Langella S, Perotti S, et al. Alcohol injection into the portal vein prior to ligation increases liver regeneration rate. HPB (Oxford). 2018;20(8):739–44.
16. Giuliante F, Ardito F, Ferrero A, et al. Tumor progression during preoperative chemotherapy predicts failure to complete 2-stage hepatectomy for colorectal liver metastases: results of an Italian multicenter analysis of 130 patients. J Am Coll Surg. 2014;219(2):285–94.
17. Werey F, Dembinski J, Michaud A, et al. Right portal vein ligation is still relevant for left hemiliver hypertrophy: results of a comparative study using a propensity score between right portal vein ligation and embolization. Langenbecks Arch Surg. 2023;409(1):25.
18. Okumura S, Goumard C, Gayet B, et al. Laparoscopic versus open two-stage hepatectomy for bilobar colorectal liver metastases: a bi-institutional, propensity score-matched study. Surgery. 2019;166(6):959–66.
19. Görgec B, Suhool A, Al-Jarrah R, et al. Surgical technique and clinical results of one- or two-stage laparoscopic right hemihepatectomy after portal vein embolization in patients with initially unresectable colorectal liver metastases: a case series. Int J Surg. 2020;77:69–75.
20. Taillieu E, De Meyere C, D'Hondt M. The role of the laparoscopic approach in two-stage hepatectomy for colorectal liver metastases: a single-center experience. Surg Endosc. 2022;36(1):559–68.

12 Two-Stage Hepatectomy

Katsunori Imai and René Adam

12.1 Introduction

Liver resection is considered to be the mainstay of curative treatment for primary hepatic malignancies, and also some secondary hepatic malignancies such as colorectal liver metastases (CRLM). Because of the recent developments in surgical techniques, optimized perioperative management, and deeper understanding of disease, hepatic resection is nowadays performed more safely over time, and its indication has been expanded dramatically. The success of hepatic resection, especially for extended multiple liver diseases, hinges on the remnant liver volume after resection. An insufficient liver future liver remnant (FLR) volume can lead to serious postoperative complications, such as post-hepatectomy liver failure.

To overcome this problem, several liver modulation techniques such as portal vein embolization (PVE)/ligation (PVL), liver venous deprivation, or two-stage hepatectomy (TSH) have been developed [1]. The concept of TSH was first introduced in 1992, and published in 2000 by Paul Brousse Hospital, to treat extensive bilobar CRLM that were diagnosed as initially unresectable [2]. TSH is nowadays considered an effective treatment for extensive CRLM patients with accepted short- and long-term outcomes. After that, associating liver partition and portal vein ligation for staged hepatectomy (ALPPS) was reported as a novel form of TSH [3]. Despite initial concerns about high morbidity and mortality, ALPPS has been

K. Imai
AP-HP, Hôpital Universitaire Paul Brousse, Unité de Recherche « Chronothérapie, Cancers et Transplantation », Université Paris-Saclay, Villejuif, France

Department of Surgery, Saiseikai Kumamoto Hospital, Kumamoto, Japan

R. Adam (✉)
AP-HP, Hôpital Universitaire Paul Brousse, Unité de Recherche « Chronothérapie, Cancers et Transplantation », Université Paris-Saclay, Villejuif, France
e-mail: rene.adam@pbr.aphp.fr

L. Aldrighetti et al. (eds.), *Liver Regeneration Techniques In Hepatic Surgery*,
https://doi.org/10.1007/978-3-032-10997-2_12

adopted by many specialized centers, and has established itself as an effective procedure that induces rapid and higher volume increase of FLR [4, 5]. In this chapter, we describe the concept of conventional TSH, especially focusing on the surgical techniques based on our experiences.

12.2 Indication of TSH

TSH is, in principle, only indicated for multiple bilobar tumors that are not amenable to complete resection by a single hepatectomy, even in combination with PVE/PVL or local ablation therapy (Fig. 12.1) [6]. When multiple tumors are unilobar and thought to be unresectable because of a small future liver remnant (FLR, usually less than 30% or 40% when patients have received prolonged chemotherapy), we perform PVE followed by one-stage hepatectomy. Even when the multiple tumors are bilobar, TSH is not indicated for cases in which all the tumors can be treated by a single hepatectomy, such as parenchyma-preserving hepatectomy, or resection combined with local ablation therapy. The presence of extrahepatic metastases is usually not considered a contraindication for TSH if these metastases are limited, resectable, and responsive or stable while on chemotherapy [7, 8].

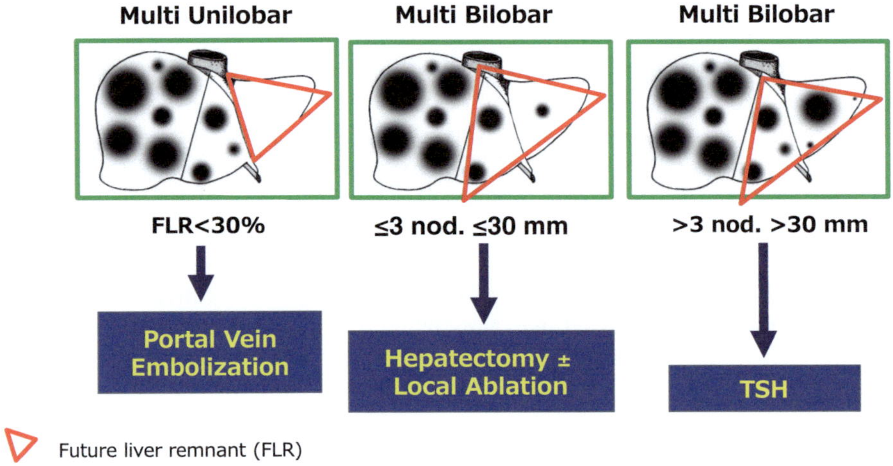

Fig. 12.1 Indication of two-stage hepatectomy (TSH) for colorectal liver metastases at Paul Brousse Hospital. (**a**) When the multiple tumors are distributed unilobar and thought to be unresectable because of small future liver remnant (FLR), portal vein embolization followed by one-stage hepatectomy is performed. (**b**) When the multiple tumors are distributed bilobar but the largest tumor size is ≤30 mm and the tumor number in the FLR is ≤3, standard one-stage hepatectomy with simultaneous local ablation therapy is performed. (**c**) When the multiple tumors are distributed bilobar, the largest tumor size is >30 mm and the tumor number in the FLR is >3, TSH or ALPPS is performed. FLR, future liver remnant; TSH, two-stage hepatectomy; ALPPS, Associating Lover Partition and Portal vein embolization for Staged hepatectomy. (From [6], with permission)

12.3 Classification of TSH

TSH is usually classified into four types (Fig. 12.2) [1].

12.3.1 Right-First Approach

The more invaded hemiliver (usually the right lobe) is resected at the first stage, leading to hypertrophy of the contralateral liver lobe. PVE or PVL is not required. At the second-stage, tumor-cleaning of the FLR is performed. In the early period of development of TSH, we sometimes chose this approach [2].

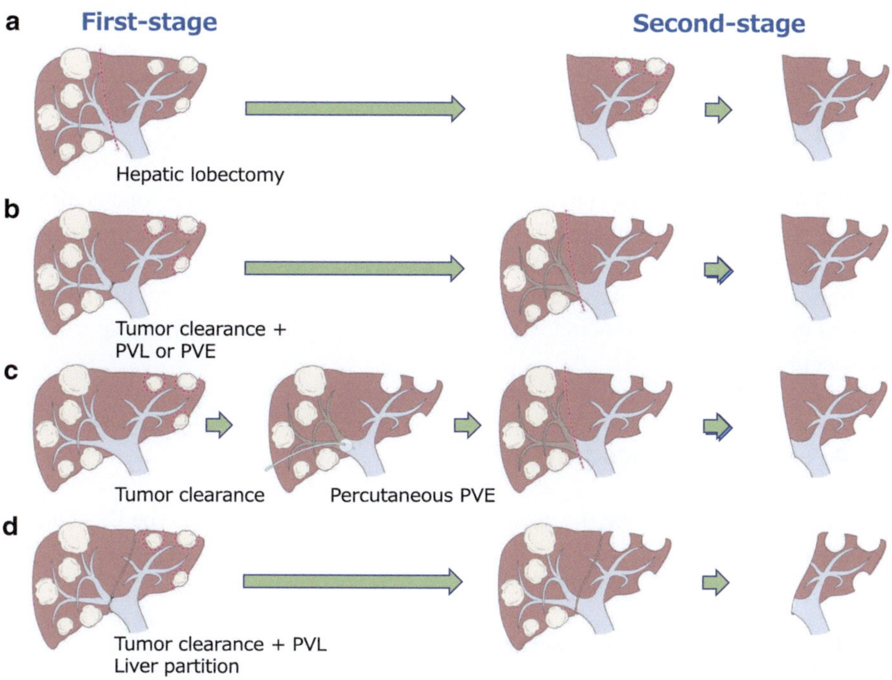

Fig. 12.2 Scheme of staged hepatectomy for colorectal liver metastases. (**a**) Right-first approach: most of the invaded hemiliver is resected at the first stage, leading to hypertrophy of the contralateral liver lobe. At the second stage, tumor cleaning of the future liver remnant (FLR) is performed, usually by nonanatomical partial resection. (**b**) Left-first approach with portal vein ligation/embolization (PVL/PVE): the less invaded liver lobe (FLR) is cleared from its metastases in combination with intraoperative PVL/PVE at the first stage. At the second stage, the tumor-bearing liver lobe (deportalized liver lobe) is anatomically removed. (**c**) Left-first approach followed by PVE: percutaneous PVE is performed between the first and second stages. (**d**) ALPPS: the less invaded liver lobe is cleared from its metastases in combination with intraoperative PVL/PVE and in situ splitting of the hemiliver at the first stage. At the second stage, usually 7–14 days later, the tumor-bearing liver lobe is removed. (From [1], with permission)

12.3.2 Left-First Approach with PVE/PVL

The less invaded liver lobe (usually the left lobe) is cleared from of its metastases in combination with intraoperative PVE/PVL at the first-stage. After confirming enough enlargement of FLR, the tumor-bearing liver lobe (deportalized liver lobe) is anatomically resected at the second stage [9].

12.3.3 Left-First Approach Followed by PVE

Percutaneous PVE is performed between the first and second stages, not during first stage. This method was pioneered by the Strasburg group [10] and popularized by the MD Anderson group. TSH in this chapter indicates the so-called classical TSH, including type A, B, and C (Fig. 12.2a–c).

12.3.4 ALPPS

ALPPS is a novel form of conventional TSH. The less invaded liver lobe is cleared from its metastases in combination with intraoperative PVL/PVE and in situ splitting of the hemiliver at the first stage. At the second stage, usually 7–14 days later, the tumor-bearing liver lobe is removed. Despite initial concerns about high mortality and morbidity rates, this innovative concept has been used by many specialized centers in the world [3–5].

12.4 Surgical Procedure of TSH

In this chapter, we describe the detailed surgical procedure of TSH type B, a current mainstream of classical TSH.

12.4.1 First-Stage Hepatectomy

First, the tumors located in the FLR are completely resected (Fig. 12.3a) (in that case, FLR does not have to be the left liver lobe). For the small tumor (usually less than 2 cm) located in the deep portion of the FLR, we sometimes perform radiofrequency ablation (RFA) in combination with hepatectomy, from the viewpoint of parenchyma-sparing strategy [11]. Subsequently, PVE or PVL is performed intraoperatively. Our method is right portal vein ligation with injection of absolute alcohol in the distal stump of the right portal vein to avoid any cavernoma reperfusion from above the ligature (Fig. 12.3b, c). Recently, another method using interventional radiology technique has been reported with safe and sufficient outcomes [12]. Briefly, the ileal vein was encircled and taped, and a catheter was inserted into the portal vein that served as a transient access tool (Fig. 12.3d). After portography, the

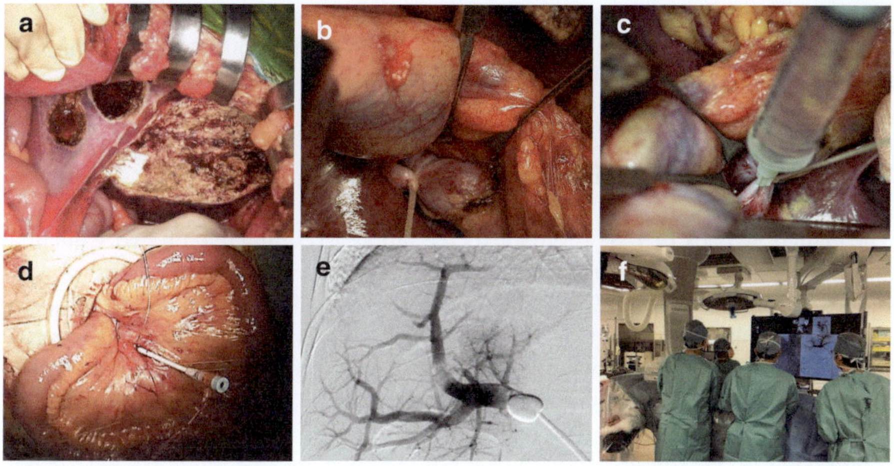

Fig. 12.3 The procedure of two-stage hepatectomy. (**a**) At the first-stage hepatectomy, the less-invaded liver lobe is cleared from its metastases, usually by nonanatomical resection. (**b**) Ligation of right portal vein. (**c**) Embolization by embolic material injection of the distal stump of the right portal vein to avoid any cavernoma reperfusion from above the ligature. (**d**) After the ileal vein was encircled and taped, a sheath is placed for the portal vein. (**e**) The embolic material was delivered through a hole in the catheter under balloon occlusion. (**f**) The embolic material was delivered through a hole in the catheter under balloon occlusion

embolic material was injected into the right branch of the portal vein under balloon occlusion (Fig. 12.3e). For this technique, a hybrid interventional radiology/operating suite seems to be very useful (Fig. 12.3f) [12]. If the primary tumor is synchronously presented, its resection is performed at the same time as the first-stage hepatectomy or after the second-stage hepatectomy (liver-first approach).

12.4.2 Second-Stage Hepatectomy

Second-stage hepatectomy should be performed after confirming that (1) curative resection (R0 or R1 by necessity) is possible, (2) sufficient FLR is secured, and (3) the remaining disease including extrahepatic diseases are controlled by chemotherapy. It is reported that the interval between the first and second stages was 32–210 days [6]. We usually perform CT volumetry 3–4 weeks after the first stage, and if the sufficient increase in FLR is not obtained, second-stage hepatectomy is postponed and interval chemotherapy using the same regimen as preoperative chemotherapy is reintroduced. We consider that it is not necessary to perform second-stage hepatectomy in hurry. We can wait until sufficient FRL and good control of the tumoral disease could be obtained under interval chemotherapy. After second-stage hepatectomy, adjuvant chemotherapy is routinely recommended if the patients' condition allows. Our previous study demonstrated that postoperative chemotherapy was an independent prognostic factor of survival after TSH [13]. However, recent update of our data failed to demonstrate the efficacy of postoperative chemotherapy on survival after TSH by multivariate analysis [7, 8]. There is little evidence supporting the routine use of postoperative chemotherapy (adjuvant setting) so far, and further study will be needed.

12.5 Drawbacks of TSH

The main drawback of TSH is obviously the failure to complete both ~~two~~ sequential procedures [8, 14]. Previous systematic review reported that dropout rate of TSH ranges 0–36% (median, 23%), and the main reason of failure was disease progression between the two stages (56–100%, median: 100%) [15]. We previously reported that among 125 patients with initially unresectable, multiple, and bilobar CRLM who were scheduled to undergo TSH, 44 patients (35.2%) could not proceed to the second stage (dropout) [8]. The reasons of failure of TSH were as follows: tumor progression in 39 patients (intrahepatic: 20, extrahepatic: 13, both: 6), insufficient volume of FLR in 3, poor general condition in 1, and postoperative mortality in 1. The overall survival (OS) after first-stage hepatectomy for patients who failed TSH were significantly lower than those who complete TSH (1-, 3-, and 5-year OS rate: 66.3%, 14.0%, and 0% vs. 95.0%, 69.0%, and 44.2%, $p < 0.0001$, Fig. 12.4). It is suggested that prevention of the failure of TSH could be crucial for patients who are planned for TSH, and this will require the inhibition of disease progression after first-stage hepatectomy.

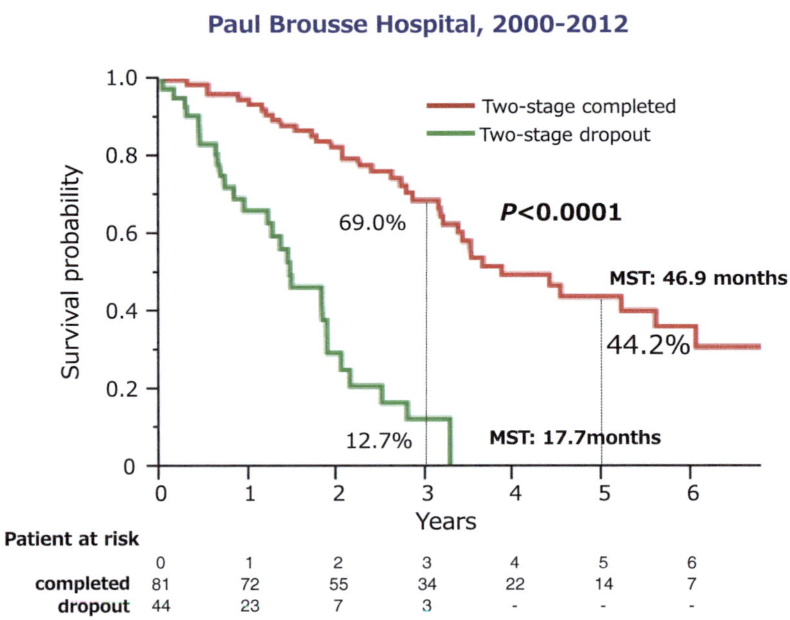

Fig. 12.4 Overall survival for patients who completed two-stage hepatectomy ($n = 91$) or dropped out ($n = 44$) between 2000 and 2012 at Paul Brousse Hospital. MST, median survival time. (From [8], with permission)

In the literature, some predictive factors for failure of TSH have been reported (Table 12.1) [6, 14]. These factors may help surgeons to predict the dropout risk for patients who are submitted to TSH. In our previous study, four independent predictive factors for failure of TSH were identified: disease progression on first-line chemotherapy, number of chemotherapy cycles >12, largest tumor size >40 mm, and carcinoembryonic antigen (CEA) at hepatectomy >30 ng/mL. Subsequently, a predictive model for failure of TSH was developed based on logistic regression (Table 12.2) [8]. For patients without any factors, the probability of dropout was 10.5%. The addition of subsequent risk factors increased the probability of dropout to 24.3–43.5% for one factor, 48.1–72.7% for two factors, 76.2–88.5% for three factors, and 95.5% for four factors. This predictive model can contribute to a better patient selection for optimal candidates for TSH.

Table 12.1 Predictive factors for dropout from the strategy of two-stage hepatectomy (Ref. [14])

Study	Year	Country	No. of patients	Dropout rate (%)	Predictive factors for dropout: Univariate	Predictive factors for dropout: Multivariate
Tsai et al.	2010	USA	45	22	Higher tumor number No preoperative chemo	ND
Narita et al.	2011	France	76	20	Age ≥ 70 ≥3 tumors in the FLR CEA >200 ng/mL before PVE	Age ≥ 70 ≥3 tumors in the FLR
Turrini et al.	2012	France	42	19	Combined resection of primary tumor Interval chemotherapy	Combined resection of primary tumor
Giuliante et al.	2014	Italy	126 (multicenter)	22	Disease progression during chemo	Disease progression during chemo
Faitot et al.	2015	France	50	24	Male gender Vascular invasion on primary >5 tumors Segment 1 metastases Need for chemo change Need for >3 curative treatments Microscopic biliary invasion	Nothing

(continued)

Table 12.1 (continued)

Study	Year	Country	No. of patients	Dropout rate (%)	Predictive factors for dropout	
					Univariate	Multivariate
Imai et al.	2015	France	125	35	CEA >30 (ng/mL) Tumor size >40 (mm) No. of chemotherapy cycles >12 No. of chemotherapy lines >1 Disease progression during first-line chemo	CEA >30 (ng/mL) Tumor size >40 (mm) No. of chemotherapy cycles >12 Disease progression during first-line chemo
Passot et al.	2016	USA	109	18	Tumor size >50 mm No. of chemotherapy cycles >6	No. of chemotherapy cycles >6
Regimbeau et al.	2017	Worldwide	869 (multicenter)	28	No repeat hepatectomy Extrahepatic metastasis Non-R0 resection at first stage No preoperative chemo	ND
Quénet et al.	2018	France	56	38	TRG 4/5 mTRG 4/5 Blazer classification 2 Tumor number > 6	Blazer classification 2 Tumor number > 6

ND not done, *FLR* future liver remnant, *CEA* carcinoembryonic antigen, *PVE* portal vein embolization, *TRG* tumor regression grade, *mTRG* modified tumor regression grade

Table 12.2 Predictive model for dropout from the strategy of two-stage hepatectomy based on four factors identified by multivariate logistic regression analysis (Ref. [8])

Factors	CEA at hepatectomy >30 (ng/mL)	Tumor size at hepatectomy >40 (mm)	Chemotherapy cycles before hepatectomy >12	Tumor progression during first-line chemotherapy	Probability (%)
0	–	–	–	–	10.5
1	+	–	–	–	25.3
	–	+	–	–	24.3
	–	–	+	–	28.9
	–	–	–	+	43.5
2	+	+	–	–	48.1
	+	–	+	–	54.0
	+	–	–	+	69.0
	–	+	+	–	52.6
	–	+	–	+	67.8
	–	–	+	+	72.7
3	+	+	+	–	76.2
	–	+	+	+	87.9
	+	–	+	+	88.5
	–	+	+	+	87.9
4	+	+	+	+	95.5

CEA carcinoembryonic antigen

12.6 Long-Term Outcome

According to our recent review, reported 5-year overall survival (OS) rate after completion of TSH ranged from 32% to 64%, with median survival time (MST) of 22–44 months [6]. We previously reported on a series of CLM patients who underwent hepatectomy, including TSH, between 1992 and 2012 [6]. A total of 1116 consecutive patients underwent initial hepatectomy for CLM at Paul Brousse Hospital. Among them, 139 patients (12.4%) were scheduled for TSH (6 patients who underwent ALPPS during this study period were excluded). Of these, 46 patients (33.1%) dropped out from the TSH strategy. On an intention-to-treat basis, the OS for patients who were scheduled for TSH was significantly worse than that for patients who underwent one-stage hepatectomy (5-year OS: 31.8% vs. 47.1%, $p = 0.0004$) (Fig. 12.5a). However, the patients who completed TSH (at least liver curative R0/R1 surgery) had comparable OS to those who underwent one-stage hepatectomy (5-year OS: 41.3% vs. 48.0%, $p = 0.40$) (Fig. 12.5b). Thus, if both sequential procedures of TSH are completed, comparable survival with one-stage hepatectomy can be expected.

In the literature review, several prognostic factors for survival after TSH have been reported (Table 12.3) [14]. As mentioned above, completion of two sequential surgery of TSH is obviously crucial for long-term outcome. Meanwhile, after completed TSH, tumor-related factors (tumor number,

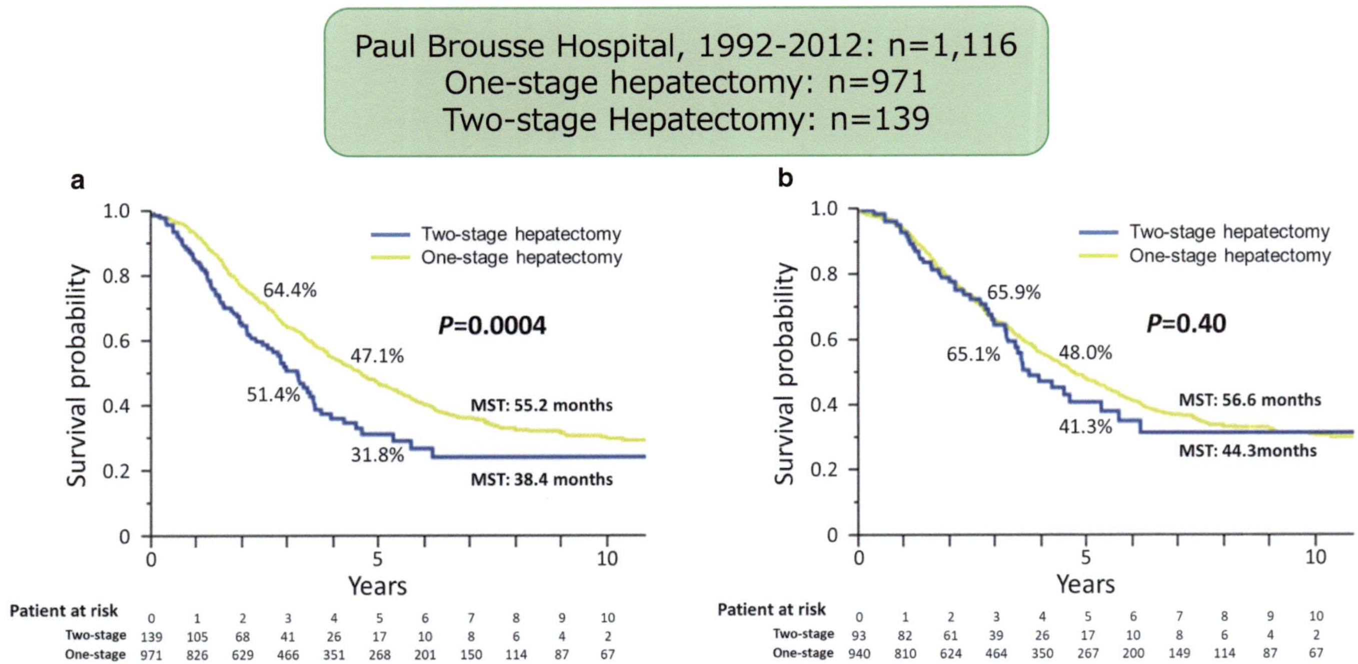

Fig. 12.5 (**a**) Overall survival for patients who were scheduled for two-stage hepatectomy ($n = 139$) and patients who underwent standard one-stage hepatectomy ($n = 971$) between 1992 and 2012 (intention-to-treat basis). (**b**) Overall survival for patients who completed two-stage hepatectomy ($n = 93$) and patients who underwent liver-curative one-stage hepatectomy ($n = 940$) between 1992 and 2012 at Paul Brousse Hospital. MST, median survival time. (From [6], with permission)

Table 12.3 Independent prognostic factors for survival after two-stage hepatectomy (Ref. [14])

Study	Year	Country	No. of patients	5-year OS	Independent prognostic factors (multivariate)	Patient cohort
Wicherts et al.	2008	France	41	42	Tumor number ≥ 6 Concomitant extrahepatic disease No postoperative chemotherapy	TSH completed cohort
Brouquet et al.	2011	USA	62	51	Major complication after first or second stage TSH failure	Whole cohort
Giuliante et al.	2014	Italy	102	32	Chemotherapy cycle ≥6	TSH completed cohort
Faitot et al.	2015	France	50	27 (3-year)	TSH failure	Whole cohort
Passot et al.	2016	USA	109	49 (completed)	Rectal primary Tumor number ≥ 6 Interval chemo after first stage *RAS* mutation	Whole cohort
Imai et al.	2019	France	93	41.3	Major complication at second stage No repeat surgery for recurrence	TSH completed cohort
Lillemoe et al.	2019	USA	83	47	No repeat surgery for recurrence First recurrence at multiple sites *RAS* mutation	TSH completed cohort (patients with recurrence)

OS overall survival, *TSH* two-stage hepatectomy

concomitant extrahepatic disease), chemotherapy-related factors (no postoperative chemotherapy, number of chemotherapy cycles), surgical factors (major complication at second stage, no repeat surgery for recurrence), recurrence-related pattern (first-recurrence at multiple sites), and molecular biomarker-related factor (*RAS* mutation) have been reported as independent prognostic factors for survival after TSH.

We have consistently argued the importance of repeat surgery for recurrence in patients with CRLM, and the TSH strategy should not be an exception. Our previous study reported that surgical intervention for recurrence after TSH significantly improved survival [7]. It is suggested that we should always perform intensive oncosurgical surveillance after TSH to avoid missing the opportunity for repeat surgery.

12.7 Future Perspective

Recently, a first randomized controlled trial (LIGRO trail) comparing ALPPS and TSH reported their oncological outcomes in patients with CRLM. After a median follow-up of 36 months, a significantly longer survival in patients allocated to ALPPS (46 months) vs. those allocated to TSH group (26 months) was observed on an intention-to-treat analysis [16]. The authors concluded that ALPPS improved survival compared with TSH in patients with CRLM. However, many arguments may question these results [17]: (1) the study was not designed for survival as an end point; (2) it was really surprising that the survival of the patients allocated to TSH arm was excessively poor (MST was only 23 months)—this poor outcome of TSH in this trial was comparable to that of TSH dropout; and (3) 90-day mortality rate of 10.7% after TSH completion was notably much higher, compared to all previous reports [6]. In this chapter, the advantages of ALPPS seem to result more from the poor results of the TSH rather than from a real superiority of ALPPS. In practice, we think that TSH and ALPPS could be complementary, and there is no rationale to make an exclusively use of one of these two procedures. ALPPS could be preferred in case of very small remnant liver as it could be the case for right extended hepatectomies. We should choose the feasible technique that offers the best outcomes on a case-by-case basis. For patients with extensive multiple bilateral liver tumors, especially CRLM, TSH is a potential treatment of choice for prolonged survival. However, not all eligible patients can benefit from this strategy. Personalized precision medicine based on molecular biology tools and multidisciplinary management will be paramount in the TSH strategy.

References

1. Imai K, Adam R, Baba H. How to increase the resectability of initially unresectable colorectal liver metastases: a surgical perspective. Ann Gastroenterol Surg. 2019;3(5):476–86. https://doi.org/10.1002/ags3.12276.
2. Adam R, Laurent A, Azoulay D, Castaing D, Bismuth H. Two-stage hepatectomy: a planned strategy to treat irresectable liver tumors. Ann Surg. 2000;232(6):777–85. https://doi.org/10.1097/00000658-200012000-00006.
3. Schnitzbauer AA, Lang SA, Goessmann H, Nadalin S, Baumgart J, Farkas SA, et al. Right portal vein ligation combined with in situ splitting induces rapid left lateral liver lobe hypertrophy enabling 2-staged extended right hepatic resection in small-for-size settings. Ann Surg. 2012;255(3):405–14. https://doi.org/10.1097/SLA.0b013e31824856f5.
4. Schadde E, Ardiles V, Robles-Campos R, Malago M, Machado M, Hernandez-Alejandro R, et al. Early survival and safety of ALPPS: first report of the International ALPPS Registry. Ann Surg. 2014;260(5):829–36.; discussion 36–8. https://doi.org/10.1097/SLA.0000000000000947.
5. Petrowsky H, Linecker M, Raptis DA, Kuemmerli C, Fritsch R, Kirimker OE, et al. First long-term oncologic results of the ALPPS procedure in a large cohort of patients with colorectal liver metastases. Ann Surg. 2020;272(5):793–800. https://doi.org/10.1097/SLA.0000000000004330.
6. Imai K, Adam R. Two-stage liver surgery. In: de Santibañes E, Ardiles V, Alvarez F, Cano Busnelli V, de Santibañes M, editors. Extreme hepatic surgery and other strategies: increasing

resectability in colorectal liver metastases. Springer International Publishing; 2017. p. 203–15. https://doi.org/10.1007/978-3-319-13896-1.
7. Imai K, Benitez CC, Allard MA, Vibert E, Cunha AS, Cherqui D, et al. Impact of surgical treatment for recurrence after 2-stage hepatectomy for colorectal liver metastases, on patient outcome. Ann Surg. 2019;269(2):322–30. https://doi.org/10.1097/SLA.0000000000002472.
8. Imai K, Benitez CC, Allard MA, Vibert E, Cunha AS, Cherqui D, et al. Failure to achieve a 2-stage hepatectomy for colorectal liver metastases: how to prevent it? Ann Surg. 2015;262(5):772–8.; discussion 8–9. https://doi.org/10.1097/SLA.0000000000001449.
9. Brouquet A, Abdalla EK, Kopetz S, Garrett CR, Overman MJ, Eng C, et al. High survival rate after two-stage resection of advanced colorectal liver metastases: response-based selection and complete resection define outcome. J Clin Oncol. 2011;29(8):1083–90. https://doi.org/10.1200/JCO.2010.32.6132.
10. Jaeck D, Oussoultzoglou E, Rosso E, Greget M, Weber JC, Bachellier P. A two-stage hepatectomy procedure combined with portal vein embolization to achieve curative resection for initially unresectable multiple and bilobar colorectal liver metastases. Ann Surg. 2004;240(6):1037–49; discussion 49–51. https://doi.org/10.1097/01.sla.0000145965.86383.89.
11. Imai K, Allard MA, Castro Benitez C, Vibert E, Sa Cunha A, Cherqui D, et al. Long-term outcomes of radiofrequency ablation combined with hepatectomy compared with hepatectomy alone for colorectal liver metastases. Br J Surg. 2017;104(5):570–9. https://doi.org/10.1002/bjs.10447.
12. Imai K, Miyamoto Y, Tamura Y, Hayashi H, Ikeda O, Yamashita YI, et al. Simultaneous portal vein embolization and colorectal resection in a hybrid interventional radiology/operating suite for synchronous colorectal liver metastases. J Gastrointest Surg. 2022;26(6):1307–10. https://doi.org/10.1007/s11605-021-05212-w.
13. Wicherts DA, Miller R, de Haas RJ, Bitsakou G, Vibert E, Veilhan LA, et al. Long-term results of two-stage hepatectomy for irresectable colorectal cancer liver metastases. Ann Surg. 2008;248(6):994–1005. https://doi.org/10.1097/SLA.0b013e3181907fd9.
14. Imai K, Allard MA, Baba H, Adam R. Optimal patient selection for successful two-stage hepatectomy of bilateral colorectal liver metastases. Ann Gastroenterol Surg. 2021;5(5):634–8. https://doi.org/10.1002/ags3.12465.
15. Chua TC, Liauw W, Chu F, Morris DL. Summary outcomes of two-stage resection for advanced colorectal liver metastases. J Surg Oncol. 2013;107(2):211–6. https://doi.org/10.1002/jso.23170.
16. Hasselgren K, Rosok BI, Larsen PN, Sparrelid E, Lindell G, Schultz NA, et al. ALPPS improves survival compared with TSH in patients affected of CRLM: survival analysis from the randomized controlled trial LIGRO. Ann Surg. 2021;273(3):442–8. https://doi.org/10.1097/SLA.0000000000003701.
17. Allard MA, Kitano Y, Imai K, Baba H, Vauthey JN, Adam R. Comment on "ALPPS improves survival compared with TSH in patients affected of CRLM: survival analysis from the randomized controlled trial LIGRO" survival benefit of ALPPS versus TSH: a proof of concept or a concept to be proved? Ann Surg. 2021;274(6):e764–e5. https://doi.org/10.1097/SLA.0000000000004539.

ALPPS: Associating Liver Partition and Portal Vein Ligation for Staged Hepatectomy

13

Victoria Ardiles, Fernando A. Alvarez, and Eduardo de Santibañes

13.1 Introduction

The concept of ALPPS (Associating Liver Partition and Portal vein ligation for Staged hepatectomy) originated from an unplanned yet insightful intraoperative decision. In September 2007, Prof. Hans J. Schlitt from Regensburg, Germany, was performing a right trisectionectomy in a 49-year-old woman with hilar cholangiocarcinoma [1]. After right portal vein ligation and complete in situ parenchymal transection along the falciform ligament, it became evident that the future liver remnant (FLR) would be insufficient to sustain postoperative liver function. Consequently, the resection was aborted. To decompress the biliary tree of segments 2 and 3, a Roux-en-Y hepaticojejunostomy was performed, and the tumor was left in situ. Unexpectedly, a CT scan performed 1 week later revealed an almost two-fold increase in FLR volume, which prompted the completion of the resection on postoperative day 9. This incidental observation of rapid hypertrophy following portal vein occlusion and liver partition led to the development of a novel approach, initially termed "in situ split liver resection." The technique was soon applied in patients with colorectal liver metastases and intrahepatic cholangiocarcinoma and gained early acceptance in several German Hepato-Pancreato-Biliary (HPB) centers.

V. Ardiles · E. de Santibañes (✉)
Department of Surgery, Division of HPB Surgery, Liver Transplant Unit, Italian Hospital of Buenos Aires, Buenos Aires, Argentina
e-mail: victoria.ardiles@hospitalitaliano.org.ar; eduardo.desantibanes@hospitalitaliano.org.ar

F. A. Alvarez
Department of Surgery, Division of HPB Surgery, Clínica Universitaria Reina Fabiola, Córdoba, Argentina
e-mail: fernandoalvarez@curf.ucc.edu.ar

L. Aldrighetti et al. (eds.), *Liver Regeneration Techniques In Hepatic Surgery*,
https://doi.org/10.1007/978-3-032-10997-2_13

By 2011, at the 9th Congress of the European-African Hepato-Pancreato-Biliary Association (E-AHPBA), the group from Mainz presented their initial experience with this approach [2]. One year later, a multicenter series involving 25 patients from five German centers was published by Schnitzbauer et al., reporting a median FLR hypertrophy of 74% within 9 days and a 100% resection rate in patients who were otherwise considered unresectable due to insufficient FLR [3]. This novel two-stage hepatectomy strategy, characterized by a short interval between stages, was subsequently named ALPPS [4].

The growing interest in the ALPPS concept, along with the enthusiasm surrounding its development, led to the creation of the International ALPPS Registry in 2012, aimed at collecting and analyzing global data on the procedure (International ALPPS Registry). Despite its rapid worldwide dissemination, ALPPS soon met with controversy due to its high morbidity and mortality rates reported in early series. Large multicenter experiences, such as the Brazilian series (39 patients) and the German series (25 patients), reported morbidity rates ranging from 59% to 68% and mortality rates of approximately 12% [3, 5]. Similarly, a collaborative Italian study describing early national experience reported morbidity above 54% and mortality reaching 20% [6].

Following the first International ALPPS Consensus Meeting held in Hamburg in February 2015, analysis of data from the International ALPPS Registry revealed that most deaths occurred after the second stage, often due to inadequate patient selection and suboptimal timing for completion of the procedure [7]. These findings prompted a paradigm shift: less invasive technical variants were developed, and stricter selection criteria were adopted, resulting in improved perioperative outcomes. Furthermore, sufficient follow-up and randomized controlled trials (RCTs) are now available, allowing more robust conclusions regarding the safety and oncologic efficacy of ALPPS [8–12]. The primary goal of techniques developed to induce FLR hypertrophy is to enable the safe completion of major liver resection by minimizing the risk of post-hepatectomy liver failure (PHLF), while maintaining low morbidity and mortality and achieving satisfactory oncologic outcomes. This chapter will focus on evaluating these key aspects in the context of ALPPS, analyzing patient selection, FLR hypertrophy, technical variations, safety, and oncological results.

13.2 FLR Hypertrophy and Feasibility to Complete Both Stages

A defining feature of ALPPS is its ability to induce rapid and marked hypertrophy of the FLR, surpassing what is typically achieved with conventional portal vein occlusion techniques in two-stage hepatectomy (TSH) strategies. This accelerated hypertrophy not only increases resectability but also reduces dropout rates in patients with marginally resectable disease [11]. The first comparative study between ALPPS and portal vein embolization (PVE) or TSH was published by Vauthey et al., who compared their historical series with the initial ALPPS experience reported by Schnitzbauer et al. [13]. Among 144 patients treated with PVE or TSH, only two-thirds underwent curative resection, with a mean hypertrophy of 62% achieved in 34 days and an R0 resection feasibility of 77%. In contrast, early data from the ALPPS Registry showed a mean hypertrophy of 80% in just 7 days, with successful completion of both stages in 98% of cases [14]. Subsequent multicentric data by Schadde et al. confirmed these findings, reporting higher resectability with ALPPS compared to PVE or portal vein ligation (PVL) (83% vs. 66%, $p = 0.027$) [15]. More recent systematic reviews and meta-analyses have found similar rates of hypertrophy between ALPPS and TSH, but ALPPS consistently achieves hypertrophy more rapidly [16, 17]. The kinetic growth rate (KGR)—defined as the percentage of hypertrophy per week—is significantly higher in ALPPS, contributing to a greater likelihood of timely resection [18]. Complete resection was achieved in approximately 90% of ALPPS patients (range: 83.3–100%) compared to 74.6% in TSH (range: 63.4–100%) [19]. The only randomized controlled trial comparing ALPPS and TSH in colorectal liver metastases (CRLM)—the LIGRO Trial—confirmed the superiority of ALPPS in terms of resection rate, with 92% of patients in the ALPPS group undergoing complete resection versus only 52% in the TSH group [11]. Another key advantage of ALPPS is its utility as a rescue strategy in patients with insufficient FLR hypertrophy following portal vein embolization or failed TSH. The first "rescue ALPPS" cases were reported by Tschuor et al., in which all patients successfully achieved adequate FLR hypertrophy and completed resection [20]. In the LIGRO Trial, among 13 patients in the TSH group with insufficient hypertrophy, 12 underwent rescue ALPPS, with successful resection in all cases within 8–16 days [11].

The rapid hypertrophy seen in ALPPS also allows for aggressive "FLR cleaning" during stage 1—including atypical resections—to ensure an oncologically safe remnant, and in selected cases, even enables monosegment ALPPS. Before ALPPS, resecting down to a single liver segment required multiple surgeries over several months. With ALPPS, this can now be achieved in a two-stage procedure within weeks, redefining the limits of resectability [21]. Despite consistent reports confirming the rapid increase in FLR volume with ALPPS, the biological mechanisms underlying this response remain incompletely understood. Early critics questioned whether the hypertrophy was due to true regeneration or simply edema. Although histological studies have shown both proliferative and architectural changes associated with the observed hypertrophy, doubts persist about whether functional improvement matches volumetric gains. Matsuo et al. [22] analyzed FLR parenchyma after ALPPS and noted signs of hepatocyte and bile canaliculi immaturity, suggesting that early volume expansion may not equate to mature, functional liver tissue. These findings align with other studies, showing a dissociation between FLR volume and function. As the technique evolved, it became clear that relying solely on FLR volume to determine readiness for stage 2 was insufficient. Several studies have demonstrated the importance of functional assessment, using tools like hepatobiliary scintigraphy (HBS) to determine the appropriate timing for stage 2, thereby reducing the risk of PHLF [23, 24]. This paradigm shift emphasizes that functional adequacy, not just volume, is critical for safe completion of ALPPS.

13.3 Patient Selection

Proper patient selection is critical for the success of ALPPS and remains one of the most important factors influencing outcomes. Initially proposed for a wide variety of liver tumors, ALPPS has evolved to be most commonly and effectively applied in cases of CRLM, which not only represent the majority of procedures in high-volume centers but also provide the most robust evidence for favorable outcomes. Data from the International ALPPS Registry indicate that patients with CRLM, particularly those under 67 years of age, are among those who benefit most from this approach [25]. The LIGRO Trial further reinforced this indication, demonstrating that ALPPS offers higher resectability, comparable safety, and superior long-term outcomes in CRLM compared to conventional TSH [11, 12].

Preoperative evaluation for ALPPS candidates involves the same rigorous imaging and volumetric analysis as for other major liver resections. Triphasic contrast-enhanced CT or MRI with 3D reconstruction, combined with liver volumetry, is essential for surgical planning. An FLR of <30% in healthy livers or <40% in patients with hepatic injury (e.g., steatosis, cholestasis, fibrosis, or prolonged chemotherapy) is considered inadequate. FLR-to-body weight ratios of <0.5% for normal liver, <0.8% for damaged liver, and <1.4% for cirrhotic liver are alternative thresholds. However, as previously mentioned, volumetric measurements do not always correlate with liver function, especially in the presence of parenchymal damage, prompting the increasing use of HBS with 99mTc-mebrofenin, which allows assessment of both segmental volume and function.

To optimize results, ALPPS should be reserved for patients with insufficient FLR and at least one of the following conditions: tumor proximity to the FLR or its vascular structures; bilobar disease not amenable to PVE or hepatic venous deprivation (HVD); need for extreme hypertrophy (>65%) in very small FLRs; failed PVE or HVD ("rescue ALPPS"). Over time, "rescue ALPPS" has become an established indication, particularly after failed volume remodeling with other strategies.

13.4 Surgical Technique and Technical Variants

13.4.1 Classic and Partial ALPPS

The original ALPPS technique consists of right portal vein ligation combined with in situ parenchymal splitting along the right side of the falciform ligament during stage 1. Once sufficient FLR hypertrophy is confirmed, usually within 2 weeks, completion hepatectomy is performed. The classic approach typically involves a right trisectionectomy, although right or left hepatectomies and extended resections have also been reported. During stage 1, the abdominal cavity is explored, the FLR is assessed by palpation and intraoperative ultrasound, and any lesions in the FLR are resected. Liver mobilization is completed, and the caudate lobe is freed from the inferior vena cava (IVC). The portal vein is ligated or transected, followed by complete parenchymal division up to the IVC. Particular attention must be paid to segment IV, whose vascularization is crucial. Portal branches to segments IVa, IVb, and I (if included in the specimen) should be divided, while preserving arterial inflow and biliary drainage to segment IV to prevent ischemia and necrosis. These refinements led to the concept of Partial ALPPS, where parenchymal transection is limited to less than 50% of the liver volume, preserving the middle hepatic vein. This approach achieves similar hypertrophy with reduced morbidity. Complete transection is now reserved for cases at high risk of tumor progression into the FLR. Biliary structures should be manipulated as little as possible during stage 1. When biliary reconstruction is necessary, it is preferably deferred to stage 2. In selected cases, such as cholestatic FLR, biliary decompression may be performed during stage 1 with careful closure of the hepatic duct stump. At the end of stage 1, vascular structures to be divided in stage 2 should be clearly marked. Hemostatic agents or barriers can be placed to reduce adhesions. Drains are placed between the transection planes and in the right subphrenic space. Stage 2 involves mobilization of the diseased liver, identification of previously marked hilar structures, and completion of the resection—usually with vascular staplers. Intraoperative bile leak testing and confirmation of FLR perfusion are strongly recommended.

13.4.2 Mini-ALPPS

Introduced by the Hospital Italiano during the first ALPPS International Consensus in 2015, Mini-ALPPS combines partial parenchymal transection, intraoperative transmesenteric PVE, and minimal liver mobilization [26]. This strategy significantly reduces the surgical impact of stage 1 without compromising FLR hypertrophy, thereby facilitating recovery and reducing complications. Unlike classic ALPPS, it avoids portal pedicle dissection, extensive liver mobilization, and disruption of the middle hepatic vein. A laparoscopic adaptation using inferior mesenteric vein cannulation has been developed, allowing the technique to be performed entirely in minimally invasive settings [27]. A variation known as Partial TIPE-ALPPS, proposed by a Japanese group, utilizes transileocecal PVE instead of transmesenteric access, although it requires an additional incision [28]. Both techniques demand a hybrid operating room equipped for interventional radiology and surgery.

13.4.3 Monosegment ALPPS

Monosegment ALPPS refers to resections where only one segment ± segment I is preserved as the FLR. First reported by the Hospital Italiano de Buenos Aires in 2014, this technique was applied in patients with extensive CRLM, preserving only segments I and IV [29]. Subsequent reports describe safe preservation of segments II, III, IV, or VI, depending on vascular anatomy. Although rare, this strategy pushes the boundaries of resectability and represents a significant innovation in liver surgery.

13.4.4 Technical Modifications (Tourniquet, Radiofrequency, Microwave, Hybrid ALPPS)

To reduce invasiveness during stage 1, several alternatives to full parenchymal transection have been proposed. Tourniquet ALPPS uses a constrictive band around the liver to functionally interrupt interlobar circulation [30]. Radiofrequency ALPPS and Microwave ALPPS rely on thermal ablation to create a necrotic groove mimicking a transection plane [31, 32]. These approaches can be performed laparoscopically or percutaneously and have shown similar hypertrophy with fewer complications. The REBIRTH trial demonstrated that Radiofrequency ALPPS induced more rapid hypertrophy than PVE without increasing morbidity [33]. Similarly, Tourniquet ALPPS has shown superior resectability with outcomes comparable to TSH [34]. Hybrid ALPPS substitutes surgical PVL with PVE during the interval between stages, avoiding portal pedicle dissection in stage 1 and facilitating stage 2 by reducing adhesions [35]. It is particularly advantageous in cases with portal vein anatomical variants. Unlike Mini-ALPPS, Hybrid ALPPS involves complete parenchymal transection as originally described.

13.4.5 Minimally Invasive ALPPS

The benefits of minimally invasive surgery have led to the adoption of laparoscopic ALPPS, performed either for one or both stages [27, 36]. Early reports suggest reduced morbidity, mortality, and hospital stay compared to open surgery. Surgical experience is essential for the safe execution of laparoscopic ALPPS. More recently, robot-assisted ALPPS has also been reported in selected centers, expanding the potential of minimally invasive approaches [37].

13.5 Interval Management and Timing of Stage 2

Patient management during the interval between stages is a critical determinant of ALPPS success. Traditionally, FLR sufficiency during the interval has been judged by volumetric criteria alone. However, this approach can be misleading, as liver function tests reflect the combined function of the entire liver, including the diseased lobe scheduled for resection. ALPPS induces rapid hypertrophy of the FLR, but functional recovery may lag behind, creating a temporal mismatch confirmed by histologic findings [22]. Consequently, reliance on volumetric thresholds alone may underestimate the risk of PHLF.

This discrepancy has driven interest in functional assessment tools, with HBS emerging as the most reliable modality. When combined with Single Photon Emission Computed Tomography-Computed Tomography (SPECT-CT), HBS provides quantitative segmental liver function. Sequential HBS studies allow dynamic monitoring of functional recovery and can guide timing for stage 2. Accepted functional thresholds include FLR uptake rate ≥2.7%/min/m^2 (AMC Group, Amsterdam) and HIBA-index ≥15% (Hospital Italiano, Buenos Aires) [23, 24, 38, 39].

The KGR, measuring volumetric hypertrophy speed, complements volumetric and functional evaluation. An ALPPS Registry study found KGR <4.1% per day predictive of PHLF [40]. Original rigid 1-week intervals have been associated with higher morbidity; thus, delaying or abandoning stage 2 should be considered based on clinical stability, complications, liver tests, and MELD score (>10) [40]. In 2016, a validated ALPPS Risk Score was introduced, aiding individualized decision-making before stage 2 [25].

13.6 Morbidity and Mortality

Morbidity and mortality were major concerns during the early experience with ALPPS, particularly in the initial series published by pioneering centers. High complication rates were attributed not only to the technical complexity of the procedure but also to insufficient experience with patient selection, perioperative management, and optimal timing of the second stage. Over time, improvements in these key areas have led to a significant reduction in adverse outcomes.

Early registry data revealed that the learning curve plays a fundamental role in the safety of ALPPS. For example, the International ALPPS Registry reported a 90-day mortality of 13% in centers with fewer than eight procedures performed, compared to just 4% in high-volume centers ($p < 0.001$) [14]. This underscores the importance of institutional experience and procedural standardization. A comprehensive analysis of 437 patients from 16 high-volume centers, each performing more than 10 ALPPS per year over a 3-year period, demonstrated a steady improvement in outcomes [8]. As indications were refined, particularly with the increasing predominance of colorectal liver metastases (CRLM) and the decline in use for biliary tumors, the 90-day mortality dropped from 17% to 4% ($p = 0.002$), and the incidence of major complications (grade ≥ IIIb according to the Clavien–Dindo classification) decreased from 10% to 3% ($p = 0.011$) [8]. This evolution was driven by both improved patient selection and technical adaptations. Indeed, 100% of surveyed centers reported modifying their selection criteria over time, and 75% reported refining surgical technique to reduce complications.

Despite these advancements, systematic reviews and meta-analyses continue to show elevated morbidity and mortality in ALPPS compared to other approaches. However, these data predominantly reflect outcomes from the early phase of the learning curve. More recent data from RCTs, such as the LIGRO Trial, show comparable safety profiles between ALPPS and TSH [11, 12].

The most comprehensive early analysis of ALPPS-related morbidity included 220 patients from 41 centers. It identified key risk factors for severe postoperative complications (Clavien–Dindo ≥IIIb), including age > 60 years, non-CRLM indications, the need for intraoperative transfusion, and prolonged operative time (>5 h) [14]. A subsequent analysis during the first International ALPPS Consensus (2015) confirmed that these same variables were also independently associated with mortality [40]. A particularly critical insight emerged from the analysis of mortality after stage 2. Approximately 93% of postoperative deaths occurred following the second operation, and 75% to PHLF. Among the predictive factors, a MELD score > 10 prior to stage 2 was identified as an independent predictor of 90-day mortality. These findings highlight the importance of assessing hepatic function—beyond volumetry—before proceeding with resection. The first stage of ALPPS may be considered a physiologic stress test of liver function. Patients who develop PHLF after stage 1 should not proceed to the second operation, and timing should be tailored to each patient rather than adhering to a routine 1-week interval. Delaying or even cancelling stage 2 should be strongly considered in patients with clinical instability, ongoing complications, elevated bilirubin or creatinine, or unfavorable MELD scores. It is important to emphasize that the initial selection of patients must remain restrictive, since once the first stage has been carried out, the quality of life and survival of the patient can be significantly compromised.

In 2016, a validated ALPPS Risk Score was developed using data from the International ALPPS Registry to predict mortality either upfront or before stage 2 [25]. The pre-stage 2 model includes the initial risk score, interstage complications ≥ Clavien–Dindo IIIb, serum bilirubin, and creatinine levels. The risk of futility rises steeply with increasing scores, from 5% (score 3.9) to 50% (score 6.9), reinforcing the need for objective decision-making tools in perioperative planning.

Finally, the severity of ALPPS and its inherent technical demands are reflected in variables such as prolonged operative time and the need for transfusions, both associated with higher risk. These findings have motivated the development of several technical modifications, including Mini-ALPPS, Hybrid ALPPS, ALTPS, RALPP, and laparoscopic approaches. All aim to reduce surgical trauma, preserve function, and improve safety. In combination with more restrictive and refined patient selection, these innovations have contributed to the steady decrease in ALPPS-related morbidity and mortality.

13.7 Oncological Results

In contemporary series from experienced centers, current outcomes are comparable to those achieved with other advanced liver resection strategies. From the early days of ALPPS, concerns were raised regarding its oncological safety, particularly in relation to early tumor recurrence due to potential manipulation during the procedure or stimulation of tumor growth by systemic factors. Despite these theoretical concerns, accumulating evidence suggests that oncological outcomes after ALPPS are largely determined by the biological aggressiveness of the underlying disease and patient selection, rather than by the procedure itself.

For patients with CRLM, the main indication for ALPPS, reported overall survival (OS), and disease-free survival (DFS) are encouraging, especially considering that these patients are often initially deemed unresectable and exhibit unfavorable prognostic features such as synchronous disease, bilobar involvement, lymph node–positive primary tumors, and extensive preoperative chemotherapy. In most series, 1- and 3-year OS after ALPPS ranges from 76% to 96% and 48% to 62%, respectively, with median DFS around 8–12 months [34, 41–47]. Postoperative recurrence remains common after ALPPS, occurring in up to 73% of patients with CRLM, most frequently within 2 years. However, this recurrence pattern is consistent with the aggressive tumor biology typically seen in the ALPPS population and should not necessarily be attributed to the surgical strategy itself. Several studies, including the analysis from the International ALPPS Registry, have shown that DFS is no longer a reliable surrogate for OS in metastatic colorectal cancer, as long-term survival is often achieved through repeat resections and multimodal treatments. In this regard, repeat liver resections after ALPPS have proven to be feasible and safe, offering survival outcomes comparable to those achieved after conventional hepatectomies.

Molecular factors, particularly KRAS and NRAS mutations, have emerged as relevant predictors of oncological outcomes after ALPPS [41, 45]. These mutations—present in 35–45% of patients with CRLM—are associated with poor response to chemotherapy, higher rates of positive margins, and reduced survival. Both registry-based analyses and institutional series have identified KRAS mutation as an independent predictor of poor prognosis following ALPPS, with shorter OS and DFS compared to wild-type tumors [41, 45]. This information is increasingly used to optimize patient selection, avoiding futile surgical interventions in high-risk molecular subtypes.

One of the most comprehensive studies to date, based on data from the International ALPPS Registry, stratified patients by markers of advanced disease (≥6 metastases, ≥2 lesions in the FLR, ≥6 segments involved) [46]. Patients with two or more of these criteria had significantly worse oncologic outcomes, including lower 2-year OS (49% vs. 72%) and shorter DFS (6 vs. 12 months). In a matched subgroup analysis comparing these high-risk ALPPS, patients with cohorts treated under palliative chemotherapy protocols (CAIRO and CAIRO2), survival outcomes were similar, raising questions about the true oncological benefit of ALPPS in patients with extensive metastatic burden. These data highlight that technical resectability alone should not guide treatment decisions; biological resectability and long-term benefit must also be considered.

Nevertheless, in well-selected patients with extensive disease but favorable biology, ALPPS remains a valuable tool. The randomized controlled LIGRO Trial demonstrated that patients randomized to ALPPS had significantly higher resection rates and longer OS (46 vs. 26 months) compared to those undergoing TSH, although this survival advantage was lost when comparing only resected patients [11, 12, 44].

An increasingly relevant outcome in oncology is quality of life (QoL). Preliminary studies, including one conducted collaboratively between two high-volume ALPPS centers, have shown that long-term QoL in patients undergoing ALPPS is comparable to population norms [42]. Using the European Organization for Research and Treatment of Cancer Quality of Life Questionnaire-Core 30 (EORTC QLQ-C30), patients reported few functional limitations or persistent symptoms, even after aggressive resections. These findings are consistent with other series showing transient postoperative QoL impairment followed by rapid recovery to baseline, further supporting the role of ALPPS in selected cases with otherwise limited therapeutic options.

In summary, oncological outcomes after ALPPS are highly dependent on careful patient selection and underlying tumor biology. The presence of high-risk features such as KRAS mutation, multiple bilobar lesions, or extensive liver involvement should be weighed cautiously when considering this strategy. While ALPPS can offer long-term survival and even cure in selected patients, ongoing randomized studies and longer follow-up are still needed to define its precise role among curative strategies for advanced CRLM.

13.8 Conclusion

ALPPS represents a significant advancement in modern liver surgery, particularly for managing patients initially considered unresectable due to an insufficient FLR volume. From its fortuitous inception to its establishment as an internationally recognized surgical technique, ALPPS has undergone substantial evolution, reflected in significant improvements in perioperative and oncological outcomes. This progress results from accumulated institutional experience, continuous technical innovations, and increasingly rigorous and evidence-based patient selection.

The distinctive capability of ALPPS to induce rapid and effective hepatic hypertrophy surpasses traditional strategies, expanding the boundaries of liver resectability. Nevertheless, the success of ALPPS largely depends on carefully evaluating not only liver volume but also liver function, using functional assessment methods such as HBS with mebrofenin and validated predictive tools such as the HIBA-index and the ALPPS Risk Score.

Although the morbidity and mortality initially associated with ALPPS generated controversy, current data demonstrate that with adequate experience and appropriate patient selection criteria, ALPPS can provide outcomes comparable to other advanced hepatic resection strategies. From an oncological perspective, ALPPS has shown promising results in properly selected patients, particularly those with colorectal liver metastases. However, molecular factors and tumor biology play decisive roles in long-term outcomes and must be carefully considered in patient selection.

In conclusion, ALPPS is currently a valuable and consolidated tool for addressing complex challenges in advanced liver surgery. Continued research, accumulation of institutional experience, and refinement of technical and patient selection criteria will be essential to further optimize outcomes and precisely define its role within the therapeutic arsenal available for patients with advanced liver disease.

References

1. Schlitt HJ, Hackl C, Lang SA. 'In-Situ Split' liver resection/ALPPS-historical development and current practice. Visc Med. 2017;33:408–12.
2. Baumgart J, Lang S, Lang H. A new method for induction of liver hypertrophy prior to right trisectionectomy: a report of three cases. HPB. 2011;13(2):1–145.
3. Schnitzbauer AA, Lang SA, Goessmann H, Nadalin S, Baumgart J, Farkas SA, et al. Right portal vein ligation combined with in situ splitting induces rapid left lateral liver lobe hypertrophy enabling two-staged extended right hepatic resection in small-for-size settings. Ann Surg. 2012;255(3):405–14.
4. de Santibañes E, Clavien PA. Playing Play-Doh to prevent postoperative liver failure: the "ALPPS" approach. Ann Surg. 2012;255(3):415–7.
5. Torres OJ, Fernandes ES, Oliveira CV, et al. Associating liver partition and portal vein ligation for staged hepatectomy (ALPPS): the Brazilian experience. Arq Bras Cir Dig. 2013;26:40–3.
6. Serenari M, Zanello M, Schadde E, et al. Importance of primary indication and liver function between stages: results of a multicenter Italian audit of ALPPS 2012-2014. HPB (Oxford). 2016;18(5):419–27.
7. Oldhafer KJ, Stavrou GA, van Gulik TM, Core Group. ALPPS–where do we stand, where do we go?: eight recommendations from the first international expert meeting. Ann Surg. 2016;263(5):839–41.
8. Linecker M, Björnsson B, Stavrou GA, et al. Risk adjustment in ALPPS is associated with a dramatic decrease in early mortality and morbidity. Ann Surg. 2017;266(5):779–86.
9. Lang H, Baumgart J, Mittler J. Associated liver partition and portal vein ligation for staged hepatectomy (ALPPS) registry: what have we learned? Gut Liver. 2020;12
10. Lang H, de Santibañes E, Schlitt HJ, et al. 10th anniversary of ALPPS-lessons learned and quo Vadis. Ann Surg. 2019;269(1):114–9.
11. Sandström P, Røsok BI, Sparrelid E, et al. ALPPS improves Resectability compared with conventional two-stage hepatectomy in patients with advanced colorectal liver metastasis: results from a Scandinavian multicenter randomized controlled trial (LIGRO trial). Ann Surg. 2018;267(5):833–40.
12. Hasselgren K, Røsok BI, Larsen PN, et al. ALPPS improves survival compared with TSH in patients affected of CRLM: survival analysis from the randomized controlled trial LIGRO. Ann Surg. 2021;273(3):442–8.
13. Shindoh J, Vauthey JN, Zimmitti G, et al. Analysis of the efficacy of portal vein embolization for patients with extensive liver malignancy and very low future liver remnant volume, including a comparison with the associating liver partition with portal vein ligation for staged hepatectomy approach. J Am Coll Surg. 2013;217(1):126–33.
14. Schadde E, Ardiles V, Robles-Campos R, et al. Early survival and safety of ALPPS: first report of the international ALPPS registry. Ann Surg. 2014;260(5):829–36.
15. Schadde E, Ardiles V, Slankamenac K, et al. ALPPS offers a better chance of complete resection in patients with primarily unresectable liver tumors compared with conventional-staged hepatectomies: results of a multicenter analysis. World J Surg. 2014;38(6):1510–9.
16. Gavriilidis P, Sutcliffe RP, Roberts KJ, et al. No difference in mortality among ALPPS, two-staged hepatectomy, and portal vein embolization/ligation: a systematic review by updated traditional and network meta-analyses. Hepatobiliary Pancreat Dis Int. 2020;19(5):411–9.
17. Bozkurt E, Sijberden JP, Kasai M, et al. Efficacy and perioperative safety of different future liver remnant modulation techniques: a systematic review and network meta-analysis. HPB (Oxford). 2024;26(4):465–75.
18. Croome KP, Hernandez-Alejandro R, Parker M, Heimbach J, Rosen C, Nagorney DM. Is the liver kinetic growth rate in ALPPS unprecedented when compared with PVE and living donor liver transplant? A multicentre analysis. HPB (Oxford). 2015;17(6):477–84.
19. Moris D, Ronnekleiv-Kelly S, Kostakis ID, et al. Operative results and oncologic outcomes of associating liver partition and portal vein ligation for staged hepatectomy (ALPPS) versus

two-stage hepatectomy (TSH) in patients with Unresectable colorectal liver metastases: a systematic review and meta-analysis. World J Surg. 2018;42(3):806–15.
20. Tschuor C, Croome KP, Sergeant G, et al. Salvage parenchymal liver transection for patients with insufficient volume increase after portal vein occlusion -- an extension of the ALPPS approach. Eur J Surg Oncol. 2013;39(11):1230–5.
21. Schadde E, Malago M, Hernandez-Alejandro R, et al. Monosegment ALPPS hepatectomy: extending resectability by rapid hypertrophy. Surgery. 2015;157(4):676–89.
22. Matsuo K, Murakami T, Kawaguchi D, Hiroshima Y, Koda K, Yamazaki K, Ishida Y, Tanaka K. Histologic features after surgery associating liver partition and portal vein ligation for staged hepatectomy versus those after hepatectomy with portal vein embolization. Surgery. 2016;159(5):1289–98.
23. Serenari M, Collaud C, Alvarez FA, et al. Interstage assessment of remnant liver function in ALPPS using hepatobiliary scintigraphy: prediction of Posthepatectomy liver failure and introduction of the HIBA index. Ann Surg. 2018;267(6):1141–7.
24. Tomassini F, D'Asseler Y, Linecker M, et al. Hepatobiliary scintigraphy and kinetic growth rate predict liver failure after ALPPS: a multi-institutional study. HPB (Oxford). 2020;22(10):1420–8.
25. Linecker M, Stavrou GA, Oldhafer KJ, et al. The ALPPS risk score: avoiding futile use of ALPPS. Ann Surg. 2016;264(5):763–71.
26. de Santibañes E, Alvarez FA, Ardiles V, et al. Inverting the ALPPS paradigm by minimizing first stage impact: the mini-ALPPS technique. Langenbecks Arch Surg. 2016;401:557–63.
27. Pekolj J, Alvarez FA, Biagiola D, et al. Totally laparoscopic mini-ALPPS using a novel approach of laparoscopic-assisted transmesenteric portal vein embolization. J Laparoendosc Adv Surg Tech A. 2018;28(10):1229–33.
28. Sakamoto Y, Matsumura M, Yamashita S, et al. Partial TIPE ALPPS for Perihilar cancer. Ann Surg. 2018;267(2):e18–20.
29. de Santibañes M, Alvarez FA, Santos FR, et al. The associating liver partition and portal vein ligation for staged hepatectomy approach using only segments I and IV as future liver remnant. J Am Coll Surg. 2014;219(2):e5–9.
30. Robles R, Parrilla P, López-Conesa A, Brusadin R, de la Peña J, Fuster M, García-López JA, Hernández E. Tourniquet modification of the associating liver partition and portal ligation for staged hepatectomy procedure. Br J Surg. 2014;101(9):1129–34.
31. Gringeri E, Boetto R, D'Amico FE, Bassi D, Cillo U. Laparoscopic microwave ablation and portal vein ligation for staged hepatectomy (LAPS): a minimally invasive first-step approach. Ann Surg. 2015;261(2):e42–3.
32. Gall TM, Sodergren MH, Frampton AE, et al. Radio-frequency-assisted liver partition with portal vein ligation (RALPP) for liver regeneration. Ann Surg. 2015;261(2):e45–6.
33. Jiao LR, Fajardo Puerta AB, Gall TMH, et al. Rapid induction of liver regeneration for major hepatectomy (REBIRTH): a randomized controlled trial of portal vein embolisation versus ALPPS assisted with radiofrequency. Cancers (Basel). 2019;11(3):302.
34. Robles-Campos R, Brusadin R, López-Conesa A, et al. Long-term outcome after conventional two-stage hepatectomy versus tourniquet-ALPPS in colorectal liver metastases: a propensity score matching analysis. World J Surg. 2019;43(9):2281–9.
35. Li J, Kantas A, Ittrich H, et al. Avoid "all-touch" by hybrid ALPPS to achieve oncological efficacy. Ann Surg. 2016;263(1):e6–7.
36. Machado MA, Makdissi FF, Surjan RC. Totally laparoscopic ALPPS is feasible and may be worthwhile. Ann Surg. 2012;256:e13.
37. Guidetti C, Müller PC, Magistri P, et al. Full robotic versus open ALPPS: a bi-institutional comparison of perioperative outcomes. Surg Endosc. 2024;38(6):3448–54.
38. Kang D, Schadde E. Hypertrophy and liver function in ALPPS: correlation with morbidity and mortality. Visc Med. 2017;33(6):426–33.
39. Truant S, Baillet C, Deshorgue AC, El Amrani M, Huglo D, Pruvot FR. Contribution of hepatobiliary scintigraphy in assessing ALPPS most suited timing. Updat Surg. 2017;69(3):411–9.

40. Schadde E, Raptis DA, Schnitzbauer AA, et al. Prediction of mortality after ALPPS Stage-1: an analysis of 320 patients from the international ALPPS registry. Ann Surg. 2015;262(5):780–5.
41. Petrowsky H, Linecker M, Raptis DA, et al. First long-term oncologic results of the ALPPS procedure in a large cohort of patients with colorectal liver metastases. Ann Surg. 2020;272(5):793–800.
42. Wanis KN, Ardiles V, Alvarez FA, et al. Intermediate-term survival and quality of life outcomes in patients with advanced colorectal liver metastases undergoing associating liver partition and portal vein ligation for staged hepatectomy. Surgery. 2018;163(4):691–7.
43. Björnsson B, Sparrelid E, Røsok B, et al. Associating liver partition and portal vein ligation for staged hepatectomy in patients with colorectal liver metastases-intermediate oncological results. Eur J Surg Oncol. 2016;42(4):531–7.
44. Björk D, Hasselgren K, Røsok BI, et al. Long-term follow-up of patients with advanced colorectal liver metastasis: a survival analysis from the randomized controlled multicenter trial LIGRO. Ann Surg Open. 2024;5(3):e455.
45. Serenari M, Alvarez FA, Ardiles V, et al. The ALPPS approach for colorectal liver metastases: impact of KRAS mutation status in survival. Dig Surg. 2018;35(4):303–10.
46. Olthof PB, Huiskens J, Wicherts DA, et al. Survival after associating liver partition and portal vein ligation for staged hepatectomy (ALPPS) for advanced colorectal liver metastases: a case-matched comparison with palliative systemic therapy. Surgery. 2017;161(4):909–19.
47. Alvarez FA, Ardiles V, Chara C, et al. Adjuvant chemotherapy is associated with better oncological outcomes after ALPPS for colorectal liver metastases. Updat Surg. 2024;76(3):855–68.

Hepatic Deprivation

14

Fabio Giannone, Gianluca Cassese, Valentina Schembri, Boris Guiu, and Fabrizio Panaro

14.1 Introduction

Liver resection represents the cornerstone treatment for most hepatic tumors. The main goal of hepatobiliary surgical oncology is to perform a R0 resection, while preserving enough future remnant liver (FRL) to ensure its functions. An important strategy is to perform a parenchymal sparing hepatectomy (PSH), which preserves as much liver parenchyma as possible [1]. Such strategy not only leaves enough FRL, but also gives the possibility to repeatedly perform the hepatectomy, potentially offering iterative therapeutical options [2]. Nonetheless, some types of primary liver tumors, as well as huge lesions or close vascular relationships, could indicate major hepatectomies. The major limitation for performing such major liver surgery is the risk of post-hepatectomy liver failure (PHLF), which still represents the main cause of mortality after major liver resection [3]. An extensive preoperative work-up is mandatory to minimize the risk for PHLF, by investigating not only the volume of the remaining parenchyma but also its function. In case of inadequate volume or function of the FRL, several techniques have been developed to induce FRL hypertrophy. Portal vein embolization (PVE), which was firstly reported in

F. Giannone
Hepato-Pancreato-Biliary, Oncologic and Robotic Unit, Azienda Ospedaliero-Universitaria SS. Antonio e Biagio e Cesare Arrigo, Alessandria, Italy

G. Cassese · F. Panaro
Hepato-Pancreato-Biliary, Oncologic and Robotic Unit, Azienda Ospedaliero-Universitaria SS. Antonio e Biagio e Cesare Arrigo, Alessandria, Italy

Department of Health Sciences, University of Eastern Piedmont "Amedeo Avogadro", Alessandria, Italy

V. Schembri · B. Guiu (✉)
Department of Radiology, St-Eloi University Hospital, Montpellier, France
e-mail: b-guiu@chu-montpellier.fr

L. Aldrighetti et al. (eds.), *Liver Regeneration Techniques In Hepatic Surgery*, https://doi.org/10.1007/978-3-032-10997-2_14

1986 by Kinoshita et al., is generally considered the standard of care for inducing hypertrophy of the FLR [4–6]. However, PVE is hampered by an important failure rate, with up to 20% of treated patients who are unable to undergo the planned liver resection due to either insufficient FLR growth or tumor progression during the post-PVE period, which may be as long as 6 weeks or more [7]. To overcome such drawbacks, other hypertrophy techniques have been developed. Associating liver partition and portal vein ligation for staged hepatectomy (ALPPS) was introduced as a surgical technique to induce greater and faster hypertrophy than PVE, but at the cost of significantly higher morbidity and mortality, as testified by the many variations introduced to the original technique [8]. Finally, in 2016, a new interventional radiological technique was proposed by Guiu et al. as a safe and effective solution: the liver venous deprivation (LVD) [9]. It consists in the simultaneous embolization of the first-order portal vein and one or two hepatic veins, together with their venous collaterals.

14.2 Physiopathology and Rationale

As previously mentioned, PVE has been used as a hypertrophy technique for more than 30 years. Following PVE, the volume of the contralateral lobe usually increases over 2–4 weeks, whereas the volume of the ipsilateral lobe decreases by almost the same amount [10, 11]. Liver regeneration is a well-known peculiar characteristic of this organ, which can be more easily observed also after liver resection. Many mechanisms have been proposed to explain the regenerative PVE effect, mainly based on the activation of inflammatory cytokines, vasoregulators, and growth factors [12]. The main drive for such an activation of the inflammatory and reparative cascade is the augmentation of the shear stress on the liver sinusoids and, ultimately, the liver damage itself. However, the underlying liver must be "healthy" to be able to have an optimal regeneration in response to the aforementioned activation mechanisms [13]. The occlusion or the resection of the hepatic vein is known to produce liver damage. In 2002, Ku et al. proposed a preoperative hepatic vein embolization (HVE) to induce the development of venous collaterals, in order to reduce the liver damage after liver resection combined with right hepatica vein (RHV) resection [14]. However, it was only in 2009 that Hwang et al. applied this principle to intentionally induce additional damage to the right liver following a PVE, in patients with limited liver growth and a consequent unsafe FLR, describing the sequential PVE + HVE [15]. Based on their living donor liver transplantation (LDLT) experience, the group from Asan Medical Center in South Korea had previously reported how the closure of the RHV system induces outflow obstruction in most of the right posterior section (RPS) and a considerable proportion of the right anterior section (RAS), with subsequent liver damage that negatively affected the outcomes in LDLT [16]. After seqquential HVE, the authors observed an almost complete reduction of the portal flow in the right lobe. Similarly, also the ipsilateral arterial flow was partially inhibited, which resulted in a further liver damage, since the arterial hyperperfusion was shown to be associated with a reduced liver damage and subsequent hypertrophy [17]. Finally, the outflow obstruction increased intrahepatic resistance to the reduced, but persistent, portal flow, observed after PVE alone, thus inducing a total deprivation of portal flow at the embolized lobe, especially in the RHV drainage territory.

Based on the TUNEL and caspase-3 assays, Hwang et al. reported an increase in the apoptotic events in the RPS, more than in the RAS, coherently with the flow obstruction and the more severe liver damage, confirming previous studies focused only on PVE [15, 18]. As a mechanism of liver hypertrophy, the hepatocytes of the non-embolized hepatic lobe have been showed to undergo both enlargement and replication in response to the liver damage, as well as the subsequent molecular signals [19]. Indeed, a higher number of PCNA-positive cellular replications was observed in the non-embolized liver. Similarly, an increased Ki-67 labeling index has been observed in the non-embolized lobe when compared to the contralateral [19]. However, many studies have shown that the hepatocyte replication is too low to explain the total regenerative response. In animal models of liver regeneration, hepatocyte replication was found to peak on day 7 and to return to baseline by day 12 [20]. Subsequently, cellular hypertrophy may partially contribute to explain the phenomenon.

The above pathophysiological substrates observed in the original sequential HVE described by Hwang et al., however, were not clinically associated with a significant clinical impact of the technique. In fact, by performing it sequentially after PVE, a double waiting time interval was observed to finally perform HVE, after which other 2–4 weeks needed to be awaited to look for clinical effectiveness. For these reasons, Guiu et al. developed the LVD technique by performing the embolization of both portal and hepatic vein flows simultaneously, together with closure of the hepatic vein collaterals. The histological findings after LVD showed extensive or at least focal necrosis in centro- and medio-lobular areas in all patients after LVD. This can explain the 2–4 times increase in transaminase levels, whereas transaminase only slightly increased after PVE [21]. Furthermore, a severe sinusoidal dilatation was reported in all LVD patients within the study from Guiu et al., testifying a higher vascular congestion. A subsequent hepatocyte atrophy was observed in the areas of sinusoidal dilatation, much greater than after PVE. It translated into an important atrophy of the venous-deprived liver, as low as −21.3% after 3–4 weeks, whereas only a −12.3% atrophy has been reported after PVE [7, 9]. Finally, the higher liver damage, together with some additional technical tips, may explain the higher liver hypertrophy rates reported for LVD, as reported below.

14.3 Technique

The LVD technique was described in 2016 by Guiu et al. as a simultaneous combined portal vein and HV embolization (Fig. 14.1). The procedure was originally performed under general anesthesia, since it can result in a long and challenging intervention. The right HV is accessed first using a "1-stick" technique by puncturing a distal part of the vein under US guidance with a dedicated introducer

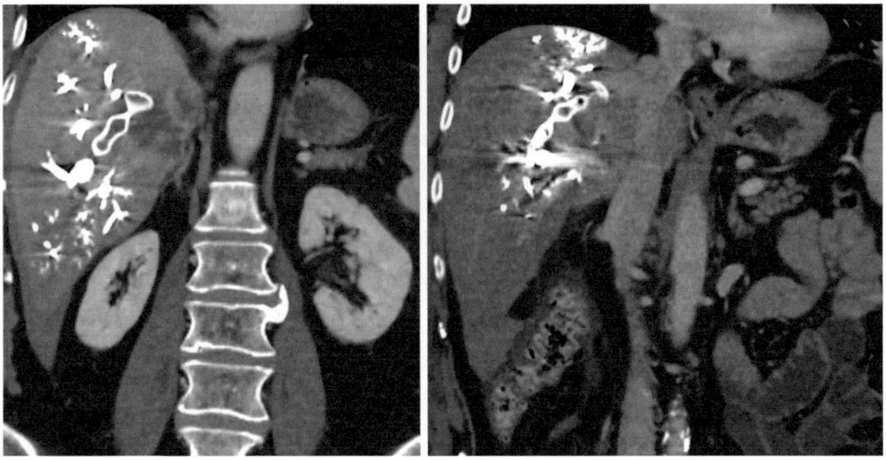

Fig. 14.1 Coronal CT view of an extended-LVD, with percutaneous right portal vein embolization, together with right and middle hepatic vein occlusion using vascular plugs type 2

needle, and then opacified. Then, using a mandril guidewire, the introducer is left in the right HV to maintain access during the PVE procedure. The same procedure must be performed in case if an accessory right HV, which may be present in up to 28% of patients. Then a right portal vein branch is accessed using the same technique under US guidance, and a portography is performed. Subsequently, the PVE procedure is performed as described elsewhere, preferably using *n*-butyl-cyanoacrylate [22]. Following PVE, the same agent is injected while retracting the catheter for the tract embolization. Then, the right HV access is used to place an Amplatzer Vascular Plug of 18–22 mm with its distal part 10 mm before the junction with the inferior vena cava to facilitate further surgical HV ligature (Fig. 14.2). Injection of the contrast medium must be used to check for correct right HV occlusion by the plug, as well as to look for patent distal branches of the right HV and potential veno-venous collateral vessels. Then, every distal branch of the right HV, as well as any collaterals (interhepatic vein communications whenever visible), are embolized. Finally, track embolization is performed using the same mixture. An intravenous antibiotic prophylaxis must be performed. During the 2 days following the procedure, pain is managed using paracetamol and/or morphine titration when necessary.

To note, the sequential HVE previously described by Hwang et al. was different from the technical point of view, since the author described a transjugular approach, without placing any vascular plug within the HV and with the use of embolization coils instead of the glue agent. Nonetheless, also other groups started to use the vascular plugs after the first cases, because of the possible migration of the caval filter that was originally placed. Indeed, some complications were reported due to migration of coils and/or filters [23]. The use of Amplatzer vascular plugs strongly reduces the risk of migration, provided the

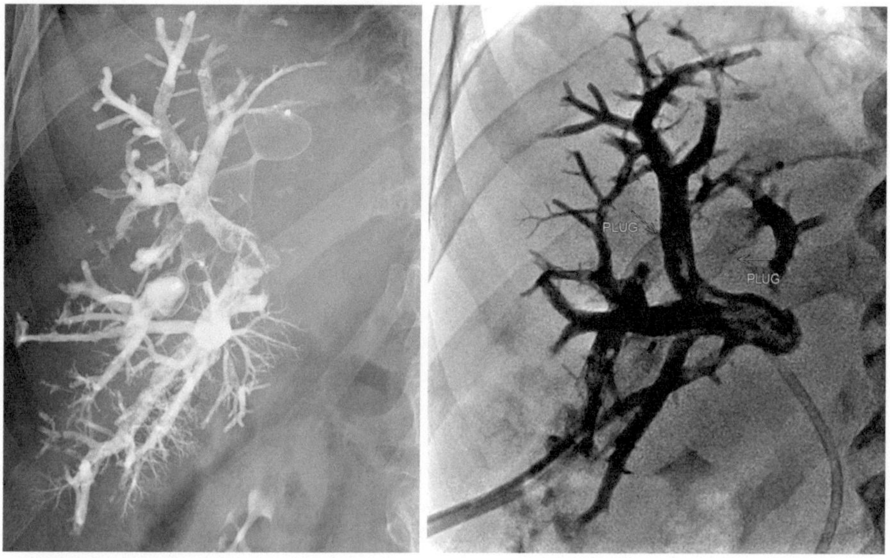

Fig. 14.2 Detail of the Amplatzer plugs in the very proximal roots of right hepatic vein and mean hepatic vein, just before the junction with the inferior vena cava

plug is oversized by at least 50%. Moreover, plugs can be recaptured if necessary and launched very precisely under both US and angiographic guidance to preserve the 10 mm safety length necessary for the surgical ligation of HV using a stapler.

The Montpellier group that firstly described the LVD technique reported some advantages also in performing it through the percutaneous access, instead of the transjugular one. First, the higher technical accessibility and catheterization of the HVs. Second, an inadvertent embolization of the middle HV can occur, as reported by Hwang et al., because right and middle HV can be confounded during catheterization. Finally, despite many literature claimed that intrahepatic veno-venous collaterals need several weeks to develop after HV ligation, the authors described the possibility to detect collaterals just several minutes after plug deployment, which can be embolized only through an intrahepatic access, since the plug must be occluded. High experience and expertise are needed to conduct embolization of intrahepatic veno-venous collaterals without inadvertent embolization of middle HV and downstream migration of glue. A recent comparison of the two types of apporoach did not show any difference in post procedural and surgical outcome, concluding that both techniques are equally safe and effective [24].

Finally, the extended-LVD (e-LVD) was also described by Guiu et al. in 2017, which consisted of the additional embolization of the median hepatic vein (MHV), in addition to the RHV, by using the same technique previously described in order to obtain an additional liver damage and a subsequent additional liver hypertrophy necessary in case of extended hepatectomies [25].

14.4 Outcomes after LVD

14.4.1 Volumetric and Functional Efficacy

One of the most important advantages emerged from the first surgical series of LVD was its effectiveness in terms of liver hypertrophy. Two of the pioneer groups compared baseline and post-LVD volumetries to those after classic PVE finding a significative higher FLR hypertrophy, degree of hypertrophy (DH), and kinetic growth rate (KGR), which translated in a faster and safer time to surgery [26, 27]. The benefit was in fact observed both in volumes achieved (FLR: 135% vs 124% in the PVE group) and in rapidity (KGR: 2.9%/week vs 1.4%/week in the PVE group). Indication varied from colorectal liver metastasis (CLRM) to hepatocellular carcinoma (HCC) and cholangiocarcinoma (CCA), including even one case of LVD for a hilar cholangiocarcinoma (HCCA). The same group of the University Hospital of Montpellier also assessed these results in terms of FLR function to confirm that the volumetric increase corresponded to a real functional gain (Fig. 14.3). Assessment through a ^{99}Tc-mebrofenin SPECT-CT confirmed better results after LVD, with an FLR functional increase of 68.2% at 21 days compared to 29.8% obtained after PVE [28]. Following these promising results, the study protocol of the HYPER-LIV01 was published, an ongoing multicentric prospective randomized trial comparing LVD and PVE before major hepatectomy for CLRM, with the aim of assessing FLR hypertrophy in the two groups at 3 weeks after the procedure [29]. Similarly, another currently recruiting trial is the Dragon 2 (NCT05428735), which will assess volumetric, perioperative, and oncologic outcomes after LVD compared to PVE for CLRM. Results of a retrospective analysis coming from this Dragon collaborative group corroborated the data that LVD could in fact result in a better hypertrophy rate than the PVE (59% versus 48%, respectively) and a higher surgical resectability (90% versus 68%, respectively) [30]. Other series later confirmed the superiority of LVD in inducing liver hypertrophy before major hepatectomies, [31, 32] and the meta-analysis published in the last years reported how LVD could become the procedure of choice for the FLR increase [33–36]. The efficacy of this

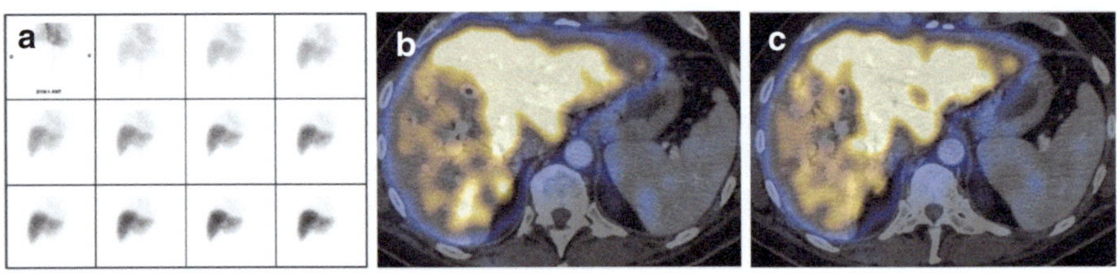

Fig. 14.3 Functional evaluation before and after E-LVD: mebrofenin extraction before E-LVD (**a**), mebrofenine distribution in the left functional liver (**b**), mebrofenin distribution in the left hypertrophic liver (**c**). In the context of a right hepatectomy extended to the middle hepatic vein, the mebrofenin extraction rate is increased and estimated at 3.7%/min/m^2, which is no longer associated with a risk of postoperative liver failure. The functional volume of the future liver remnant is estimated at 32.2%

technique was recently confirmed also in specific setting of patients, as in cirrhotic patients after trans-arterial chemoembolization [37] in patients with risk factors for FLR inadequacy as low baseline FLR or previous chemotherapy [38] and in HCCA [39, 40]. Volumetric and functional results after LVD have been also compared to another type of technique, the ALLPS procedure. One of the largest cohorts come from a French multicenter study that reported similar volumetric increase in the two techniques but with a higher KGR in the ALLPS group [41]. Similar volumetric outcomes are generally reported in other series, [42] while a potential volumetric advantage for LVD cases in terms of FLR/body weight ratio and DH is evocated in the most recent meta-analysis [33, 34].

14.4.2 LVD Safety and Resectability Rate

Data on safety and efficacy of LVD come from the recently published Dragon 1 trial, a prospective, multicentric phase II study evaluating morbidity, mortality, and resection rates after this procedure [23]. A total of 102 patients with CRLM were recruited across 43 centers, with no post-procedure mortality, only two major complications and a 90% rate of surgical resection. LVD safety seems confirmed in different series in literature, both with the transhepatic and the transjugular approach, even in cirrhotic and high-morbidity patients [24, 27, 37]. Two recent meta-analysis comparing PVE and LVD morbidity show comparable short-term outcomes while similar level of evidence for procedural safety do not exist to our knowledge against ALPPS [35, 43]. in terms of resection rate, LVD shows generally higher surgical completion than the more common PVE, with rates of subsequent liver resection generally reaching the 85–90% in literature. A lower rate of drop-out is sometimes observed when an ALPPS is performed, although this is typically at the expense of a higher risk of liver failure [33, 36, 38, 44, 45]. In HCCA, where biliary-related morbidities commonly lower the likely of performing a safe hepatectomy, LVD has been reported as a viable option to PVE [39]. A collaboration between the EuroLVD registry and the Dragon collaborative group in fact reported interesting volumetric outcomes associated to a 70% rate of resectability, with only a few patients experiencing insufficient liver growth, and exclusively cholangitis-related post-LVD morbidities [46].

14.4.3 Perioperative Outcomes

One of the reasons for exploring potential alternatives to liver hypertrophy techniques is to not compromise perioperative and postoperative safety, a major concern raised for ALPPS. Although it was not investigated as a primary outcome, the Dragon 1 trial reported a 22% of grade B or C PHLF and a related postoperative mortality rate of 6.2% following LVD [23]. Compared to PVE and ALPPS, patients undergoing LVD generally experience significantly lower rates of post-hepatectomy liver failure (PHLF), mainly due to the higher and faster DH and KGR obtained, along with a parallel rapid functional increase [33, 34, 43]. Similar favorable postoperative outcomes were observed after hepatectomy for HCCA, with acceptable rates of liver failure and a low mortality, highlighting the functional gain achieved by the FLR with this type of technique even in complex cases and damaged livers [39, 46]. There were no differences in other type of liver-specific morbidities, as perioperative hemorrhage or bile leak were observed in patients undergoing LVD in the different series.

14.4.4 Oncologic Adequacy

Long-term outcomes are generally less explored in literature when assessing LVD global safety, and only a few studies reported risk of recurrence and oncologic-related mortality compared to other techniques. In a Dragon collaborative study, LVD group showed similar recurrence/progression-free survival to patients undergoing PVE, but better survival curves were observed with the simultaneous embolization of the hepatic and portal vein [45]. This data, however, is partially biased by the higher resectability rate observed after LVD (92% against 68% after PVE), in addition to the fact that different pathologies were included in the analysis. In surgical series specifically assessing CRLM, the two techniques appear to be associated with similar oncologic outcomes [47]. The same authors later compared DFS and OS after surgical resection for patients previously undergoing LVD or ALPPS, finding a slightly better survival in the first group, although not significative, and comparable recurrence rates [42]. A recent meta-analysis focused on long-term outcomes differences in resected patients after LVD or PVE found similar survival rates but higher 3 years DFS curves [35]. Once again, heterogeneity was high and level of evidence was very low, with no meta regression for each pathology. There is no evidence, however, that this type of technique could somehow promote tumor progression, as was previously hypothesized for the ALPPS procedure.

References

1. Deng G, Li H, Jia G, Fang D, Tang Y, Xie J, et al. Parenchymal-sparing versus extended hepatectomy for colorectal liver metastases: a systematic review and meta-analysis. Cancer Med. 2019;8:6165–75. https://doi.org/10.1002/cam4.2515.
2. Oba M, Hasegawa K, Shindoh J, Yamashita S, Sakamoto Y, Makuuchi M, et al. Survival benefit of repeat resection of successive recurrences after the initial hepatic resection for colorectal liver metastases. Surgery. 2016;159:632–40. https://doi.org/10.1016/j.surg.2015.09.003.
3. Pulitano C, Crawford M, Joseph D, Aldrighetti L, Sandroussi C. Preoperative assessment of postoperative liver function: the importance of residual liver volume. J Surg Oncol. 2014;110:445–50. https://doi.org/10.1002/jso.23671.
4. Kinoshita H, Sakai K, Hirohashi K, Igawa S, Yamasaki O, Kubo S. Preoperative portal vein embolization for hepatocellular carcinoma. World J Surg. 1986;10:803–8. https://doi.org/10.1007/BF01655244.

5. Makuuchi M, Thai BL, Takayasu K, Takayama T, Kosuge T, Gunvén P, et al. Preoperative portal embolization to increase safety of major hepatectomy for hilar bile duct carcinoma: a preliminary report. Surgery. 1990;107:521–7.
6. Glantzounis GK, Tokidis E, Basourakos S-P, Ntzani EE, Lianos GD, Pentheroudakis G. The role of portal vein embolization in the surgical management of primary hepatobiliary cancers. A systematic review. Eur J Surg Oncol J Eur Soc Surg Oncol Br Assoc Surg Oncol. 2017;43:32–41. https://doi.org/10.1016/j.ejso.2016.05.026.
7. van Lienden KP, van den Esschert JW, de Graaf W, Bipat S, Lameris JS, van Gulik TM, et al. Portal vein embolization before liver resection: a systematic review. Cardiovasc Intervent Radiol. 2013;36:25–34. https://doi.org/10.1007/s00270-012-0440-y.
8. Edmondson MJ, Sodergren MH, Pucher PH, Darzi A, Li J, Petrowsky H, et al. Variations and adaptations of associated liver partition and portal vein ligation for staged hepatectomy (ALPPS): many routes to the summit. Surgery. 2016;159:1058–72. https://doi.org/10.1016/j.surg.2015.11.013.
9. Guiu B, Chevallier P, Denys A, Delhom E, Pierredon-Foulongne M-A, Rouanet P, et al. Simultaneous trans-hepatic portal and hepatic vein embolization before major hepatectomy: the liver venous deprivation technique. Eur Radiol. 2016;26:4259–67. https://doi.org/10.1007/s00330-016-4291-9.
10. Imamura H, Matsuyama Y, Tanaka E, Ohkubo T, Hasegawa K, Miyagawa S, et al. Risk factors contributing to early and late phase intrahepatic recurrence of hepatocellular carcinoma after hepatectomy. J Hepatol. 2003;38:200–7. https://doi.org/10.1016/s0168-8278(02)00360-4.
11. Hemming AW, Reed AI, Howard RJ, Fujita S, Hochwald SN, Caridi JG, et al. Preoperative portal vein embolization for extended hepatectomy. Ann Surg. 2003;237:686–91.; discussion 691–3. https://doi.org/10.1097/01.SLA.0000065265.16728.C0.
12. Rauchfuss F, Lambeck S, Claus RA, Ullmann J, Schulz T, Weber M, et al. Sustained liver regeneration after portal vein embolization—a human molecular pilot study. Dig Liver Dis. 2012;44:681–8. https://doi.org/10.1016/j.dld.2012.04.002.
13. Cassese G, Han H-S, Al Farai A, Guiu B, Troisi RI, Panaro F. Future remnant liver optimization: preoperative assessment, volume augmentation procedures and management of PVE failure. Minerva Surg. 2022;77:368–79. https://doi.org/10.23736/S2724-5691.22.09541-7.
14. Ku Y, Tominaga M, Sugimoto T, Iwasaki T, Fukumoto T, Takahashi T, et al. Preoperative hepatic venous embolization for partial hepatectomy combined with segmental resection of major hepatic vein. Br J Surg. 2002;89:63–9. https://doi.org/10.1046/j.0007-1323.2001.01955.x.
15. Hwang S, Lee S-G, Ko G-Y, Kim B-S, Sung K-B, Kim M-H, et al. Sequential preoperative ipsilateral hepatic vein embolization after portal vein embolization to induce further liver regeneration in patients with hepatobiliary malignancy. Ann Surg. 2009;249:608–16. https://doi.org/10.1097/SLA.0b013e31819ecc5c.
16. Hwang S, Lee S-G, Park K-M, Kim K-H, Ahn C-S, Lee Y-J, et al. Hepatic venous congestion in living donor liver transplantation: preoperative quantitative prediction and follow-up using computed tomography. Liver Transpl. 2004;10:763–70. https://doi.org/10.1002/lt.20178.
17. Kito Y, Nagino M, Nimura Y. Doppler sonography of hepatic arterial blood flow velocity after percutaneous transhepatic portal vein embolization. AJR Am J Roentgenol. 2001;176:909–12. https://doi.org/10.2214/ajr.176.4.1760909.
18. Harada H, Imamura H, Miyagawa S, Kawasaki S. Fate of the human liver after hemihepatic portal vein embolization: cell kinetic and morphometric study. Hepatol Baltim Md. 1997;26:1162–70. https://doi.org/10.1053/jhep.1997.v26.pm0009362357.
19. Komori K, Nagino M, Nimura Y. Hepatocyte morphology and kinetics after portal vein embolization. Br J Surg. 2006;93:745–51. https://doi.org/10.1002/bjs.5332.
20. Duncan JR, Hicks ME, Cai SR, Brunt EM, Ponder KP. Embolization of portal vein branches induces hepatocyte replication in swine: a potential step in hepatic gene therapy. Radiology. 1999;210:467–77. https://doi.org/10.1148/radiology.210.2.r99fe10467.

21. Imamura H, Shimada R, Kubota M, Matsuyama Y, Nakayama A, Miyagawa S, et al. Preoperative portal vein embolization: an audit of 84 patients. Hepatology. 1999;29:1099–105. https://doi.org/10.1002/hep.510290415.
22. Guiu B, Bize P, Gunthern D, Demartines N, Halkic N, Denys A. Portal vein embolization before right hepatectomy: improved results using n-butyl-cyanoacrylate compared to microparticles plus coils. Cardiovasc Intervent Radiol. 2013;36:1306–12. https://doi.org/10.1007/s00270-013-0565-7.
23. Korenblik R, James S, Smits J, Díaz-Nieto R, Davis R, Chan BKY, et al. Safety and efficacy of combined portal and hepatic vein embolisation in patients with colorectal liver metastases (DRAGON1): a multicentre, single-arm clinical trial. Lancet Reg Health Eur. 2025;53:101284. https://doi.org/10.1016/j.lanepe.2025.101284.
24. Della Corte A, Santangelo D, Augello L, Ratti F, Cipriani F, Canevari C, et al. Single-center retrospective study comparing double vein embolization via a trans-jugular approach with liver venous deprivation via a trans-hepatic approach. Cardiovasc Intervent Radiol. 2023;46:1703–12. https://doi.org/10.1007/s00270-023-03538-3.
25. Guiu B, Quenet F, Escal L, Bibeau F, Piron L, Rouanet P, et al. Extended liver venous deprivation before major hepatectomy induces marked and very rapid increase in future liver remnant function. Eur Radiol. 2017;27:3343–52. https://doi.org/10.1007/s00330-017-4744-9.
26. Kobayashi K, Yamaguchi T, Denys A, Perron L, Halkic N, Demartines N, et al. Liver venous deprivation compared to portal vein embolization to induce hypertrophy of the future liver remnant before major hepatectomy: a single center experience. Surgery. 2020;167:917–23. https://doi.org/10.1016/j.surg.2019.12.006.
27. Panaro F, Giannone F, Riviere B, Sgarbura O, Cusumano C, Deshayes E, et al. Perioperative impact of liver venous deprivation compared with portal venous embolization in patients undergoing right hepatectomy: preliminary results from the pioneer center. Hepatobiliary Surg Nutr. 2019;8:329–37. https://doi.org/10.21037/hbsn.2019.07.06.
28. Guiu B, Quenet F, Panaro F, Piron L, Cassinotto C, Herrerro A, et al. Liver venous deprivation versus portal vein embolization before major hepatectomy: future liver remnant volumetric and functional changes. Hepatobiliary Surg Nutr. 2020;9:564–76. https://doi.org/10.21037/hbsn.2020.02.06.
29. Deshayes E, Piron L, Bouvier A, Lapuyade B, Lermite E, Vervueren L, et al. Study protocol of the HYPER-LIV01 trial: a multicenter phase II, prospective and randomized study comparing simultaneous portal and hepatic vein embolization to portal vein embolization for hypertrophy of the future liver remnant before major hepatectomy for colorectal liver metastases. BMC Cancer. 2020;20:574. https://doi.org/10.1186/s12885-020-07065-z.
30. Heil J, Korenblik R, Heid F, Bechstein WO, Bemelmans M, Binkert C, et al. Preoperative portal vein or portal and hepatic vein embolization: DRAGON collaborative group analysis. Br J Surg. 2021;108:834–42. https://doi.org/10.1093/bjs/znaa149.
31. Gadani S, Chansangrat J, Kapoor B, McBride A, Partovi S, Obuchowski N, et al. Liver vein deprivation versus portal vein embolization: retrospective review of safety and effectiveness. J Vasc Interv Radiol. 2025;36:31–39.e2. https://doi.org/10.1016/j.jvir.2024.09.025.
32. Boubaddi M, Marichez A, Pecquenard F, Maulat C, Buc E, Sulpice L, et al. Liver venous deprivation (LVD) before extended hepatectomy: a French multicentric retrospective cohort. Hepatobiliary Surg Nutr. 2024;13:937–49. https://doi.org/10.21037/hbsn-24-315.
33. Bozkurt E, Sijberden JP, Kasai M, Abu HM. Efficacy and perioperative safety of different future liver remnant modulation techniques: a systematic review and network meta-analysis. HPB. 2024;26:465–75. https://doi.org/10.1016/j.hpb.2024.01.002.
34. Gavriilidis P, Marangoni G, Ahmad J, Azoulay D. Simultaneous portal and hepatic vein embolization is better than portal embolization or ALPPS for hypertrophy of future liver remnant before major hepatectomy: a systematic review and network meta-analysis. Hepatobiliary Pancreat Dis Int HBPD INT. 2023;22:221–7. https://doi.org/10.1016/j.hbpd.2022.08.013.
35. Chaouch MA, Mazzotta A, da Costa AC, Hussain MI, Gouader A, Krimi B, et al. A systematic review and meta-analysis of liver venous deprivation versus portal vein embolization before

hepatectomy: future liver volume, postoperative outcomes, and oncological safety. Front Med. 2024;10:1334661. https://doi.org/10.3389/fmed.2023.1334661.
36. Korenblik R, van Zon JFJA, Olij B, Heil J, Dewulf MJL, Neumann UP, et al. Resectability of bilobar liver tumours after simultaneous portal and hepatic vein embolization versus portal vein embolization alone: meta-analysis. BJS Open. 2022;6:zrac141. https://doi.org/10.1093/bjsopen/zrac141.
37. Sy T-V, Dung LT, Giang B-V, Nghia NQ, Viet Khai N, Manh Thau C, et al. Safety and efficacy of liver venous deprivation following Transarterial chemoembolization before major hepatectomy for hepatocellular carcinoma. Ther Clin Risk Manag. 2023;19:425–33. https://doi.org/10.2147/TCRM.S411080.
38. Haddad A, Khavandi MM, Lendoire M, Acidi B, Chiang Y-J, Gupta S, et al. Propensity score-matched analysis of liver venous deprivation and portal vein embolization before planned hepatectomy in patients with extensive colorectal liver metastases and high-risk factors for inadequate regeneration. Ann Surg Oncol. 2025;32:1752–61. https://doi.org/10.1245/s10434-024-16558-1.
39. Marino R, Ratti F, Della Corte A, Santangelo D, Clocchiatti L, Canevari C, et al. Comparing liver venous deprivation and portal vein embolization for Perihilar Cholangiocarcinoma: is it time to shift the focus to hepatic functional reserve rather than hypertrophy? Cancer. 2023;15:4363. https://doi.org/10.3390/cancers15174363.
40. Hocquelet A, Sotiriadis C, Duran R, Guiu B, Yamaguchi T, Halkic N, et al. Preoperative portal vein embolization alone with biliary drainage compared to a combination of simultaneous portal vein, right hepatic vein embolization and biliary drainage in Klatskin tumor. Cardiovasc Intervent Radiol. 2018;41:1885–91. https://doi.org/10.1007/s00270-018-2075-0.
41. Chebaro A, Buc E, Durin T, Chiche L, Brustia R, Didier A, et al. Liver venous deprivation or associating liver partition and portal vein ligation for staged hepatectomy?: a retrospective multicentric study. Ann Surg. 2021;274:874–80. https://doi.org/10.1097/SLA.0000000000005121.
42. Cassese G, Troisi RI, Khayat S, Quenet F, Tomassini F, Panaro F, et al. Liver venous deprivation versus associating liver partition and portal vein ligation for staged hepatectomy for colo-rectal liver metastases: a comparison of early and late kinetic growth rates, and perioperative and oncological outcomes. Surg Oncol. 2022;43:101812. https://doi.org/10.1016/j.suronc.2022.101812.
43. Yang L, Yang M, Wang T, Qiu Y, Yang Y, Wang W. Comparison of liver venous deprivation with portal vein embolization alone in patients undergoing major liver resection: a systematic review and meta-analysis. HPB. 2024;26:1329–38. https://doi.org/10.1016/j.hpb.2024.07.409.
44. Yi F, Zhang W, Feng L. Efficacy and safety of different options for liver regeneration of future liver remnant in patients with liver malignancies: a systematic review and network meta-analysis. World J Surg Oncol. 2022;20:399. https://doi.org/10.1186/s12957-022-02867-w.
45. Korenblik R, Heil J, Smits J, James S, Olij B, Bechstein WO, et al. Liver regeneration after portal and hepatic vein embolization improves overall survival compared with portal vein embolization alone: mid-term survival analysis of the multicentre DRAGON 0 cohort. Br J Surg. 2024;111:znae087. https://doi.org/10.1093/bjs/znae087.
46. Smits J, Chau S, James S, Korenblik R, Tschögl M, Arntz P, et al. Combined portal and hepatic vein embolisation in perihilar cholangiocarcinoma. HPB. 2024;26:1458–66. https://doi.org/10.1016/j.hpb.2024.07.407.
47. Cassese G, Troisi RI, Khayat S, Benoudifa B, Quenet F, Guiu B, et al. Liver venous deprivation versus portal vein embolization before major hepatectomy for colorectal liver metastases: a retrospective comparison of short- and medium-term outcomes. J Gastrointest Surg. 2023;27:296–305. https://doi.org/10.1007/s11605-022-05551-2.

Radioembolization 15

Cristina Mosconi, Alberta Cappelli, Domenico Santangelo, and Francesco De Cobelli

15.1 Introduction

Hepatic resection outcomes have dramatically improved over the last 20–30 years; however, they remain heavily dependent on the future liver remnant volume (FLR) and function [1, 2]. Thus, multiple techniques have been devised to increase the FLR and improve the safety profile of hepatic resection. The mainstay of techniques available includes portal vein embolization (PVE), associated liver partition and portal vein ligation (ALPPS), and radiation lobectomy (RL) obtained with transarterial radioembolization (TARE). Each of these techniques has its own merits and pitfalls.

TARE, a newer intra-arterial embolotherapy, has become the main therapy for patients with liver tumor and liver metastasis at some institutions [3]. In TARE,

C. Mosconi (✉)
Department of Radiology, IRCCS Azienda Ospedaliero-Universitaria di Bologna, Bologna, Italy

Department of Medical and Surgical Sciences (DIMEC), Alma Mater Studiorum – University of Bologna, Bologna, Italy
e-mail: cristina.mosconi@aosp.bo.it

A. Cappelli
Department of Radiology, IRCCS Azienda Ospedaliero-Universitaria di Bologna, Bologna, Italy

D. Santangelo
Department of Radiology, IRCCS San Raffaele Hospital, Milan, Italy

Department of Advanced Biomedical Sciences, University of Naples Federico II, Naples, Italy

F. De Cobelli
Department of Radiology, IRCCS San Raffaele Hospital, Milan, Italy

Vita-Salute San Raffaele University, Milan, Italy

L. Aldrighetti et al. (eds.), *Liver Regeneration Techniques In Hepatic Surgery*,
https://doi.org/10.1007/978-3-032-10997-2_15

radioembolic microspheres carry an isotope, yttrium 90 (90Y), to liver tumors through the hepatic artery, where they lodge at the arteriolar level and serve as a point of radiation through beta decay; the intent is microembolic with the preservation of blood flow to the targeted liver segments to promote radiation injury.

TARE is currently used as a palliative treatment for malignant liver diseases. It allows for selective radiation therapy of hypervascular lesions [4]. As a result, local tumor control and downsizing can be achieved, possibly leading to resectability of the lesions. Several studies have shown that PVE induces more pronounced contralateral hypertrophy [5] and TARE-induced hypertrophy of the untreated liver lobe seems to take longer than after PVE [6], but there is little data on the effect of cirrhosis on hypertrophy after TARE.

TARE has historically been performed in a lobar or sequential lobar fashion with palliative intent for patients with advanced disease or for those in whom other therapies have failed. The evolution of TARE has led to new applications in earlier-stage disease. RL derived from the observation that unilobar radioembolization was effective in treating the hepatic tumor and resulted in an atrophy–hypertrophy complex, in which the treated hepatic lobe with tumor atrophies and there is compensatory hypertrophy of the future liver remnant (FLR). RL can facilitate surgical resection in those patients initially diagnosed with disease unresectable secondary to inadequate FLR. Radiation segmentectomy (RS) goes further by delivering high radiation doses selectively (typically up to two Couinaud segments) to patients with limited disease burden. This approach delivers ablative 90Y dosing while also sparing non-tumor-bearing hepatic parenchyma. The combined technique of a modified RL approach exploits the segmental high-dose therapy of RS with the capacity of RL to hypertrophy the FLR.

15.2 Technical Aspects

15.2.1 Physics

TARE permits the use of particles loaded with two kinds of isotopes: Y90 or Holmium (Ho166). Physical characteristics of radionuclides are shown in [7]. Y90 is a β-emitter with an average radiation energy of 0.94 MeV, an average tissue penetration depth of 2.5 mm, and a maximum penetration capability of up to 11 mm [8]. Ho166 is both a β- and γ-emitter, which relies a β_{max} energy of 1.85 MeV and a penetration that ranges from 2.5 to 9 mm [9]. Ho166 also releases primary gamma photons suitable for scintigraphy imaging. Additionally, as a lanthanide, its paramagnetic properties allow for visualization through MRI, facilitating the assessment of its distribution within the liver and the quantification of the absorbed tumor dose [10, 11]. Therapeutic effects of both isotopes involve the ability of high-energy β-particles to induce lethal damage to tumor cells by causing DNA double-strand breaks [12]. The microspheres used in TARE are classified into resin and glass-based types for Y90 and poly-L-lactic acid (PLLA)-based type for Ho166. Characteristics of all three microspheres are described in [7]. Resin microspheres contain a lower radiation dose per sphere (50 Bq), but they are delivered in high quantities (13 × 106 per GBq). Glass microspheres are highly radioactive (2500 Bq per sphere), but limited in number compared to others (0.4 × 106 per GBq). Finally, PLLA microspheres, though less common, offer intermediate dose per sphere (450 Bq), but quantity of sphere injected similar to resin spheres (10 × 106 per GBq) [7].

Considering their physical differences, resin, glass, and PLLA exhibit different tumor dose thresholds for tumor target and liver required to achieve optimal therapeutic responses [13]. Despite that, it has been proven that these differences does not influence overall survival (OS) and toxicity [14–16]. Furthermore, adverse events (AE) associated with microspheres differ in frequency between resin and glass types. When comparing resin to glass microspheres, reported rates were 1.4% vs. 0.1% for gastrointestinal ulceration, 5% vs. 1.9% for cholecystitis, 22.2% vs. 6.9% for hepatic abnormalities, and 8% vs. 2.8% for hepatic encephalopathy, respectively [17].

15.2.2 Procedure

TARE is a multistep procedure that requires extensive pretreatment planning to ensure safety and efficacy. The process begins with an angiographic study of the aorta, superior mesenteric artery, and celiac trunk for detecting any arterio-portal shunting and mapping the hepatic vascular anatomy to identify the vessels supplying the tumor, both intrahepatic and extrahepatic, and the potential extrahepatic blood flow to other organs [18]. The injection of microspheres into nontarget vessels can result in AEs. While coil embolization of nontarget vessels was once a routine practice, it is no longer recommended as a standard procedure [19]. A cone beam CT (CBCT) is often performed during this step to better assess the hepatic vessels feeding the lesion and tumor perfusion. In addition, it could be useful in evaluating extrahepatic arterial perfusion, differentiating segmental liver area of perfusion and confirming full tumor coverage from the injection position [20, 21]. During mapping study, a calibrated amount of technetium macroaggregates (99mTc-MAA) is administered at the selected site within the hepatic vasculature to simulate the distribution of microspheres. Since macroaggregates (MAA) degrades rapidly in the liver, a planar scintigraphy scan is performed <1 h after the injection to assess lung shunting, evaluate potentially extrahepatic nontarget accumulation of spheres, and confirm adequate tumor targeting [22]. Single photon emission computed tomography/CT (SPECT/CT) should be used instead of planar imaging to assess the intrahepatic 99mTc-MAA distribution [23, 24]. After treatment administration, bremsstrahlung SPECT/CT or Y90-PET can also be performed to correlate sites of dose administration and identify sites of nontarget dose deposition [13]. TARE can be tailored to specific disease presentations through advanced techniques such as RS and RL. RS involves delivering a high radiation dose (>190 Gy) to a single or maximum two Couinaud hepatic segments [25]. This approach is particularly effective for patients with tumors localized to small regions of the liver, as it minimizes radiation-induced toxicity and preserves the maximum amount of healthy liver parenchyma [26]. Thus, it should be used for small lesions, which are not achievable from ablation such as hepatic dome, caudate lobe or zone near vessels or bile ducts [27, 28]. RL targets an entire hepatic lobe and is often used to downstage the disease. In fact, RL offers double effect: inducing tumor response and necrosis and promoting FLR hypertrophy to facilitate bridge to liver resection (LR) [27, 29].

15.3 TARE Dosimetry

TARE follows the same radiobiological principles as those applied in radiation oncology: the absorbed dose must exceed a specific threshold to produce an observable (deterministic) effect and higher absorbed doses result in increasingly severe effect [30]. In hepatocellular carcinoma (HCC), microsphere composition has impact on dose: data on radiation segmentectomy with glass microspheres suggest aiming for dose thresholds of at least 400 Gy while recommended target dose thresholds in resin microspheres are typically in the range of 190–200 Gy [31]. To quantify the delivered dose, two dosimetry algorithms have been proposed: standard dosimetry models (body surface area (BSA) and medical internal radiation dose (MIRD)), as well as personalized dosimetry models (partition models and image-based models).

15.3.1 Body Surface Area (BSA) Model

This model calculates the prescribed activity based only on the BSA and the tumor burden, using the following formula [32]:

$$A(\mathrm{GBq}) = (\mathrm{BSA} - 0.2) + \frac{Vt}{Vt + Vn}$$

where A (GBq) is the activity within the tissue targeted, V_t represents the tumor volume, and V_n is the normal tissue (liver) volume. BSA is calculated with the following formula [33]:

$$\mathrm{BSA}(\mathrm{m}^2) = \mathrm{kg}^{0.425} \times \mathrm{cm}^{0.725} \times 0.007184$$

The main advantage of this model is its simplicity. The BSA model offers limited personalization and does not permit adjustments to account for the absorbed radiation dose in tumor tissue relative to the surrounding nontumor liver tissue. For large treatment areas, this model may lead to underestimation of activity due to its imposed restriction of ^{90}Y activity between 1.0 and 3.0 GBq [34]. Additionally, the correlation between BSA and liver volume is weak [35], which can result in substantially lower activity concentrations in patients with larger livers. Conversely, the model may lead to overdosing in obese patients with a comparatively smaller normal liver volume relative to their body size [32].

15.3.2 Medical Internal Radiation Dose (MIRD) Model

This model calculates the delivered activity as it follows [32]:

$$A(\mathrm{GBq}) = \frac{D(\mathrm{Gy}) \times \text{liver mass}(\mathrm{kg})}{50 \times \left(1 - \frac{\mathrm{LSF}}{100}\right)}$$

where D (Gy) is the delivered dose to the treated segment/lobe, 50 is a constant derived from the characteristics of the ^{90}Y isotope, and LSF is the lung shunt fraction. The MIRD model is a single-compartment approach based on the assumption of a uniform activity distribution within the targeted tissue. However, the targeted region includes both tumor and nontumor liver parenchyma, which constitutes the primary limitation of this model. In cases of severe cirrhosis or emphysema, the model may underestimate the dose delivered to the liver or lungs, assuming equivalent radiation absorption as in normal liver or lung tissue [36], resulting in patient overtreatment [37]. Despite these limitations, the MIRD model offers advantages, such as simplicity of calculation and the ability to provide consistent and reproducible dose estimations [38].

15.3.3 Partition Model

This model is a more advanced method based on 99-Tc-MAA SPECT, which incorporates tumor, nontumor liver, and lung compartments. This approach is thought to reduce the risk of radiation-induced hepatotoxicity compared to the BSA and MIRD models [39]. The partition model is technically more intricate due to the presence of multiple compartments (tumor, nontumor liver, and lung), which also explain its accuracy. It enables individualized activity administration by separately calculating and applying dose thresholds for each compartment. Its limitations include reliance on Tc-MAA-SPECT, which exhibits variability in biodistribution compared to Y90 microspheres, as well as the influence of catheter positioning during dose delivery [40]. It assumes uniform distribution of activity within each compartment, not truly reflecting the real-life conditions. CBCT is playing an increasingly important role in TARE planning and in partition model, particularly, recent study shown CBCT to be more accurate than contrast-enhanced CT and Tc-MAA-SPECT in predicting tumor and perfused liver volumes, better correlating with posttreatment Y90 PET, used as a reference standard [41]. In patients with multiple tumors, classic partition model consider all tumors as one aggregated compartment; the multitumor partition model (MTPM) overcome this problem, considering each tumor as one compartment to account for them heterogeneity, with dose estimation more aligned with advanced image-based techniques compared to those obtained from the classic partition model [31].

15.3.4 Image-Based Models

This model includes local deposition model (LDM) and dose point kernel (DPK) convolution, both based on the pretreatment Tc-MAA-SPECT and CT. These methods divide SPECT and CT images into defined voxels, after which volumes of interest (VOIs) are delineated based on CT data. Tissue density is assumed to be uniform within each VOI, implying homogeneity within the corresponding structure. Tc-MAA SPECT images are then used to calculate the activity within each voxel. The LDM model assumes that the energy released by each Y90 β-particle is confined to the voxel where the decay occurs, with minimal interaction between adjacent voxels due to the relatively small irradiation radius compared to voxel size. In contrast, DPK convolution accounts for the possibility that β-particles within a voxel may also irradiate neighboring voxels, thus incorporating activity from surrounding regions when estimating voxel-level activity [31]. Both LDM and DPK convolution exhibit superior dosimetric accuracy compared to standard models and classic partition models [42]. Although image-based methods offer improved dosimetric precision, they were traditionally more time-intensive and complex to apply [31], although several software solutions have been introduced, producing reliable and reproducible inter-user measurements and demonstrate satisfactory performance [43].

Dosimetry and dosimetric models can significantly impact TARE outcome. Several studies have failed to demonstrate the superiority in terms of overall survival of TARE vs. Sorafenib in patients with advanced HCC, most likely due to the use of standard dosimetry [44–46]. The DOSISPHERE-01 study [47], a randomized, multicenter, open-label phase 2 trial compared standard dosimetry versus personalized dosimetry in Y90 glass microspheres TARE in 60 patients with Barcelona Clinic Liver Cancer (BCLC) B and C stage hepatocellular carcinoma (HCC). Patients in the standard dosimetry received 120 ± 20 Gy to the perfused lobe; personalized dosimetry group includes patients receiving ≥205 Gy or higher delivered to the target lesion, and less than 120 Gy to the liver nontumor tissue. Overall response rate (ORR) was 71% and 36% for personalized and standardized dosimetry groups, respectively; OS rates were 26.6 and 10.7 months for the personalized and standard dosimetry, respectively, in the intention-to-treat analysis with fewer adverse events. The use of personalized dosimetry was further validated by the global TARGET study [48], a multicenter retrospective study in 207 patients with BCLC B-C HCC treated with increased tumor-absorbed doses. Patients receiving an increased tumor-absorbed dose were associated with improved ORR and OS.

In the past, whole-liver or lobar TARE was the standard approach; however, current trends have shifted toward more selective catheterization and personalized dosimetry. It has been noted that lobar TARE leads to atrophy of the treated lobe, accompanied by compensatory hypertrophy of the contralateral lobe, configuring a phenomenon known as the "atrophy–hypertrophy complex" [49]. Grisanti et al. [50] investigated the dosimetric and clinical parameters influencing liver volume changes after lobar radioembolization with Y90-loaded resin microspheres. In this study, FLR hypertrophy was strongly associated with dosimetric parameters specific to the nontumoral liver tissue dose. In particular, the fraction of non-tumoral liver volume receiving ≥30 Gy (NTL-V30) was a significant predictor of FLR increase, particularly in patients with a baseline FLR <30%. The study found no significant correlation between tumor dose or size and hypertrophy, nor were specific dosimetric parameters predictive of atrophy in the treated liver lobe. These findings underscore the importance of voxel-based dosimetry in optimizing TARE treatment planning to balance therapeutic efficacy and liver regeneration.

15.4 Scientific Evidence

15.4.1 Characteristics of the Studies

Many studies published between 2008 and 2020 reported that radioembolization with Y90-microspheres is able to induce contralateral liver hypertrophy with simultaneous ipsilateral control of tumor growth. The concept of radioembolization-induced liver hypertrophy, also termed as RL, was first described in 2008 in patients with colorectal liver metastases (CRLM) and in 2009 in patients with hepatocellular carcinoma (HCC) [51, 52].

The most robust data from cholangiocellular carcinoma (CCC) derive from the review of Cucchetti et al. [53] and include results from nine studies [54–62]. The interest for this treatment has been growing during the years, also considering the results for Associating Liver Partitioning and Portal vein ligation for Staged hepatectomy (ALPPS) in patients with primary liver malignancies have been disappointing, as this treatment offers local tumor control with high perioperative morbidity and mortality rates and simultaneous hypertrophy of the contralateral lobe [63, 64].

In the review of Birgin [65], a total of 189 studies were identified by the search criteria, but finally, 16 studies, comprising 602 patients, remained eligible because considered the most significant studies in terms of results [51, 52, 66–79] All studies were retrospective, except for one that is a nonrandomized and not controlled study [75]. The only available prospective study was published in a small cohort of 24 patients with palliative treatment of advanced HCC [66].

Notwithstanding the prospective design, this study lacks information on the effect of radioembolization on inducing hypertrophy in subgroups of patients at high risk of poor hypertrophy, such as patients with diabetes, advanced cirrhosis, and portal vein thrombosis (PVT).

15.4.2 Characteristics of the Study Population

In the review of Birgin [65], the median age of the patients was 68 (range: 59–79) with a prevalence of men (76%). Pathological findings revealed 490 (81%) primary liver malignancies: of these, 462 (94%) patients had HCC and 28 (6%) patients had CCC. A total of 136 (22%) patients suffered from secondary liver malignancies, of which 86 (77%) patients had CRLM. Underlying liver cirrhosis was present in 375 cases (62%). Only eight studies, included 42 patients, reported the presence of portal hypertension (PHTN) and nine studies (73 patients) included PVT. Prior to radioembolization, a total of 136 patients received other therapies: 102 patients (17%) had prior chemotherapy, 24 patients (4%) had prior local ablative therapy, and 10 patients (2%) had prior resection (hepatectomy). The local tumor control was 84%.

Ten studies provided data on liver surgery following radioembolization in primarily unresectable liver tumors, showing that 109 out of 362 patients (30%) underwent subsequent surgery. The time interval of surgery after the last treatment of radioembolization was reported in three studies within a time range between 2 and 30 weeks after intra-arterial treatment [69, 73, 74].

15.4.3 Contralateral Lobe Hypertrophy

Data from the literature reported that a median kinetic growth rate (KGR) per week of the contralateral liver lobe was 0.7%, but it is reported to decline slowly over time. These data demonstrated a significant amount of contralateral lobe hypertrophy following radioembolization: up to 84% of the treated patients showed a local tumor control following the treatment and a 30% of patients with primarily unresectable liver malignancies finally underwent hepatic resection with acceptable postoperative morbidity and mortality rates. The most commonly used modality of radioembolization was Y90-glass-microspheres (435 patients, 72%), whereas Y90-resin-microspheres were used in 167 (28%) patients. The median KGR between types of microspheres showed a similar distribution: 0.8% (range: 0.3–3%) for glass-microspheres only and 0.8% (range: 0.4–1.3%) for resin-microspheres only. Only one study used both glass and resin microspheres for a total of 34 patients [67].

With regard to the underlying malignancy, the median KGR was 0.7% (range: 0.3–2.5%) in primary malignancies, 0.8% (range: 0.7–1.3%) in secondary malignancies, and 0.8% (range: 0.7–1.7%) in both primary and secondary malignancies. Three studies assessed entirely cirrhotic patients in a cohort of HCC [67, 76, 79]. Interesting, patients with HCC and underlying cirrhosis had a similar KGR of 0.7% per week (range: 0.6–1.1%) compared to patients without liver cirrhosis with a KGR per week of 0.7% (range: 0.3–1.3%). Although the impact of underlying liver cirrhosis on the induction of contralateral hypertrophy following radioembolization remains controversial with comparable KGR compared to patients without liver cirrhosis, additional studies need to investigate more precise information on the regenerative potential of this treatment. In the majority of cases (97%; 585 patients), the treatment was unilobar; on the other hand, bilobar treatment was conducted in 17 patients. Only patients who received unilobar treatment were assessed for measurements of contralateral liver lobe hypertrophy.

Three studies reported on RS in 15 out of 169 patients (9%) The median applied activity of yttrium was 2.1 GBq, with a median administered dose of 121 Gy [68, 73, 76]. The mean follow-up (FU) was 5 months and ranged between 4 weeks and 18 months. An important aim analyzed by the papers was the ratio between future liver remnant and total liver volume (FLR/TLV): at the baseline it ranged between 23.4% and 49.6% and after radioembolization between 27.0% and 68.6%. However, after a period of observation of 9 months, the maximum degree of relative contralateral hypertrophy exceeding 40% was achieved. Further subgroup analysis of patients with PVT, PHTN, previous chemotherapy, previous local ablative treatment, or previous hepatectomy was not feasible due to heterogeneous data patient into the studies. A case of post-TARE FLR hypertrophy is shown in Fig. 15.1.

15.4.4 Oncological Outcome

Regarding the oncological outcome of these studies, we found that 57 out of 360 patients (16%) developed tumor progression during a median follow-up (FU) period of 11 months (range: 1–49 months).

Tumor progression was reported in the majority of patients (42 patients) in the contralateral liver lobe whereas a total of 11 patients had progressive disease in the ipsilateral liver lobe and 3 patients suffered from distant extrahepatic metastases. Tumor response following radioembolization was analyzed in six studies (118 patients). According to response evaluation criteria in solid tumors (RECIST) criteria, complete and/or partial response was observed in 36 patients

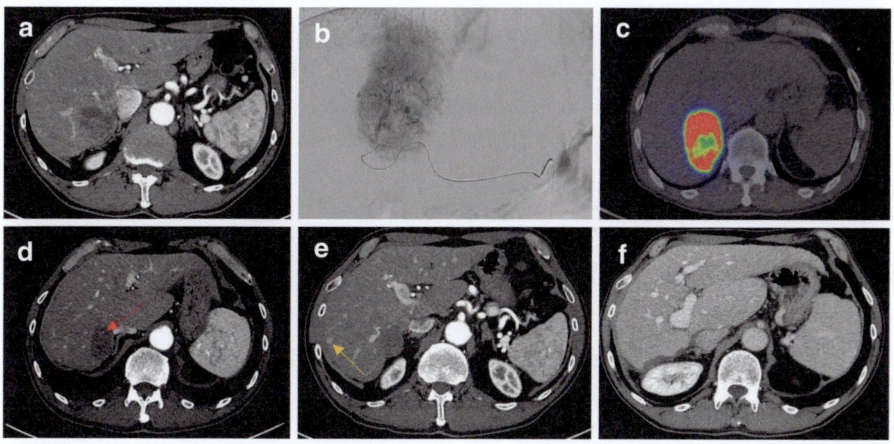

Fig. 15.1 (**a**) Seventy-year-old man with HCC in segments VII–VIII and an additional lesion in the caudate lobe (not shown). The patient was initially not a surgical candidate due to disease extension and insufficient future liver remnant (FLR). (**b**, **c**) The multidisciplinary board decided to proceed with selective ablative-dose TARE for the lesion in segment VII–VIII followed by systemic therapy with Atezolizumab–Bevacizumab. (**d**) One-year after TARE, local tumor progression was observed in the anterior portion of the treated tumor (red arrow) and (**e**) another satellite lesion appeared in the same segment (yellow arrow). At this point, the treated HCC mass was reduced in size and confined within the VII segment, the lesion in the caudate lobe was stable, and the left lobe remained disease free. (**f**) The patient subsequently underwent right dorsal sectorectomy with microwave ablation (MWA) of the caudate lesion. This approach was feasible due to the significant hypertrophy of the left and caudate lobes

(31%), stable disease in 65 patients (55%), and a total of 17 patients showed progressive disease (14%). According to the European Association for the Study of the Liver (EASL) and the World Health Organization (WHO) criteria, two studies (44 patients) reported data from tumor response: complete response was depicted in 9 patients, partial response in 14 patients, and stable disease in 21 patients [69, 74].

According to the WHO criteria, partial response was demonstrated in 11 patients, stable disease in 30 patients, and progressive disease in 3 patients. Cucchetti et al. [53] suggest that even if incomplete response is reached after radioembolization, a partial response may also be sufficient to disengage the tumor from normal vital structures, allowing for subsequent surgical resection.

15.4.5 Comparison of Techniques

Data from the literature [80–82] compared the different techniques to induce liver hypertrophy and concluded that although FLR hypertrophy is generally slower after radioembolization than PVE, TARE produces a high rate of tumor response.

This prolonged time of the radiation lobectomy could be a longer time for observation as a sort of "neoadjuvant radioembolization," which may facilitate a careful assessment of initially occult intrahepatic and extrahepatic disease while also providing an opportunity to consolidate disease.

Charles et al. [81] suggested that TARE in combination with PVE may be more advantageous than chemoembolization with PVE. They hypothesized that the smaller particle sizes used in radioembolization relative to chemoembolization allow for more distal and selective embolization. In addition, TARE + PVE is safer than chemoembolization in patients with PVT [83, 84]. Finally, they proposed that radioembolization + PVE may work synergistically in inducing FLR hypertrophy through radioembolization's atrophy of the treated liver lobe, thereby further promoting compensatory regeneration of the FLR segments [85].

15.4.6 Post-radioembolization Treatment and Complications

When we go to analyze post-TARE treatment and complications, a total of 326 patients in 12 studies disclosed TARE-related adverse effects as follows: fatigue (78 patients), abdominal pain (41 patients), hyperbilirubinemia (22 patients), fever without infection (9 patients), lack of appetite (8 patients), weight loss (5 patients), ascites (3 patients), encephalopathy (1 patients), leukopenia (1 patients), acute cholecystitis (1 patients), and pseudoaneurysm at the puncture site (1 patients).

Lewandowski et al. [74] were the only to grade the adverse effects in line with the Radiation-Lobectomy Clinical Toxicity (RLCT) grade.

In comparison to transarterial chemoembolization, a post-embolization syndrome or radioembolization-induced liver disease is rare [86]. In the literature, the incidence of radioembolization-induced liver disease (REILD) is up to 10% [87]. However, the definition of REILD is currently not well finalized and data of adverse effects is highly variable: globally the related hepatotoxicity was below 10% [88]. Four studies reported on postoperative complications after radioembolization following surgery according to Clavien–Dindo classification, showing a postoperative morbidity rate (Clavien–Dindo grade III–IVb) of 15% (16 patients) and a 3% of cases (3 patients) died postoperatively within 90 days after hepatectomy (Clavien–Dindo grade V) [69, 73, 74, 77].

15.4.7 Controversial Issues

A controversial issue is the optimal FLR volume for safe hepatectomy: an FLR and TLV ratio of 20–30% has been suggested as a threshold for patients with normal liver parenchyma and 40–45% for patients with liver cirrhosis [89]. More recently, the impact of radioembolization-induced contralateral liver hypertrophy has been assessed in two systematic reviews, including seven and eight studies, respectively [6, 64]. In both reviews, the small number of patients and the different time points of volume assessments resulted in a huge range of relative degrees of liver hypertrophy between 7–62% and 26–42%, respectively.

However, in the daily practice, the ratio of FLR and TLV rather than the relative degree of liver lobe hypertrophy is the indicator of a safe resectability. No differences in clinical response were reported regarding the need of larger injection volumes and subsequent higher microembolic effects for resin-based microspheres due to lower relative activity [90]. To report, radioembolization does not result in macrovascular embolization, suggesting that the liver lobe hypertrophy is probably due to the radiation effects [51, 67, 91]. Moreover, due to the lack of strong data, the impact of dose-dependent and activity-related hypertrophy effects of microspheres remains unclear.

15.5 Conclusion

The available literature shows a considerable degree of radioembolization-induced contralateral lobe hypertrophy with good tumor control even when subsequent surgery was performed. However, the missing of randomized trial and registry to collect data from different centers comparing radioembolization with standard therapies makes the role of radioembolization in the treatment algorithm of liver tumors unclear. Therefore, the promising potential of radioembolization in the multimodal approach of liver malignancies needs to be investigated. Multidisciplinary committees including expert hepatobiliary surgeons not only to judge the unresectability of liver malignancies but also the possibility of performing hepatectomy once downsizing of the tumor (as well as hypertrophy of the contralateral lobe) is achieved.

References

1. Belghiti J, Hiramatsu K, Benoist S, Massault PP, Sauvanet A, Farges O. Seven hundred forty-seven hepatectomies in the 1990s: an update to evaluate the actual risk of liver resection1. J Am Coll Surg. 2000;191:38–46.
2. Farges O, Belghiti J, Kianmanesh R, Marc Regimbeau J, Santoro R, Vilgrain V, Denys A, Sauvanet A. Portal vein embolization before right hepatectomy: prospective clinical trial. Ann Surg. 2003;237:208–17.
3. Salem R, Gabr A, Riaz A, et al. Institutional decision to adopt Y90 as primary treatment for hepatocellular carcinoma informed by a 1,000-patient 15-year experience. Hepatology. 2018;68:1429–40.
4. Cardarelli-Leite L, Chung J, Klass D, et al. Ablative Transarterial Radioembolization improves survival in patients with HCC and portal vein tumor thrombus. Cardiovasc Intervent Radiol. 2020;43:411–22.
5. Garlipp B, Amthauer H, Kupitz D, et al. The impact of unilateral 90Y-radioembolization on functional changes in the contralateral hepatic lobe: the prospective, open-label RadioEmbolization, Volumetry, and liver FuncTion measurements (REVoluTion) study. Ann Surg Open. 2021;2:e095.
6. Teo J-Y, Allen JC, Ng DC, Choo S-P, Tai DWM, Chang JPE, Cheah F-K, Chow PKH, Goh BKP. A systematic review of contralateral liver lobe hypertrophy after unilobar selective internal radiation therapy with Y90. HPB. 2016;18:7–12.
7. d'Abadie P, Hesse M, Louppe A, Lhommel R, Walrand S, Jamar F. Microspheres used in liver Radioembolization: from conception to clinical effects. Molecules. 2021;26:3966.
8. Tong AKT, Kao YH, Too CW, Chin KFW, Ng DCE, Chow PKH. Yttrium-90 hepatic radioembolization: clinical review and current techniques in interventional radiology and personalized dosimetry. Br J Radiol. 2016;89:20150943.
9. Stella M, Braat AJAT, Van Rooij R, De Jong HWAM, Lam MGEH. Holmium-166 Radioembolization: current status and future prospective. Cardiovasc Intervent Radiol. 2022;45:1634–45.
10. Smits MLJ, Elschot M, Van Den Bosch MAAJ, et al. In vivo dosimetry based on SPECT and MR imaging of^{166} Ho-microspheres for treatment of liver malignancies. J Nucl Med. 2013;54:2093–100.
11. Van De Maat GH, Seevinck PR, Elschot M, et al. MRI-based biodistribution assessment of holmium-166 poly(L-lactic acid) microspheres after radioembolisation. Eur Radiol. 2013;23:827–35.
12. Kennedy A, Coldwell D, Sangro B, Wasan H, Salem R. Radioembolization for the treatment of liver tumors: general principles. Am J Clin Oncol. 2012;35:91–9.
13. Weber M, Lam M, Chiesa C, et al. EANM procedure guideline for the treatment of liver cancer and liver metastases with intra-arterial radioactive compounds. Eur J Nucl Med Mol Imaging. 2022;49:1682–99.
14. Bozkurt M, Eldem G, Bozbulut UB, Bozkurt MF, Kılıçkap S, Peynircioğlu B, Çil B, Lay Ergün E, Volkan-Salanci B. Factors affecting the response to Y-90 microsphere therapy in the cholangiocarcinoma patients. Radiol Med (Torino). 2021;126:323–33.
15. Buettner S, Braat AJAT, Margonis GA, et al. Yttrium-90 Radioembolization in intrahepatic Cholangiocarcinoma: a multicenter retrospective analysis. J Vasc Interv Radiol. 2020;31:1035–1043.e2.
16. Cheng B, Villalobos A, Sethi I, Wagstaff W, Galt J, Brandon D, Schuster DM, Bercu Z, Majdalany B, Kokabi N. Determination of tumor dose response thresholds in patients with Chemorefractory intrahepatic Cholangiocarcinoma treated with resin and glass-based Y90 Radioembolization. Cardiovasc Intervent Radiol. 2021;44:1194–203.
17. Kallini JR, Gabr A, Thorlund K, Balijepalli C, Ayres D, Kanters S, Ebrahim S, Mills E, Lewandowski RJ, Salem R. Comparison of the adverse event profile of TheraSphere® with

SIR-spheres® for the treatment of Unresectable hepatocellular carcinoma: a systematic review. Cardiovasc Intervent Radiol. 2017;40:1033–43.
18. Liu DM, Salem R, Bui JT, et al. Angiographic considerations in patients undergoing liver-directed therapy. J Vasc Interv Radiol. 2005;16:911–35.
19. Kallini JR, Gabr A, Salem R, Lewandowski RJ. Transarterial Radioembolization with Yttrium-90 for the treatment of hepatocellular carcinoma. Adv Ther. 2016;33:699–714.
20. Louie JD, Kothary N, Kuo WT, Hwang GL, Hofmann LV, Goris ML, Iagaru AH, Sze DY. Incorporating cone-beam CT into the treatment planning for Yttrium-90 Radioembolization. J Vasc Interv Radiol. 2009;20:606–13.
21. Wong KM, Tan BS, Taneja M, Wong SY, Loke JS, Lin SE, Lo RH, Teo KB, Tay KH. Cone beam computed tomography for vascular interventional radiology procedures: early experience. Ann Acad Med Singap. 2011;40:308–14.
22. Grosser OS, Ruf J, Kupitz D, et al. Pharmacokinetics of ^{99m} Tc-MAA- and ^{99m} Tc-HSA-microspheres used in preradioembolization dosimetry: influence on the liver–lung shunt. J Nucl Med. 2016;57:925–7.
23. Sancho L, Rodriguez-Fraile M, Bilbao JI, Beorlegui Arteta C, Iñarrairaegui M, Moran V, Sangro B. Is a technetium-99m macroaggregated albumin scan essential in the workup for selective internal radiation therapy with Yttrium-90? An analysis of 532 patients. J Vasc Interv Radiol. 2017;28:1536–42.
24. Ilhan H, Goritschan A, Paprottka P, Jakobs TF, Fendler WP, Todica A, Bartenstein P, Hacker M, Haug AR. Predictive value of ^{99m} Tc-MAA SPECT for ^{90} Y-labeled resin microsphere distribution in Radioembolization of primary and secondary hepatic tumors. J Nucl Med. 2015;56:1654–60.
25. Riaz A, Gates VL, Atassi B, et al. Radiation segmentectomy: a novel approach to increase safety and efficacy of radioembolization. Int J Radiat Oncol Biol Phys. 2011;79:163–71.
26. Gabr A, Entezari P, Riaz A, Salem R, Lewandowski RJ. Contemporary techniques and applications of Radioembolization in patients with hepatocellular carcinoma. Adv Clin Radiol. 2020;2:113–25.
27. Miller FH, Lopes Vendrami C, Gabr A, Horowitz JM, Kelahan LC, Riaz A, Salem R, Lewandowski RJ. Evolution of Radioembolization in treatment of hepatocellular carcinoma: a pictorial review. Radiographics. 2021;41:1802–18.
28. Vouche M, Habib A, Ward TJ, et al. Unresectable solitary hepatocellular carcinoma not amenable to radiofrequency ablation: multicenter radiology-pathology correlation and survival of radiation segmentectomy. Hepatology. 2014;60:192–201.
29. Gabr A, Polineni P, Mouli SK, Riaz A, Lewandowski RJ, Salem R. Neoadjuvant radiation lobectomy as an alternative to portal vein embolization in hepatocellular carcinoma. Semin Nucl Med. 2019;49:197–203.
30. Garin E, Palard X, Rolland Y. Personalised dosimetry in Radioembolisation for HCC: impact on clinical outcome and on trial design. Cancer. 2020;12:1557.
31. Knight GM, Gordon AC, Gates V, Talwar A, Riaz A, Salem R, Lewandowski R. Evolution of personalized dosimetry for Radioembolization of hepatocellular carcinoma. J Vasc Interv Radiol. 2023;34:1214–25.
32. Webster LA, Villalobos A, Majdalany BS, Bercu ZL, Gandhi RT, Kokabi N. Standard radiation dosimetry models: what interventional radiologists need to know. Semin Interv Radiol. 2021;38:405–11.
33. Du Bois D, Du Bois EF. A formula to estimate the approximate surface area if height and weight be known. 1916. Nutr Burbank Los Angel Cty Calif. 1989;5:303–11. discussion 312–3
34. Kao YH, Tan EH, Ng CE, Goh SW. Clinical implications of the body surface area method versus partition model dosimetry for yttrium-90 radioembolization using resin microspheres: a technical review. Ann Nucl Med. 2011;25:455–61.
35. Grosser OS, Ulrich G, Furth C, Pech M, Ricke J, Amthauer H, Ruf J. Intrahepatic activity distribution in Radioembolization with Yttrium-90–labeled resin microspheres using the body surface area method—a less than perfect model. J Vasc Interv Radiol. 2015;26:1615–21.

36. Toohey RE, Stabin MG, Watson EE. The AAPM/RSNA physics tutorial for residents: internal radiation dosimetry: principles and applications (CME available in print version and on RSNA link). Radiographics. 2000;20:533–46.
37. Sarwar A, Kudla A, Weinstein JL, Ali A, Malik R, Bullock A, Khwaja KO, Curry M, Faintuch S, Ahmed M. Yttrium-90 radioembolization using MIRD dosimetry with resin microspheres. Eur Radiol. 2021;31:1316–24.
38. Gulec SA, Mesoloras G, Stabin M. Dosimetric techniques in 90Y-microsphere therapy of liver cancer: the MIRD equations for dose calculations. J Nucl Med Off Publ Soc Nucl Med. 2006;47:1209–11.
39. Gnesin S, Canetti L, Adib S, Cherbuin N, Silva Monteiro M, Bize P, Denys A, Prior JO, Baechler S, Boubaker A. Partition model–Based^{99m} Tc-MAA SPECT/CT predictive dosimetry compared with^{90} Y TOF PET/CT Posttreatment dosimetry in Radioembolization of hepatocellular carcinoma: a quantitative agreement comparison. J Nucl Med. 2016;57:1672–8.
40. Thomas MA, Mahvash A, Abdelsalam M, Kaseb AO, Kappadath SC. Planning dosimetry for^{90} Y radioembolization with glass microspheres: evaluating the fidelity of^{99m} Tc-MAA and partition model predictions. Med Phys. 2020;47:5333–42.
41. Di Gaeta E, Olivieri M, Savi A, et al. Radioembolization for hepatocellular carcinoma: a comparison on dual-phase cone-beam CT, contrast-enhanced CT (CECT) and 99mTc-macroaggregated albumin-SPECT/CT in predicting final distribution volumes and dosimetry of the post-embolization 90Y PET/CT. Radiol Med (Torino). 2024; https://doi.org/10.1007/s11547-024-01946-0.
42. Mikell JK, Mahvash A, Siman W, Baladandayuthapani V, Mourtada F, Kappadath SC. Selective internal radiation therapy with Yttrium-90 glass microspheres: biases and uncertainties in absorbed dose calculations between clinical dosimetry models. Int J Radiat Oncol. 2016;96:888–96.
43. Meyers N, Jadoul A, Bernard C, Delwaide J, Lamproye A, Detry O, Honoré P, Gerard L, Hustinx R. Inter-observer variability of 90Y PET/CT dosimetry in hepatocellular carcinoma after glass microspheres transarterial radioembolization. EJNMMI Phys. 2020;7:29.
44. Vilgrain V, Pereira H, Assenat E, et al. Efficacy and safety of selective internal radiotherapy with yttrium-90 resin microspheres compared with sorafenib in locally advanced and inoperable hepatocellular carcinoma (SARAH): an open-label randomised controlled phase 3 trial. Lancet Oncol. 2017;18:1624–36.
45. Chow PKH, Gandhi M, Tan S-B, et al. SIRveNIB: selective internal radiation therapy versus Sorafenib in Asia-Pacific patients with hepatocellular carcinoma. J Clin Oncol. 2018;36:1913–21.
46. Ricke J, Klümpen HJ, Amthauer H, et al. Impact of combined selective internal radiation therapy and sorafenib on survival in advanced hepatocellular carcinoma. J Hepatol. 2019;71:1164–74.
47. Garin E, Tselikas L, Guiu B, et al. Personalised versus standard dosimetry approach of selective internal radiation therapy in patients with locally advanced hepatocellular carcinoma (DOSISPHERE-01): a randomised, multicentre, open-label phase 2 trial. Lancet Gastroenterol Hepatol. 2021;6:17–29.
48. Lam M, Garin E, Maccauro M, et al. A global evaluation of advanced dosimetry in transarterial radioembolization of hepatocellular carcinoma with Yttrium-90: the TARGET study. Eur J Nucl Med Mol Imaging. 2022;49:3340–52.
49. Najafi A, Binkert CA. Transarterial Radioembolization to impact liver volumetry: when and how. Cardiovasc Intervent Radiol. 2022;45:1646–50.
50. Grisanti F, Prieto E, Bastidas JF, Sancho L, Rodrigo P, Beorlegui C, Iñarrairaegui M, Bilbao JI, Sangro B, Rodríguez-Fraile M. 3D voxel-based dosimetry to predict contralateral hypertrophy and an adequate future liver remnant after lobar radioembolization. Eur J Nucl Med Mol Imaging. 2021;48:3048–57.
51. Jakobs TF, Hoffmann R-T, Dehm K, Trumm C, Stemmler H-J, Tatsch K, La Fougere C, Murthy R, Helmberger TK, Reiser MF. Hepatic Yttrium-90 radioembolization of chemotherapy-refractory colorectal cancer liver metastases. J Vasc Interv Radiol. 2008;19:1187–95.

52. Gaba RC, Lewandowski RJ, Kulik LM, et al. Radiation lobectomy: preliminary findings of hepatic volumetric response to lobar Yttrium-90 Radioembolization. Ann Surg Oncol. 2009;16:1587–96.
53. Cucchetti A, Cappelli A, Ercolani G, Mosconi C, Cescon M, Golfieri R, Pinna AD. Selective internal radiation therapy (SIRT) as conversion therapy for unresectable primary liver malignancies. Liver Cancer. 2016;5:303–11.
54. Soydal C, Kucuk ON, Bilgic S, Ibis E. Radioembolization with 90Y resin microspheres for intrahepatic cholangiocellular carcinoma: prognostic factors. Ann Nucl Med. 2016;30:29–34.
55. Filippi L, Pelle G, Cianni R, Scopinaro F, Bagni O. Change in total lesion glycolysis and clinical outcome after 90Y radioembolization in intrahepatic cholangiocarcinoma. Nucl Med Biol. 2015;42:59–64.
56. Camacho JC, Kokabi N, Xing M, Prajapati HJ, El-Rayes B, Kim HS. Modified response evaluation criteria in solid tumors and European Association for the Study of the liver criteria using delayed-phase imaging at an early time point predict survival in patients with Unresectable intrahepatic Cholangiocarcinoma following Yttrium-90 Radioembolization. J Vasc Interv Radiol. 2014;25:256–65.
57. Rafi S, Piduru SM, El-Rayes B, Kauh JS, Kooby DA, Sarmiento JM, Kim HS. Yttrium-90 radioembolization for unresectable standard-chemorefractory intrahepatic Cholangiocarcinoma: survival, efficacy, and safety study. Cardiovasc Intervent Radiol. 2013;36:440–8.
58. Mouli S, Memon K, Baker T, Benson AB, Mulcahy MF, Gupta R, Ryu RK, Salem R, Lewandowski RJ. Yttrium-90 radioembolization for intrahepatic cholangiocarcinoma: safety, response, and survival analysis. J Vasc Interv Radiol. 2013;24:1227–34.
59. Hoffmann R-T, Paprottka PM, Schön A, et al. Transarterial hepatic Yttrium-90 Radioembolization in patients with Unresectable intrahepatic Cholangiocarcinoma: factors associated with prolonged survival. Cardiovasc Intervent Radiol. 2012;35:105–16.
60. Haug AR, Heinemann V, Bruns CJ, Hoffmann R, Jakobs T, Bartenstein P, Hacker M. 18F-FDG PET independently predicts survival in patients with cholangiocellular carcinoma treated with 90Y microspheres. Eur J Nucl Med Mol Imaging. 2011;38:1037–45.
61. Saxena A, Bester L, Chua TC, Chu FC, Morris DL. Yttrium-90 radiotherapy for unresectable intrahepatic cholangiocarcinoma: a preliminary assessment of this novel treatment option. Ann Surg Oncol. 2010;17:484–91.
62. Ibrahim SM, Mulcahy MF, Lewandowski RJ, Sato KT, Ryu RK, Masterson EJ, Newman SB, Benson A, Omary RA, Salem R. Treatment of unresectable cholangiocarcinoma using yttrium-90 microspheres: results from a pilot study. Cancer. 2008;113:2119–28.
63. Gulec SA, Pennington K, Hall M, Fong Y. Preoperative Y-90 microsphere selective internal radiation treatment for tumor downsizing and future liver remnant recruitment: a novel approach to improving the safety of major hepatic resections. World J Surg Oncol. 2009;7:6.
64. Braat MNGJA, Samim M, Van Den Bosch MAAJ, Lam MGEH. The role of 90Y-radioembolization in downstaging primary and secondary hepatic malignancies: a systematic review. Clin Translat Imaging. 2016;4:283–95.
65. Birgin E, Rasbach E, Seyfried S, Rathmann N, Diehl SJ, Schoenberg SO, Reissfelder C, Rahbari NN. Contralateral liver hypertrophy and oncological outcome following Radioembolization with 90Y-microspheres: a systematic review. Cancer. 2020;12:294.
66. Teo JY, Allen JC, Ng DCE, et al. Prospective study to determine early hypertrophy of the contra-lateral liver lobe after unilobar, Yttrium-90, selective internal radiation therapy in patients with hepatocellular carcinoma. Surgery. 2018;163:1008–13.
67. Edeline J, Lenoir L, Boudjema K, et al. Volumetric changes after 90Y Radioembolization for hepatocellular carcinoma in cirrhosis: an option to portal vein embolization in a preoperative setting? Ann Surg Oncol. 2013;20:2518–25.
68. Fernández-Ros N, Silva N, Bilbao JI, Iñarrairaegui M, Benito A, D'Avola D, Rodriguez M, Rotellar F, Pardo F, Sangro B. Partial liver volume radioembolization induces hypertrophy in the spared hemiliver and no major signs of portal hypertension. HPB. 2014;16:243–9.

69. Gabr A, Abouchaleh N, Ali R, Baker T, Caicedo J, Katariya N, Abecassis M, Riaz A, Lewandowski RJ, Salem R. Outcomes of surgical resection after Radioembolization for hepatocellular carcinoma. J Vasc Interv Radiol. 2018;29:1502–1510.e1.
70. Garlipp B, De Baere T, Damm R, et al. Left-liver hypertrophy after therapeutic right-liver radioembolization is substantial but less than after portal vein embolization. Hepatology. 2014;59:1864–73.
71. Goebel J, Sulke M, Lazik-Palm A, Goebel T, Dechêne A, Bellendorf A, Mueller S, Umutlu L, Theysohn J. Factors associated with contralateral liver hypertrophy after unilateral radioembolization for hepatocellular carcinoma. PLoS One. 2017;12:e0181488.
72. Vouche M, Lewandowski RJ, Atassi R, et al. Radiation lobectomy: time-dependent analysis of future liver remnant volume in unresectable liver cancer as a bridge to resection. J Hepatol. 2013;59:1029–36.
73. Justinger C, Kouladouros K, Gärtner D, Tatsch K, Reimer P, Rüdiger T, Binnenhei M, Bentz M, Schön MR. Liver resection after selective internal radiotherapy (SIRT): proof of concept, initial survival, and safety. J Surg Oncol. 2015;112:436–42.
74. Lewandowski RJ, Donahue L, Chokechanachaisakul A, Kulik L, Mouli S, Caicedo J, Abecassis M, Fryer J, Salem R, Baker T. ^{90}Y radiation lobectomy: outcomes following surgical resection in patients with hepatic tumors and small future liver remnant volumes. J Surg Oncol. 2016;114:99–105.
75. Orcutt ST, Abuodeh Y, Naghavi A, Frakes J, Hoffe S, Kis B, Anaya DA. Kinetic analysis of contralateral liver hypertrophy after radioembolization of primary and metastatic liver tumors. Surgery. 2018;163:1020–7.
76. Palard X, Edeline J, Rolland Y, et al. Dosimetric parameters predicting contralateral liver hypertrophy after unilobar radioembolization of hepatocellular carcinoma. Eur J Nucl Med Mol Imaging. 2018;45:392–401.
77. Rayar M, Sulpice L, Edeline J, Garin E, Levi Sandri GB, Meunier B, Boucher E, Boudjema K. Intra-arterial Yttrium-90 Radioembolization combined with systemic chemotherapy is a promising method for downstaging unresectable huge intrahepatic Cholangiocarcinoma to surgical treatment. Ann Surg Oncol. 2015;22:3102–8.
78. Teo JY, Goh BKP, Cheah FK, et al. Underlying liver disease influences volumetric changes in the spared hemiliver after selective internal radiation therapy with^{90}Y in patients with hepatocellular carcinoma. J Dig Dis. 2014;15:444–50.
79. Theysohn JM, Ertle J, Müller S, Schlaak JF, Nensa F, Sipilae S, Bockisch A, Lauenstein TC. Hepatic volume changes after lobar selective internal radiation therapy (SIRT) of hepatocellular carcinoma. Clin Radiol. 2014;69:172–8.
80. Kim D, Cornman-Homonoff J, Madoff DC. Preparing for liver surgery with "alphabet soup": PVE, ALPPS, TAE-PVE, LVD and RL. Hepatobiliary Surg Nutr. 2020;9:136–51.
81. Charles J, Nezami N, Loya M, Shube S, Davis C, Hoots G, Shaikh J. Portal vein embolization: rationale, techniques, and outcomes to maximize remnant liver hypertrophy with a focus on contemporary strategies. Life. 2023;13:279.
82. Ahmed A, Stauffer JA, LeGout JD, Burns J, Croome K, Paz-Fumagalli R, Frey G, Toskich B. The use of neoadjuvant lobar radioembolization prior to major hepatic resection for malignancy results in a low rate of post hepatectomy liver failure. J Gastrointest Oncol. 2021;12:751–61.
83. Kulik LM, Carr BI, Mulcahy MF, et al. Safety and efficacy of 90Y radiotherapy for hepatocellular carcinoma with and without portal vein thrombosis. Hepatology. 2008;47:71–81.
84. Riaz A, Lewandowski RJ, Kulik LM, Mulcahy MF, Sato KT, Ryu RK, Omary RA, Salem R. Complications following Radioembolization with Yttrium-90 microspheres: a comprehensive literature review. J Vasc Interv Radiol. 2009;20:1121–30.
85. Salem R, Mazzaferro V, Sangro B. Yttrium 90 radioembolization for the treatment of hepatocellular carcinoma: biological lessons, current challenges, and clinical perspectives. Hepatology. 2013;58:2188–97.

86. Sangro B, Gil-Alzugaray B, Rodriguez J, Sola I, Martinez-Cuesta A, Viudez A, Chopitea A, Iñarrairaegui M, Arbizu J, Bilbao JI. Liver disease induced by radioembolization of liver tumors: description and possible risk factors. Cancer. 2008;112:1538–46.
87. Gil-Alzugaray B, Chopitea A, Iñarrairaegui M, et al. Prognostic factors and prevention of radioembolization-induced liver disease. Hepatology. 2013;57:1078–87.
88. Braat MNGJA, Van Erpecum KJ, Zonnenberg BA, Van Den Bosch MAJ, Lam MGEH. Radioembolization-induced liver disease: a systematic review. Eur J Gastroenterol Hepatol. 2017;29:144–52.
89. Khan AS, Garcia-Aroz S, Ansari MA, Atiq SM, Senter-Zapata M, Fowler K, Doyle MB, Chapman WC. Assessment and optimization of liver volume before major hepatic resection: current guidelines and a narrative review. Int J Surg. 2018;52:74–81.
90. Van Der Gucht A, Jreige M, Denys A, et al. Resin versus glass microspheres for ^{90}Y transarterial radioembolization: comparing survival in unresectable hepatocellular carcinoma using pretreatment partition model dosimetry. J Nucl Med. 2017;58:1334–40.
91. Sato K, Lewandowski RJ, Bui JT, et al. Treatment of Unresectable primary and metastatic liver cancer with Yttrium-90 microspheres (TheraSphere®): assessment of hepatic arterial embolization. Cardiovasc Intervent Radiol. 2006;29:522–9.

Part IV

Liver Hypertrophy in Different Settings of Disease

Rationale and Techniques for Liver Hypertrophy in Colorectal Liver Metastases

16

Ernesto Sparrelid

16.1 Introduction

A majority of patients with colorectal liver metastases (CRLM)—about 80%—are considered to be unresectable when they are first diagnosed [1]. Selecting the best treatment strategy for these patients presents significant challenges in modern hepatobiliary clinical praxis. This is partly due to the lack of standardized criteria for determining resectability, but also caused by the fact that this field has been rapidly evolving during the last decades with the introduction of several new treatment concepts. Even among highly experienced liver surgeons, there is considerable disagreement regarding these definitions and the optimal treatment options [2], and there is also a risk that patients are never offered a curative intent treatment if not discussed at a hepatobiliary multidisciplinary team conference [3]. Since complete local treatment of CRLM is the only therapeutic option with the potential of long-term survival or cure, efforts are being put into converting unresectable patients to resection candidates. The concept of resectability has evolved substantially over the past decades, largely due to our enhanced understanding of liver regeneration and the development of several techniques for modulating the future liver remnant (FLR). In this chapter, several aspects on these techniques and associated considerations with specific regards to patients with initially unresectable CRLM will be discussed.

E. Sparrelid (✉)
Division of Surgery and Oncology, Department of Clinical Science, Intervention and Technology, Karolinska Institutet, Karolinska University Hospital, Stockholm, Sweden
e-mail: ernesto.sparrelid@ki.se

L. Aldrighetti et al. (eds.), *Liver Regeneration Techniques In Hepatic Surgery*,
https://doi.org/10.1007/978-3-032-10997-2_16

16.2 Surgery and Other Techniques for Modulation of the FLR in Patients with CRLM

16.2.1 Aspects on FLR and PHLF

Emanating from the setting of CRLM, there has been a paradigm shift in the last decades regarding the assessment of resectability, which in turn has affected the entire field of hepatobiliary surgery. In the past, tumor factors such as size and number of metastases, as well as bilobar distribution, decided if a patient was considered resectable [4]. Currently, however, the limit of resectability is defined by the amount of functional liver left behind after a planned resection [5]. Even if the level of evidence on the safe extent of resection is not the highest, many observational studies report increased post-hepatectomy liver failure (PHLF) if the volume of remaining liver after a resection is small [6]. In the setting of CRLM with an otherwise healthy background liver, studies support resection of about 70–80% as generally being safe, leaving behind an FLR of only 20–30% [7]. However, in modern treatment of CRLM, many patients will have received neoadjuvant chemotherapy prior to resection, leading to chemotherapy-associated liver injury and impaired liver function. Also here observational studies and expert consensus recommend an FLR of over 30% in order to avoid PHLF [8]. Even if PHLF is less frequent after resection for CRLM (compared to primary hepatobiliary tumors), it is still the main reason for postoperative mortality also for these patients, making it the highest priority to avoid this feared complication for which we still lack effective treatment [9].

16.2.2 Classical Two-Stage Hepatectomy and the Addition of Portal Vein Occlusion

The effort to increase resectability in CRLM has been the main driver of the development of two-stage hepatectomies. Initially, two-stage hepatectomy was introduced as a concept to enable resection in patients with bilobar CRLM and metastases in the FLR where the remaining liver was considered inadequately small for a one-stage procedure [10]. Here, the regenerative ability of the liver was used by resecting all lesions in the FLR and waiting for a general hypertrophy (also in the FLR) before performing the completion hepatectomy. Soon after, this concept was combined with selective portal vein occlusion (by either ligation or embolization) to induce more hypertrophy in the FLR [11]. Even if no strong evidence supports the superiority of portal vein embolization (PVE) over ligation, PVE is today the main method for inducing hypertrophy of the FLR in all settings, including CRLM, and can be performed in both two-stage hepatectomy and prior to one-stage procedures [12].

16.2.3 Associating Liver Partition and Portal Vein Ligation for Staged Hepatectomy

After its initial hype, associating liver partition and portal vein ligation for staged hepatectomy has recently been used more selectively and some even completely abandoned this technique due to high morbidity and mortality [13]. However, studies demonstrated lower morbidity and mortality when applied to patients with CRLM [14], and the only randomized controlled trials have also been performed in this subset of patients [15]. To date, no FLR modulation technique is superior to associating liver partition and portal vein ligation for staged hepatectomy in terms of speed and degree of hypertrophy, as well as resectability rates.

16.2.4 Combined Portal and Hepatic Vein Embolization

Even if the described high morbidity (mainly PHLF) and mortality associated with associating liver partition and portal vein ligation for staged hepatectomy is lower in patients with CRLM, and in parity with many studies on TSH, efforts have been made to find alternatives to this procedure. One is the simultaneous combination of selective PVE and hepatic vein embolization (PVE/HVE), demonstrating increased and more rapid hypertrophy compared to PVE alone in observational studies [16]. This concept is currently being investigated in several prospective trials including only patients with CRLM (ClinicalTrials.gov ID: NCT05428735) [17].

16.2.5 Parenchymal-Sparing Resections

Another concept that is being employed increasingly in patients with CRLM is parenchymal-sparing surgery [18]. This method is preferred by many hepatobiliary surgeons to enable increased resectability, but mainly because up to 70% of the patients resected for CRLM will experience recurrence [19] and performing a major hepatectomy many times precludes subsequent additional resections. Some dedicated proponents of this strategy have further pushed the technical limits of this approach, enabling very advanced parenchymal resections and claiming that major hepatectomies are rarely needed, and hence neither preoperative modulation of the FLR [20].

16.3 The Effect of Chemotherapy in Unresectable CRLM with Modulation of the FLR

Previously, arguments were raised against administration of chemotherapy shortly before or after PVE due to its claimed hampering effect on hypertrophy of the FLR. Even if the results in several studies are conflicting, many recent reports do not support this apprehension and claim, not only that hypertrophy is unaffected by periprocedural chemotherapy, but also that progression of the metastases is stopped by administrating chemotherapy after PVE, while waiting for its hypertrophic effect [21]. This concept of administrating chemotherapy after PVE has been challenged by other studies, demonstrating that the effect of preprocedural chemotherapy seem to remain after PVE, without support of growing metastases in the waiting period [22].

Regarding the potential effect of preoperative treatment in inducing chemotherapy-induced liver injury, there is a lack of consensus in several aspects. One is whether it should be administered close to the resection as mentioned above, another is what thresholds that should be applied depending on the extent of presumed liver injury. Most apply the rule of thumb that an FLR of more than 30% should be aimed for [8], but others claim the need of an even higher FLR (about 40%), and some disregard FLR volume completely and opt for functional assessment solely [23]. In the recently published multi-societal consensus guidelines on preoperative assessment of liver function prior to liver surgery, some kind of liver function test is recommended prior to major resections in patients subjected to preoperative chemotherapy [24]. However, many still employ only volumetry of the FLR (if even that) as the main determinant of resectability.

16.4 Ablation

The use of thermal ablation in CRLM has not been as strongly supported as its use to treat small hepatocellular carcinoma, and hence resection has remained the mainstay in the treatment of CRLM. In recent years, several observational studies have reported promising outcome after microwave ablation with curative intent for CRLM. Recurrence rates are indeed still higher than for resection, but overall survival seem to be equal [25]. This is further supported in the just published randomized controlled trial COLLISION, challenging the assumption that ablation is inferior to resection as treatment for small CRLM [26]. When patients present with extensive bilobar distribution of CRLM, combining thermal ablation with resection can potentially preserve the FLR and have been reported to achieve 5-year overall survival of 56%, at least comparable to that of a two-stage hepatectomy but with improved perioperative outcomes [27]. A sequential treatment strategy has also been proposed, with planned incomplete resection followed by postoperative image-guided completion ablation of intentionally untreated metastases, potentially providing improved local tumor control compared to intraoperative ultrasound-guided ablations [28].

16.5 Additional Considerations and Strategies in Bilobar and Synchronous Disease

In bilobar disease, the most described approach is to use two-stage hepatectomy with clearance of the FLR metastases in the first stage (combined with PVE), and then complete resection in the second stage after hypertrophy of the FLR. However, as we have seen above, this concept is being challenged. An additional strategy is to use preoperative PVE even in the presence of bilobar disease with metastases in the FLR, and then performed a one-stage hepatectomy with local resections in the FLR, thus sparing the patient one surgical procedure. In one small observational study reporting the results of this strategy, the metastases in the FLR did not grow after PVE and could be resected at the subsequent one-stage procedure [22]. This concept is currently being investigated in a Nordic multicenter setting (ClinicalTrials.gov ID: NCT04182386).

Another consideration is how to handle the primary tumor, since extensive CRLM are almost always a synchronous disease. In the recent multi-societal consensus guidelines, synchronous resection of both primary tumor and liver metastases are recommended only if the liver resection is minor [29], excluding all patients discussed in this chapter from being treated in the bowel and liver simultaneously. Another claim that this could be challenged in selected patients, where major hepatectomy can safely be performed together with resection of the primary colorectal tumor [30].

References

1. Adam R, Wicherts DA, de Haas RJ, Ciacio O, Levi F, Paule B, et al. Patients with initially unresectable colorectal liver metastases: is there a possibility of cure? J Clin Oncol. 2009;27(11):1829–35.
2. Ignatavicius P, Oberkofler CE, Chapman WC, DeMatteo RP, Clary BM, D'Angelica MI, et al. Choices of therapeutic strategies for colorectal liver metastases among expert liver surgeons: a throw of the dice? Ann Surg. 2020;272(5):715–22.
3. Young AL, Adair R, Culverwell A, Guthrie JA, Botterill ID, Toogood GJ, et al. Variation in referral practice for patients with colorectal cancer liver metastases. Br J Surg. 2013;100(12):1627–32.
4. Ekberg H, Tranberg KG, Andersson R, Lundstedt C, Hagerstrand I, Ranstam J, et al. Determinants of survival in liver resection for colorectal secondaries. Br J Surg. 1986;73(9):727–31.
5. Pawlik TM, Schulick RD, Choti MA. Expanding criteria for resectability of colorectal liver metastases. Oncologist. 2008;13(1):51–64.
6. Shoup M, Gonen M, D'Angelica M, Jarnagin WR, DeMatteo RP, Schwartz LH, et al. Volumetric analysis predicts hepatic dysfunction in patients undergoing major liver resection. J Gastrointest Surg. 2003;7(3):325–30.
7. Kishi Y, Abdalla EK, Chun YS, Zorzi D, Madoff DC, Wallace MJ, et al. Three hundred and one consecutive extended right hepatectomies: evaluation of outcome based on systematic liver volumetry. Ann Surg. 2009;250(4):540–8.
8. Abdalla EK, Adam R, Bilchik AJ, Jaeck D, Vauthey JN, Mahvi D. Improving resectability of hepatic colorectal metastases: expert consensus statement. Ann Surg Oncol. 2006;13(10):1271–80.

9. Baumgartner R, Gilg S, Bjornsson B, Hasselgren K, Ghorbani P, Sauter C, et al. Impact of post-hepatectomy liver failure on morbidity and short- and long-term survival after major hepatectomy. BJS Open. 2022;6(4)
10. Adam R, Laurent A, Azoulay D, Castaing D, Bismuth H. Two-stage hepatectomy: a planned strategy to treat irresectable liver tumors. Ann Surg. 2000;232(6):777–85.
11. Jaeck D, Bachellier P, Nakano H, Oussoultzoglou E, Weber JC, Wolf P, et al. One or two-stage hepatectomy combined with portal vein embolization for initially nonresectable colorectal liver metastases. Am J Surg. 2003;185(3):221–9.
12. Imai K, Allard MA, Baba H, Adam R. Optimal patient selection for successful two-stage hepatectomy of bilateral colorectal liver metastases. Ann Gastroenterol Surg. 2021;5(5):634–8.
13. Schnitzbauer AA, Lang SA, Goessmann H, Nadalin S, Baumgart J, Farkas SA, et al. Right portal vein ligation combined with in situ splitting induces rapid left lateral liver lobe hypertrophy enabling 2-staged extended right hepatic resection in small-for-size settings. Ann Surg. 2012;255(3):405–14.
14. Schadde E, Raptis DA, Schnitzbauer AA, Ardiles V, Tschuor C, Lesurtel M, et al. Prediction of mortality after ALPPS Stage-1: an analysis of 320 patients from the international ALPPS registry. Ann Surg. 2015;262(5):780–5. discussion 5–6
15. Sandstrom P, Rosok BI, Sparrelid E, Larsen PN, Larsson AL, Lindell G, et al. ALPPS improves resectability compared with conventional two-stage hepatectomy in patients with advanced colorectal liver metastasis: results from a Scandinavian multicenter randomized controlled trial (LIGRO trial). Ann Surg. 2018;267(5):833–40.
16. Guiu B, Chevallier P, Denys A, Delhom E, Pierredon-Foulongne MA, Rouanet P, et al. Simultaneous trans-hepatic portal and hepatic vein embolization before major hepatectomy: the liver venous deprivation technique. Eur Radiol. 2016;26(12):4259–67.
17. Korenblik R, Olij B, Aldrighetti LA, Hilal MA, Ahle M, Arslan B, et al. Dragon 1 protocol manuscript: training, accreditation, implementation and safety evaluation of portal and hepatic vein embolization (PVE/HVE) to accelerate future liver remnant (FLR) hypertrophy. Cardiovasc Intervent Radiol. 2022;45(9):1391–8.
18. Gold JS, Are C, Kornprat P, Jarnagin WR, Gonen M, Fong Y, et al. Increased use of parenchymal-sparing surgery for bilateral liver metastases from colorectal cancer is associated with improved mortality without change in oncologic outcome: trends in treatment over time in 440 patients. Ann Surg. 2008;247(1):109–17.
19. Buisman FE, Galjart B, van der Stok EP, Balachandran VP, Boerner T, Drebin JA, et al. Recurrence patterns after resection of colorectal liver metastasis are modified by perioperative systemic chemotherapy. World J Surg. 2020;44(3):876–86.
20. Torzilli G. Parenchyma-sparing vessel-guided major hepatectomy: nonsense or new paradigm in liver surgery? Br J Surg. 2021;108(2):109–11.
21. Fischer C, Melstrom LG, Arnaoutakis D, Jarnagin W, Brown K, D'Angelica M, et al. Chemotherapy after portal vein embolization to protect against tumor growth during liver hypertrophy before hepatectomy. JAMA Surg. 2013;148(12):1103–8.
22. Spelt L, Sparrelid E, Isaksson B, Andersson RG, Sturesson C. Tumour growth after portal vein embolization with pre-procedural chemotherapy for colorectal liver metastases. HPB (Oxford). 2015;17(6):529–35.
23. Olthof PB, Arntz P, Truant S, El Amrani M, Dasari BVM, Tomassini F, et al. Hepatobiliary scintigraphy to predict postoperative liver failure after major liver resection; a multicenter cohort study in 547 patients. HPB (Oxford). 2023;25(4):417–24.
24. Primavesi F, Maglione M, Cipriani F, Denecke T, Oberkofler CE, Starlinger P, et al. E-AHPBA-ESSO-ESSR Innsbruck consensus guidelines for preoperative liver function assessment before hepatectomy. Br J Surg. 2023;110(10):1331–47.
25. Tinguely P, Ruiter SJS, Engstrand J, de Haas RJ, Nilsson H, Candinas D, et al. A prospective multicentre trial on survival after microwave ablation VErsus resection for resectable colorectal liver metastases (MAVERRIC). Eur J Cancer. 2023;187:65–76.
26. van der Lei S, Puijk RS, Dijkstra M, Schulz HH, Vos DJW, De Vries JJJ, et al. Thermal ablation versus surgical resection of small-size colorectal liver metastases (COLLISION): an international, randomised, controlled, phase 3 non-inferiority trial. Lancet Oncol. 2025;26:187.

27. Karanicolas PJ, Jarnagin WR, Gonen M, Tuorto S, Allen PJ, DeMatteo RP, et al. Long-term outcomes following tumor ablation for treatment of bilateral colorectal liver metastases. JAMA Surg. 2013;148(7):597–601.
28. Okuno M, Kawaguchi Y, De Bellis M, Vega EA, Huang SY, Ahrar K, et al. A new sequential treatment strategy for multiple colorectal liver metastases: planned incomplete resection and postoperative completion ablation for intentionally-untreated tumors under guidance of cross-sectional imaging. Eur J Surg Oncol. 2021;47(2):311–6.
29. Siriwardena AK, Serrablo A, Fretland AA, Wigmore SJ, Ramia-Angel JM, Malik HZ, et al. Multisocietal European consensus on the terminology, diagnosis, and management of patients with synchronous colorectal cancer and liver metastases: an E-AHPBA consensus in partnership with ESSO, ESCP, ESGAR, and CIRSE. Br J Surg. 2023;110(9):1161–70.
30. Sijberden JP, Zimmitti G, Conci S, Russolillo N, Masetti M, Cipriani F, et al. Simultaneous resection of colorectal cancer and synchronous liver metastases: what determines the risk of unfavorable outcomes? An international multicenter retrospective cohort study. Int J Surg. 2023;109(3):244–54.

Rationale and Techniques for Liver Hypertrophy in Hepatocellular Carcinoma

17

Miu-Yee Chan and Albert Chi-Yan Chan

17.1 Introduction

Liver regeneration is a complex biological process crucial for maintaining hepatic homeostasis, particularly in the context of liver diseases such as hepatocellular carcinoma (HCC). The liver possesses a remarkable ability to regenerate in response to injury, a feature that is both an advantage and a challenge in the management of HCC. Understanding the various techniques employed to induce liver hypertrophy is essential for developing effective therapeutic strategies for patients with HCC.

This chapter will explore the rationale for inducing hypertrophy in the setting of HCC and the various techniques currently utilized in clinical practice. By integrating insights from recent research and clinical studies, we aim to provide a comprehensive overview of how liver regeneration strategies can be optimized to improve outcomes for patients with HCC.

17.2 Challenges of Liver Regeneration in Patients with Hepatocellular Carcinoma

Unlike liver remnant augmentation in other pathologies such as colorectal liver metastases, patients with HCC often suffer from concomitant chronic hepatitis to various degrees. Cirrhotic liver is known to have less predictable results in liver regeneration or hypertrophy.

Supplementary Information The online version contains supplementary material available at https://doi.org/10.1007/978-3-032-10997-2_17.

M.-Y. Chan · A. C.-Y. Chan (✉)
Division of Hepatobiliary and Pancreatic Surgery and Liver Transplantation, Department of Surgery, The University of Hong Kong, Hong Kong, China
e-mail: acchan@hku.hk

L. Aldrighetti et al. (eds.), *Liver Regeneration Techniques In Hepatic Surgery*,
https://doi.org/10.1007/978-3-032-10997-2_17

Cirrhosis is a diffuse fibrosing condition secondary to liver injury, which is usually a low-grade injury [1]. As the injury becomes chronic, the parenchyma is overtaken by a meshwork of fibrosing tissue made up of collagen and elastin fibers [2], thus hindering complete resolution of injury and regeneration.

Albeit in a lesser extent, it is possible for the cirrhotic liver to grow to a certain degree so that resection is considered feasible and safe. Vennarecci et al. [3] reported a median future liver remnant (FLR) volume increase was 18.7% within 1 week after the first step of ALPPS and 38.6% after the second stage. In another series studied by D'Haese et al. [4], patients with HCC were compared with patients with colorectal liver metastases (CRLM). It was shown that although not as much as patients with CRLM, patients with HCC does have significant increase in FLR volume (46% vs. 76%; $p < 0.001$). It was also demonstrated that hypertrophy correlated directly with degree of fibrosis. The more severe the fibrosis, the less percentage of hypertrophy was achieved. In a review by Lopez-Lopez et al. [5], four studies were found to report an increase of volume ranging between 24.4% and 38.4% in cirrhosis versus 39.4–49.6% in non-cirrhosis at a median of 36 days after initial PVE. In cirrhotic patients, the drop-out rate of PVE was 20% with a resection rate of 96%.

However, the growth in liver volume does not always translate into an adequate functional growth. It was observed that there is a discrepancy up to 50% between volume and functional growth of the liver as shown in hepatobiliary scintigraphy in between stages [2]. In rat models, it was shown that the functional maturity lagged behind the volume increase. Whether this discrepancy would be greater in patients with cirrhosis is still a question yet to be answered.

17.3 Different Methods of Future Remnant Augmentation

17.3.1 Portal Vein Embolization

Portal vein embolization is one of the most widespread methods of future remnant augmentation due to its relatively lower risk involved [3]. The overall morbidity rate for PVE was 2.2% without immediate mortality in meta-analysis [6]. Resection rate was 85% after 4 weeks of waiting period. 0.8% of patients developed liver failure after operation and died, whereas 2.5% of patients had transient liver failure following resection. Major reasons leading to drop out before or during resection are inadequate remnant growth (1.7%), tumor progression (e.g., severe invasion to porta, gross tumor extension), leading to inoperability (0.9%) or distant metastases (1.6%). In another review that looked into only patients with HCC, the mortality rate for PVE ranges from 0% to 11.5% and morbidity from 24% to 56% [7]. Among the patients who successfully received resection, the long-term outcomes were satisfactory when compared to major resections without PVE [8–11]. The mean FLR hypertrophy was 30.9% over a mean interval of 40.3 days in another meta-analysis in 2021 [12].

Indeed, the relatively long waiting time of 4–6 weeks before the resection is one of the drawbacks of PVE, especially tumors that require future remnant augmentation are often either large HCC or tumors neighboring major pedicle. Another theory was that after PVE, the compensatory increase in hepatic artery flow to ipsilateral lobe may lead to rapid tumor progression and insufficient FLR hypertrophy [13]. It was reported that the median tumor growth rate increased from 0.59 cm^3/day (range: 0.22–6.01 cm^3/day) to 2.37 cm^3/day (range: 0.29–13.97 cm^3/day) [14]. It was why some advocated adding transarterial chemoembolization (TACE) on top of PVE in order to improve survival [3, 13].

On top of PVE, there is recent advocation in using both PVE and hepatic vein embolization (PVE/HVE) to enhance remnant hypertrophy. By embolizing both the inflow and outflow of the ipsilateral lobe, it aims at increasing the FLR rapidly and effectively, while preserving liver function. This method was called by multiple names, such as radiological simultaneous portohepatic vein embolization (RASPE) and liver venous deprivation (LVD). In 2021, the DRAGON collaborative group published a multicenter retrospective study comparing PVE and PVE/HVE [15]. It was shown that the resectability in PVE/HVE was significantly higher than in PVE group (hypertrophy rate: 59% vs. 48%; $p = 0.020$). The complication and mortality rate after the procedure were similar in both groups. This technique so far was mainly used in patients with colorectal liver metastasis (1% of patients in PVE/HVE group in aforementioned study). Its efficacy and safety in patients with cirrhosis was still yet to be proven. It is also technically more demanding and its reproducibility is still in question.

17.3.2 Associated Liver Partition and Portal Vein Ligation for Staged Hepatectomy

ALPPS is known for its rapid FLR growth within a short period of time and a higher resectability for higher tumor load. Similar to PVE, patients with chronic hepatitis were shown to undergo less rapid and less extensive hypertrophy. From the international registry [4] and a tertiary center in Singapore [6], HCC patients consistently underwent less rapid (5–19% FLR per day vs. 9–35% FLR per day) and less extensive hypertrophy (40–47% vs. 76–138% increase in FLR) when compared to patients with normal liver.

ALPPS did receive skepticisms since it was first described by Schnitzbauer et al. [7], mainly due to its relatively higher mortality, and especially so for cirrhotic patients. At its early years, ALPPS for HCC patients were reported to have 31% 90-day mortality and 57.6% morbidity [4]. The mortality rate was significantly higher than that of patients with CRLM (31% vs. 7%; $p < 0.0001$). The morbidity rate did not differ significantly from CRLM group. The most common complications included intra-abdominal abscess, bile leak, and pleural effusion, while the most common cause leading to mortality being post-hepatectomy liver failure. Nonetheless, with careful patient selection and in experienced hands, the 90-day mortality rate could be as low as 7.1% [6, 8, 9]. In a systemic review in 2020 [10], the 90-day mortality ranged from 0% to 50%, with an average of 17.6%. Such wide range implied a large room for improvement on safety, but it was not impossible to achieve.

With the data from LIGRO Trial [11], it was concluded that there was no difference between ALPPS and PVE with regards to perioperative complication (Clavien–Dindo grade III–IV) and 90-day mortality, while improving the resectability of patients with CRLM. However, similar randomized controlled trial in HCC is still lacking. From the comparative study by our center in 2021 [16], ALPPS conferred a higher resection rate in cirrhotic patients (97.8% vs. 67.7%; $p < 0.001$) and had a comparable long-term outcome to PVE (5-year overall survival 46.8% vs. 64.1%; $p = 0.234$).

As for oncological outcomes, despite initial concerns about whether the compensatory increase in arterial flow after stage I operation would enhance tumor growth, more recent studies have shown promising results (Table 17.1). The 3-year survival from various studies [16–18] reported to be 57.4–60.2%. The long-term outcome of ALPPS was also comparable to upfront hepatectomy and two-stage hepatectomy with PVE [16].

17.3.3 Variations of ALPPS

Several variations have been proposed for ALPPS, trying to minimize the mortality and morbidity rates. To minimize the aggressiveness of stage I operation, surgeons have tried to replace in situ split of parenchyma by ablation to create an avascular plane. Means of ablation includes microwave and radiofrequency ablation [19], and these might be carried out in laparoscopic [20] or even percutaneous means [21]. Wang et al. reported an encouraging result of 53% median percentage FLR increase [19]. When compared to ALPPS, laparoscopic ablation with radiofrequency with portal vein ligation as first stage operation was found to have lower morbidity but a slower hypertrophy rate in a series by Chan et al. [22].

Another alternative to ablation was the use of tourniquet. Campos et al. described the method of tightening a tourniquet at the intended plane of transection to occlude the blood flow in between [23]. The method was attempted in HCC patients, but the results were variable. Cai et al. reported a mortality rate of 50% as well as failure to achieve an adequate FLR hypertrophy [24]. However, in the study by Lopez-Lopez et al. [25], adequate FLR hypertrophy with a median of 76% (range: 50–187.5%) was achieved. Hospital mortality rate was 11.1%. This might be explained by the difference in patient population, as the latter study had only 44% of patients with HCC.

There were also other reports on combining partial split-ALPPS with PVE, namely mini-ALPPS and hybrid-ALPPS. These methods reduced the morbidity rate by reducing the magnitude of parenchymal transection, while allowing more liberal use of minimally-invasive approach. The effectiveness of partial ALPPS shall be discussed in the latter part of the chapter.

Most of the above studies on these variation from ALPPS consisted of small series. More data were needed to determine their safety and efficacy when compared to ALPPS.

Table 17.1 Oncological outcomes of ALPPS for HCC

	N	FLR/ESLV (%)		Relative hypertrophy (%)	Days between stages	Morbidity[a] (%)	PHLF[b] (%)	90-day mortality (%)	Overall survival (%)	
		Stage I	Stage II						3-year	5-year
Ye et al. (2024) [17]	44 (pure HCC subgroup)	34.5 ± 7.6	53.7 ± 9.4	19.4 (3.6–42.1)	11 (3–50)	Stage I: 11.4 Stage II: 20	N/A	2.9	40	14.3
Chan et al. (2021) [11]	46	24.5	37.4	48	7	8.7	4.3	6.5	60.2	46.8
Deng et al. (2021) [16]	20	36.6 (19.0–47.4)	57.6 (43.7–85.1)	64.5	18	N/A	N/A	5	57.4	N/A
Peng et al. (2019) [18]	20	36.8 ± 10.7	54.5 ± 10.9	52.4 ± 26.9	15.3	25	N/A	10%	58.9	N/A

[a]Clavien–Dindo classification III or above
[b]Post-hepatectomy liver failure by 50–50 criteria

17.4 Patient Selection for ALPPS

Patient selection is especially crucial in patients with HCC. Patient factors affecting outcomes in CRLM would also be applicable in patients with HCC. Advanced age had consistently been proven to be one of the risk factors for morbidity and mortality. From early data of the international registry in 2014, patients older than 60 years of age had more severe complications (Clavien–Dindo IIIb or above) (OR = 3.76, $p = 0.007$) [26] and higher mortality (OR = 14.3, $p = 0.001$) [27]. A study by D'Haese et al. comparing the outcomes of ALPPS in patients with CRLM vs. HCC demonstrated that only patients less than 60 years old with low-grade fibrosis in HCC can undergo ALPPS with a higher risk–benefit ratio [4]. From an international survey for surgeons participating in ALPPS in 2016 [28], only 4% would impose strict age limitation during patient selection. Most respondents based the decision on functional status, requiring patients receiving ALPPS to be a least ambulatory.

Child A cirrhosis, indocyanine green clearance rate <20% at 15 min, platelet count over 100×10^9/L were preferred for undergoing ALPPS in our center [8, 16]. Patients with signs of portal hypertension including ascites and/or intra-abdominal varices were excluded. These criteria were mostly derived from our practice in performing major hepatectomy. Further studies would be needed to validate these criteria for ALPPS in HCC. Furthermore, ALPPS is usually considered when FLR is less than 30% as a substantial gain in volume is needed. For patients with FLR of 30–35%, PVE is preferred as less gain in volume is enough in a one-stage procedure.

17.5 Operative Techniques of ALPPS

Operative techniques of ALPPS in HCC is in general the same as in other cases. Our center advocates the use of anterior approach in most cases, i.e., leaving most of the attachments to the right lobe intact during stage I operation. This method can minimize adhesions and facilitate stage II operation [29]. Such approach also provides another advantage of preventing iatrogenic tumor rupture during the mobilization, which may happen especially when the tumor is large [29].

It was found that the completeness in the parenchymal splitting procedure had an impact on FLR hypertrophy. In the study from our center in 2016 [30], a complete split (i.e., a full parenchymal split down to the surface of retrohepatic IVC, Fig. 17.1) was shown to have a more rapid FLR hypertrophy rate than partial split in cirrhotic liver (hypertrophy rate 32.2 mL/day vs. 16.9 mL/day, $p = 0.086$). Such difference was less obvious in cirrhotic livers though (FLR/ ESLV% increment: 14.8% vs. 11.0%, $p = 0.668$), whereas in chronic hepatitis the increment in volume was significantly greater for complete split (FLR/ESLV% increment: 18.1% vs. 11.3%, $p = 0.042$). Although some surgeons favor partial split (i.e., 50–80% of total thickness) in the hope of lowering the mortality rate, and claiming a similar FLR hypertrophy, most of these data focused on CRLM rather than HCC [31–33]. Unless the transection is deemed too challenging, a complete split can enhance FLR

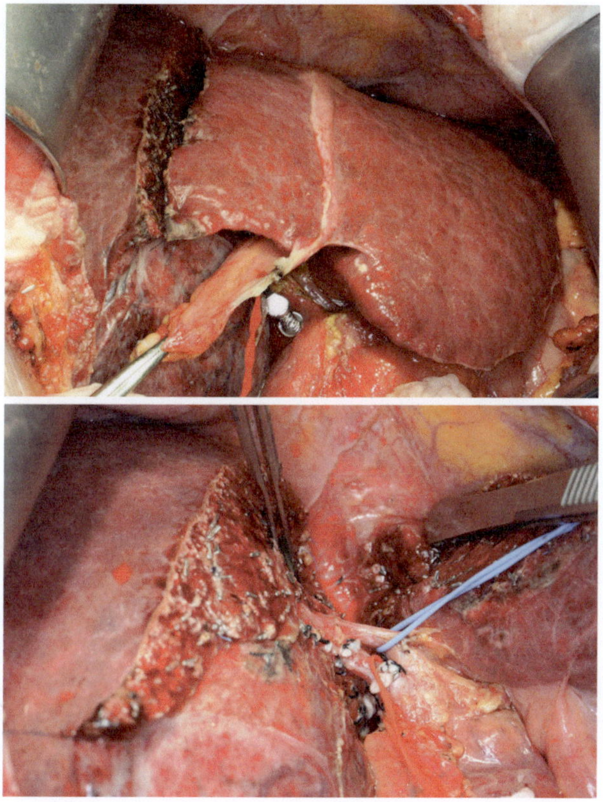

Fig. 17.1 (Top) Open ALPPS procedure in a patient with cirrhosis; (bottom) complete split achieved in the same patient with exposure of IVC

hypertrophy and ensure a better shot for second-stage operation, especially in the presence of chronic hepatitis or cirrhosis.

To facilitate the transection of the deep parenchymal tissue layer when performing a complete split, a right-angled instrument can be introduced to the avascular plane between the retrohepatic inferior vena cava (IVC) and the posterior surface of liver (Fig. 17.2). This plane is the same plane as described in the hanging maneuver by Belghiti et al. [34], but the tape used for the "hanging" was replaced by the right-angled instrument, as it would be challenging to pass a tape without fully mobilizing the right lobe. Such maneuver can help avoid injury to the retrohepatic IVC and minimize blood loss.

Some other techniques are also applicable in the case of HCC. Preservation of the middle hepatic vein (MHV) was found to be beneficial, as it helps prevent the ischemia of segment IV and bile leak. It also reduces the incidence of functional impairment due to obstruction to venous outflow [35]. Another way to preserve segment IV blood supply is by limiting the hilar dissection to only exposing the right-side pedicle. Although up to 39% of surgeons practicing ALPPS believed that skeletonizing the hepaticoduodenal ligament was indicated [28], there is no consensus on whether it is always necessary, especially in cases of HCC where lymphatic spread is not common.

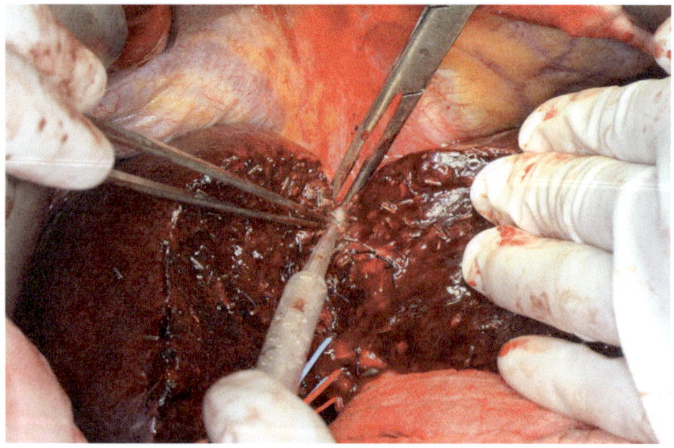

Fig. 17.2 Right-angled instrument introduced between the retrohepatic IVC and the posterior surface of liver to facilitate splitting of deep layer of parenchyma

Extra care should be given to avoid any complications, which may impede the recovery and growth of FLR. The use of ultrasonic dissection device is preferred in our center, as it provides clear delineation of vascular and ductal structures and allows definitive control of such structures [36–38]. This is especially important in cirrhotic patients, as any bile leakage will have detrimental effect on subsequent FLR hypertrophy. Bile leak test should be performed upon completion of both stage I and II operations.

Minimally-invasive approach to ALPPS is possible to reduce adhesions and overall inflammatory response associated with laparotomy. Both laparoscopic and robotic approaches were reported in the literature, but mostly on indications other than HCC. According to the review by Baili et al. [39], FLR hypertrophy of laparoscopic ALPPS for a variety of indications ranged from 50.3% to 120%, while only one patient (16.7%) experienced a major complication and no in-hospital mortality. Minimally-invasive ALPPS in cirrhotic liver would usually be more challenging than in normal liver, and such data on feasibility, safety, and outcomes is still lacking. From the preliminary data in our center [40], the overall complication rates (33% vs. 40%, $p = 0.64$) and Grade B/C post-hepatectomy liver failure rates (36% vs. 20%, $p = 0.34$) were similar in open and laparoscopic ALPPS for HCC patients. The open group had a higher percentage gain in FLR (51% vs. 35%). It was found that laparoscopic approach was feasible and associated with less blood loss but might require a longer waiting time before stage II operation.

17.6 Conclusion

Liver hypertrophy in patients with chronic hepatitis or early cirrhosis is not only possible but is also an essential component in the management of HCC. This can only be achieved by careful patient selection and meticulous operation techniques [41]. With more understanding in the underlying mechanisms and accumulation in evidence, let us hope that a more clearly defined guideline on FLR augmentation techniques could be available in the near future for surgeons worldwide.

References

1. Tampi C. Pathology for the HPB Surgeon. Indian J Surg. 2012;74(1):67–72.
2. Kang D, Schadde E. Hypertrophy and liver function in ALPPS: correlation with morbidity and mortality. Visc Med. 2017;33(6):426–33.
3. Shao Z, Liu X, Peng C, Wang L, Xu D. Combination of transcatheter arterial chemoembolization and portal vein embolization for patients with hepatocellular carcinoma: a review. World J Surg Oncol. 2021;19(1):293.
4. D'Haese JG, Neumann J, Weniger M, Pratschke S, Björnsson B, Ardiles V, et al. Should ALPPS be used for liver resection in intermediate-stage HCC? Ann Surg Oncol. 2016;23(4):1335–43.
5. Lopez-Lopez V, Robles-Campos R, Brusadin R, Lopez-Conesa A, de la Peña J, Caballero A, et al. ALPPS for hepatocarcinoma under cirrhosis: a feasible alternative to portal vein embolization. Ann Transl Med. 2019;7(22):691.
6. Chia DKA, Yeo Z, Loh SEK, Iyer SG, Madhavan K, Kow AWC. ALPPS for hepatocellular carcinoma is associated with decreased liver remnant growth. J Gastrointest Surg. 2018;22(6):973–80.
7. Schnitzbauer AA, Lang SA, Goessmann H, Nadalin S, Baumgart J, Farkas SA, et al. Right portal vein ligation combined with in situ splitting induces rapid left lateral liver lobe hypertrophy enabling 2-staged extended right hepatic resection in small-for-size settings. Ann Surg. 2012;255(3):405–14.
8. Chan AC, Poon RT, Chan C, Lo CM. Safety of ALPPS procedure by the anterior approach for hepatocellular carcinoma. Ann Surg. 2016;263(2):e14–6.
9. Vennarecci G, Grazi GL, Sperduti I, Busi Rizzi E, Felli E, Antonini M, et al. ALPPS for primary and secondary liver tumors. Int J Surg. 2016;30:38–44.
10. Zhang J, Huang H, Bian J, Sang X, Xu Y, Lu X, et al. Safety, feasibility, and efficacy of associating liver partition and portal vein ligation for staged hepatectomy in treating hepatocellular carcinoma: a systematic review. Ann Transl Med. 2020;8(19):1246.
11. Sandström P, Røsok BI, Sparrelid E, Larsen PN, Larsson AL, Lindell G, et al. ALPPS improves resectability compared with conventional two-stage hepatectomy in patients with advanced colorectal liver metastasis: results from a Scandinavian Multicenter Randomized Controlled Trial (LIGRO Trial). Ann Surg. 2018;267(5):833–40.
12. Charalel RA, Sung J, Askin G, Jo J, Mitry M, Chung C, et al. Systematic reviews and meta-analyses of portal vein embolization, associated liver partition and portal vein ligation, and radiation lobectomy outcomes in hepatocellular carcinoma patients. Curr Oncol Rep. 2021;23(11):135.
13. Zhang CW, Dou CW, Zhang XL, Liu XQ, Huang DS, Hu ZM, et al. Simultaneous transcatheter arterial chemoembolization and portal vein embolization for patients with large hepatocellular carcinoma before major hepatectomy. World J Gastroenterol. 2020;26(30):4489–500.
14. Hayashi S, Baba Y, Ueno K, Nakajo M, Kubo F, Ueno S, et al. Acceleration of primary liver tumor growth rate in embolized hepatic lobe after portal vein embolization. Acta Radiol. 2007;48(7):721–7.
15. Heil J, Korenblik R, Heid F, Bechstein WO, Bemelmans M, Binkert C, et al. Preoperative portal vein or portal and hepatic vein embolization: DRAGON collaborative group analysis. Br J Surg. 2021;108(7):834–42.
16. Chan A, Zhang WY, Chok K, Dai J, Ji R, Kwan C, et al. ALPPS versus portal vein embolization for hepatitis-related hepatocellular carcinoma: a changing paradigm in modulation of future liver remnant before major hepatectomy. Ann Surg. 2021;273(5):957–65.
17. Peng C, Li C, Liu C, Wen T, Yang J, Li B, et al. The outcome of the HCC patients underwent ALPPS: retrospective study. Medicine (Baltimore). 2019;98(38):e17182.
18. Deng Z, Jin Z, Qin Y, Wei M, Wang J, Lu T, et al. Efficacy of the association liver partition and portal vein ligation for staged hepatectomy for the treatment of solitary huge hepatocellular carcinoma: a retrospective single-center study. World J Surg Oncol. 2021;19(1):95.

19. Wang Q, Yan J, Feng X, Chen G, Xia F, Li X, et al. Safety and efficacy of radiofrequency-assisted ALPPS (RALPPS) in patients with cirrhosis-related hepatocellular carcinoma. Int J Hyperthermia. 2017:1–7.
20. Gringeri E, Boetto R, D'Amico FE, Bassi D, Cillo U. Laparoscopic microwave ablation and portal vein ligation for staged hepatectomy (LAPS): a minimally invasive first-step approach. Ann Surg. 2015;261(2):e42–e3.
21. Zhang YB, Peng SY, Huang DS. Percutaneous microwave ablation liver partition and portal vein embolization for rapid liver regeneration: a minimally invasive first step of ALPPS for hepatocellular carcinoma. Ann Surg. 2016;264(1):e1–2.
22. Chen Z, Shen S, Xie W, Liao J, Feng S, Li S, et al. Comparison of clinical efficacy between LAPS and ALPPS in the treatment of hepatitis B virus-related hepatocellular carcinoma. Gastroenterol Rep (Oxf). 2023;11:goad060.
23. Campos RR, Brusadin R, Conesa AL, Paricio PP. Staged liver resection for perihilar liver tumors using a tourniquet in the umbilical fissure and sequential portal vein embolization on the fourth postoperative day (a modified ALTPS). Cirugía Española (English Edition). 2014;92(10):682–6.
24. Cai X, Tong Y, Yu H, Liang X, Wang Y, Liang Y, et al. The ALPPS in the treatment of Hepatitis B – related hepatocellular carcinoma with cirrhosis: a single-center study and literature review. Surg Innov. 2017;24(4):358–64.
25. López-López V, Robles-Campos R, Brusadin R, López-Conesa A, Navarro Á, Arevalo-Perez J, et al. Tourniquet-ALPPS is a promising treatment for very large hepatocellular carcinoma and intrahepatic cholangiocarcinoma. Oncotarget. 2018;9(46):28267.
26. Schadde E, Ardiles V, Robles-Campos R, Malago M, Machado M, Hernandez-Alejandro R, et al. Early survival and safety of ALPPS: first report of the International ALPPS Registry. Ann Surg. 2014;260(5):829–36. discussion 36–8
27. Brouquet A, Abdalla EK, Kopetz S, Garrett CR, Overman MJ, Eng C, et al. High survival rate after two-stage resection of advanced colorectal liver metastases: response-based selection and complete resection define outcome. J Clin Oncol. 2011;29(8):1083–90.
28. Buac S, Schadde E, Schnitzbauer AA, Vogt K, Hernandez-Alejandro R. The many faces of ALPPS: surgical indications and techniques among surgeons collaborating in the international registry. HPB (Oxford). 2016;18(5):442–8.
29. Chan ACY, Poon RTP, Lo CM. Modified anterior approach for the ALPPS procedure: how we do it. World J Surg. 2015;39(11):1.
30. Chan ACY, Chok K, Dai JWC, Lo CM. Impact of split completeness on future liver remnant hypertrophy in associating liver partition and portal vein ligation for staged hepatectomy (ALPPS) in hepatocellular carcinoma: complete-ALPPS versus partial-ALPPS. Surgery. 2017;161(2):357–64.
31. de Santibañes E, Alvarez FA, Ardiles V, Pekolj J, de Santibañes M. Inverting the ALPPS paradigm by minimizing first stage impact: the Mini-ALPPS technique. Langenbecks Arch Surg. 2016;401(4):557–63.
32. Huang HC, Bian J, Bai Y, Lu X, Xu YY, Sang XT, et al. Complete or partial split in associating liver partition and portal vein ligation for staged hepatectomy: a systematic review and meta-analysis. World J Gastroenterol. 2019;25(39):6016–24.
33. Petrowsky H, Györi G, de Oliveira M, Lesurtel M, Clavien PA. Is partial-ALPPS safer than ALPPS? A single-center experience. Ann Surg. 2015;261(4):e90–2.
34. Belghiti J, Guevara OA, Noun R, Saldinger PF, Kianmanesh R. Liver hanging maneuver: a safe approach to right hepatectomy without liver mobilization. J Am Coll Surg. 2001;193(1):109–11.
35. Donati M, Basile F, Oldhafer KJ. Present status and future perspectives of ALPPS (Associating liver partition and portal vein ligation for staged hepatectomy). Fut Oncol. 2015;11(16):2255–8.
36. Fan S-T, Lo C-M, Liu C-L, Lam C-M, Yuen W-K, Yeung C, et al. Hepatectomy for hepatocellular carcinoma: toward zero hospital deaths. Ann Surg. 1999;229(3):322.
37. Fan ST, Lai EC, Lo CM, Chu KM, Liu CL, Wong J. Hepatectomy with an ultrasonic dissector for hepatocellular carcinoma. Br J Surg. 1996;83(1):117–20.
38. Singh SV, Techniques and energy sources for liver resection: when and how? 2018.

39. Baili E, Tsilimigras DI, Moris D, Sahara K, Pawlik TM. Technical modifications and outcomes after Associating Liver Partition and Portal Vein Ligation for Staged Hepatectomy (ALPPS) for primary liver malignancies: a systematic review. Surg Oncol. 2020;33:70–80.
40. Chan A, Keith AKP. Chapter 12 – ALPPS for cirrhotic liver. In: Makuuchi M, Sakamoto Y, editors. Safe major hepatectomy after preoperative liver regeneration. Academic; 2024. p. 167–81.
41. Ye C, Ou M, Wen Z, Xu B, Lu T, Guo Y, et al. Efficacy of associating liver partition and portal vein ligation for staged hepatectomy (ALPPS) in hepatocellular carcinoma with macrovascular invasion: a single-center retrospective analysis. World J Surg Oncol. 2024;22(1):260.

Rationale and Techniques for Liver Hypertrophy in Cholangiocarcinoma

18

Shoji Kawakatsu, Takashi Mizuno, Shunsuke Onoe, Nobuyuki Watanabe, Mihoko Yamada, and Tomoki Ebata

18.1 Introduction

Cholangiocarcinoma is an epithelial cell malignancy originating from the biliary tree and is categorized into three groups [1]: intrahepatic, perihilar, and distal. Among them, perihilar cholangiocarcinoma (PHCC) is the most common type, accounting for the majority of cholangiocarcinomas [1, 2]. The standard surgery for this disease requires major hepatectomy combined with caudate lobectomy and extrahepatic bile duct resection. Although surgical resection is the only curative treatment, the high mortality rate after this invasive hepatectomy is a global issue [3]. Most surgical mortalities are associated with postoperative liver failure, and preventive measures are crucial because no effective treatment is available after onset. Insufficient liver remnant volume is closely associated with postoperative liver failure and preoperative portal vein embolization (PVE) has substantially improved the safety of this surgery. In this section, we will discuss the evolution of surgical treatment for perihilar cholangiocarcinoma, including preoperative liver hypertrophy, and refer to our clinical practices at Nagoya University Hospital.

18.2 Historical Shift in Surgical Treatment for Perihilar Cholangiocarcinoma

Since the groundbreaking report by Bismuth et al. [4], the standard surgical procedure for this disease has shifted from local excision to major hepatectomy. PHCC easily invades the biliary branches of the caudate lobe because most of them merge

S. Kawakatsu · T. Mizuno · S. Onoe · N. Watanabe · M. Yamada · T. Ebata (✉)
Division of Surgical Oncology, Department of Surgery, Nagoya University Graduate School of Medicine, Nagoya, Japan
e-mail: ebata.tomoki.n1@f.mail.nagoya-u.ac.jp

L. Aldrighetti et al. (eds.), *Liver Regeneration Techniques In Hepatic Surgery*,
https://doi.org/10.1007/978-3-032-10997-2_18

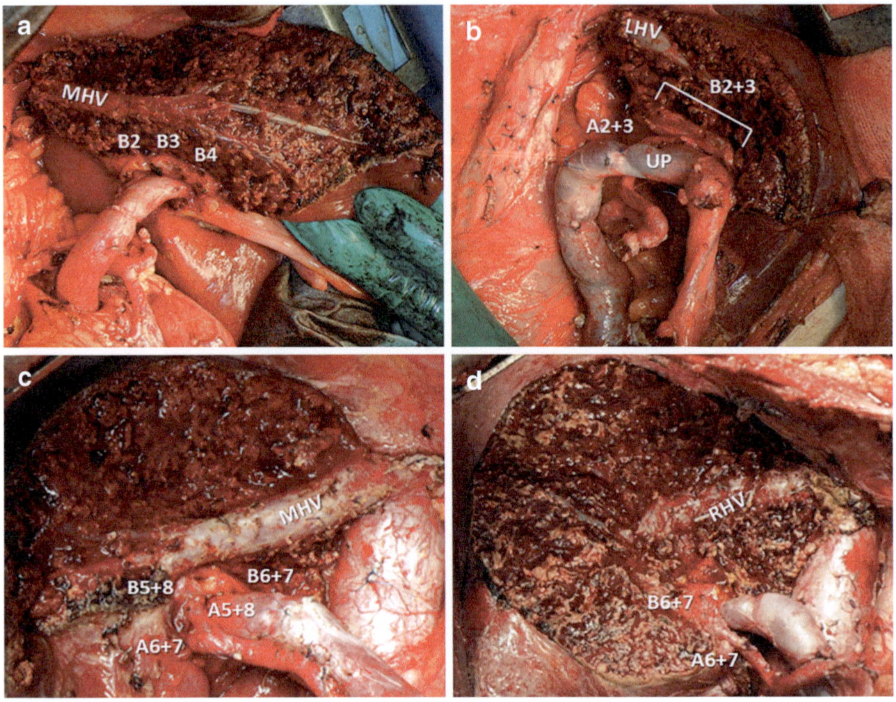

Fig. 18.1 Intraoperative view after resection: (**a**) right hemihepatectomy (H15678), (**b**) right trisectionectomy (H145678), (**c**) left hemihepatectomy (H1234), (**d**) left trisectionectomy (H123458)

into the right or left hepatic duct at the hepatic hilus. Thus, Nimura et al. introduced routine caudate lobectomy to obtain a wide surgical margin [5], which became the preferred treatment method. Consequently, major hepatectomy combined with caudate lobectomy and extrahepatic bile duct resection was considered the standard procedure for PHCC. The types of hepatectomy have been organized into four standard major hepatectomies: right hemihepatectomy (H15678, according to the New World Terminology [6]), right trisectionectomy (H145678), left hemihepatectomy (H1234), and left trisectionectomy (H123458) (Fig. 18.1). The possibility of performing safe major hepatectomy largely depends on the future liver remnant volume to maintain functional recovery to meet metabolic demand after surgery.

18.3 Portal Vein Embolization

PVE, introduced by Makuuchi and Kinoshita in the 1980s [7, 8], can induce liver hypertrophy of the nonembolized lobe. A previous meta-analysis involving 37 highly selected studies supported the benefit of PVE [9]. PVE can be performed via three approaches: the transileocolic venous approach, the transhepatic contralateral approach [8], and the transhepatic ipsilateral approach [10]. The third approach in which the portal branch of the liver on the resection side is punctured was established by Nagino et al. in the 1990s [10] and is globally used as the current standard. A distinct advantage of this approach is the minimized risk of vascular injury in the future remnant liver. Additionally, the risk of portal bleeding after catheter sheath removal is low because the punctured portal branch is embolized. Another advantage is straightforward catheterization of the segment 4 portal branches, allowing for trisegment PVE [11–13]. H145678 and H123458 are the most extensive hepatectomies, with average resection rates of 81% and 67%, respectively [13]. Therefore, preoperative liver hypertrophy is more critical.

18.3.1 Indication

In previous reports, the safety limit of the future remnant liver volume ranged from 20% to 40% in the normal liver [14–18]. Given its extended nature, the indications for PVE before hepatobiliary resection for PHCC should be distinguished from those before simple hepatectomy. Extrahepatic bile duct resection perturbs early liver regeneration [19] and has an adverse impact on the postoperative outcome after major hepatectomy [20]. Moreover, major hepatectomy for PHCC is often associated with combined pancreatoduodenectomy, portal vein resection, and hepatic artery resection. The influence of such combined resection on liver regeneration is unknown. A recent meta-analysis [21] revealed that a future liver remnant less than 40% was the most common indication for PVE prior to hepatectomy for PHCC.

18.3.2 Liver Regeneration

In recent systematic reviews, the mean future remnant liver hypertrophy rates were reported to be 37.9–49.4% [9, 22–24]. PVE induces hypertrophy in the nonembolized lobe within 14 days [25]. However, liver regeneration is negatively influenced by coexisting liver disease [26]. In patients with obstructive jaundice or cholangitis, liver hypertrophy is severely impaired [27], and a longer interval period after PVE may be required to achieve a sufficient future liver remnant volume [28]. Ebata et al. reported liver hypertrophy after PVE in patients with biliary cancer [29]. In this study, the volume ratio of the nonembolized lobe increased from 33% to 43%, the volume of the nonembolized lobe increased from 361 to 460 mL, and the volume of the embolized lobe decreased from 688 to 581 mL.

18.3.3 Adverse Events

PVE can be performed safely with a major complication rate between 2.2% to 3.9% [9, 22, 23, 30]. Although infrequent, portal vein thrombosis, pneumothorax, hemoperitoneum, subcapsular hematoma, or arterial puncture [31, 32] can occur after

PVE. In particular, if the embolic material migrates to the portal branch of the future remnant liver, critical deterioration in hepatic function will occur [25], and the patient may not be able to undergo resection [33].

Another important limitation of PVE is the potential for disease progression during the interval period before hepatectomy [34]. Tumor progression may be accelerated by the release of circulating growth factors in response to PVE [35–37]. In general, PHCC is a slow-growing cancer, as already described in the earliest report by Klatskin [38], so there is time to wait until enough hypertrophy has been achieved through PVE. However, in patients with more advanced disease, the acceleration of disease progression due to PVE may render them inoperable [25].

18.4 Additional Strategies for Increasing the Incidence of Hypertrophy

A sufficient increase in the volume of the nonembolized lobe is not always achieved after PVE [25]. In these patients, hepatic artery embolization [39, 40] or hepatic vein embolization [41, 42] may be proposed as the next steps. Although its usefulness has been reported [39, 40], subsequent hepatic artery embolization strongly increases the risk of liver abscess. Hepatic vein embolization can also induce a certain increase in future liver remnant volume after PVE, but only a few small retrospective series are available to date [41–44]. Because these optional interventions are still experimental, their indications should be strictly selective.

Associating liver partition and portal vein ligation for staged hepatectomy (ALPPS) [45] may present another strategy. However, in patients with PHCC, bile is colonized and infected through preoperative biliary drainage [24], leading to frequent postoperative infectious complications. Moreover, the primary tumor is left in situ in the first stage, and leakage of bile that contains floating cancer cells [46, 47] could be a source of peritoneal dissemination. Under the present circumstances, the indications for ALPPS for PHCC may be limited [48].

18.5 Clinical Practice at Nagoya University Hospital

We have focused on the surgical treatment of PHCC since the beginning of the 1980s. Changes in the surgical procedure at our institution between 1977 and 2023 are shown in Fig. 18.2. PVE is principally indicated when the estimated percentage of future liver remnant is less than 40% [49]. All PVE procedures were performed via the ipsilateral approach [10, 12, 13], and the right anterior portal branch was routinely targeted for access unless it was obstructed by tumor involvement. The left trisegment PVE helped the identification of hepatic dissection lines [50, 51] and was more actively used before H123458.

Since 2012, at our institute, PVE has been performed using gelatin sponge particles and metal coils [52]. Between 2012 and 2015, a total of 136 patients

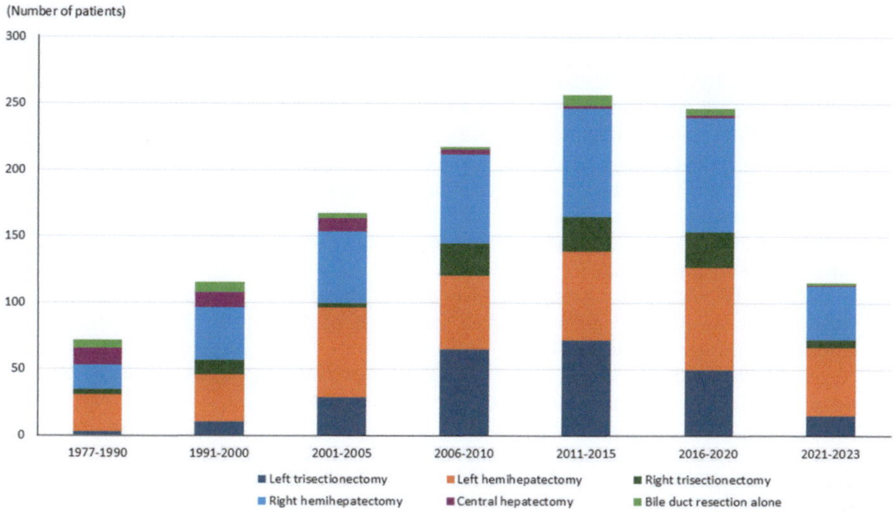

Fig. 18.2 Changes in types of hepatectomy between 1977 and 2023 at Nagoya University Hospital (n = 1194)

underwent PVE prior to major hepatectomy. The following complications occurred in 5 (3.7%) patients: hepatic artery injury in 3 (2.2%) patients, hemothorax in 1 (0.7%) patient, and subcapsular biloma in 1 (0.7%) patient. Recanalization of the targeted portal vein was observed in 2 (1.5%) patients; therefore, additional PVE was performed.

When sufficient hypertrophy could not be achieved after complete PVE, the operation was postponed by 1–2 months. Next, sequential hepatic artery embolization [52] or hepatic vein embolization [56] was considered, although their indications are strictly selective. Unfortunately, in our small series, hepatic vein embolization did not result in any significant additional liver hypertrophy.

18.6 Conclusion

Surgical treatment of PHCC has steadily evolved through a series of small advances in the past few decades [53]. Among them, preoperative PVE for patients who need major hepatectomy may be one of the most effective breakthroughs. Although immune therapies have remarkably improved the systemic therapy and outcomes of PHCC in the last decade, surgical challenges remain the cornerstone for this disease and should not be quickly abandoned. There remains controversy as to the best preoperative liver hypertrophy method, and further study will be necessary before definitive conclusions can be drawn.

References

1. Nakeeb A, Pitt HA, Sohn TA, et al. Cholangiocarcinoma. A spectrum of intrahepatic, perihilar, and distal tumors. Ann Surg. 1996;224(4):463–73. discussion 73–5
2. DeOliveira ML, Cunningham SC, Cameron JL, et al. Cholangiocarcinoma: thirty-one-year experience with 564 patients at a single institution. Ann Surg. 2007;245(5):755–62.
3. Mueller M, Breuer E, Mizuno T, et al. Perihilar cholangiocarcinoma: novel benchmark values for surgical and oncological outcomes from 24 expert centers. Ann Surg. 2021;274(5):780–8.
4. Bismuth H, Nakache R, Diamond T. Management strategies in resection for hilar cholangiocarcinoma. Ann Surg. 1992;215(1):31–8.
5. Nimura Y, Hayakawa N, Kamiya J, Kondo S, Shionoya S. Hepatic segmentectomy with caudate lobe resection for bile duct carcinoma of the hepatic hilus. World J Surg. 1990;14(4):535–43. discussion 44
6. Nagino M, DeMatteo R, Lang H, et al. Proposal of a new comprehensive notation for hepatectomy: the "New World" terminology. Ann Surg. 2021;274:1.
7. Kinoshita H, Sakai K, Hirohashi K, Igawa S, Yamasaki O, Kubo S. Preoperative portal vein embolization for hepatocellular carcinoma. World J Surg. 1986;10(5):803–8.
8. Makuuchi M, Thai BL, Takayasu K, et al. Preoperative portal embolization to increase safety of major hepatectomy for hilar bile duct carcinoma: a preliminary report. Surgery. 1990;107(5):521–7.
9. Abulkhir A, Limongelli P, Healey AJ, et al. Preoperative portal vein embolization for major liver resection: a meta-analysis. Ann Surg. 2008;247(1):49–57.
10. Nagino M, Nimura Y, Kamiya J, Kondo S, Kanai M. Selective percutaneous transhepatic embolization of the portal vein in preparation for extensive liver resection: the ipsilateral approach. Radiology. 1996;200(2):559–63.
11. Madoff DC, Abdalla EK, Gupta S, et al. Transhepatic ipsilateral right portal vein embolization extended to segment IV: improving hypertrophy and resection outcomes with spherical particles and coils. J Vasc Interv Radiol. 2005;16(2 Pt 1):215–25.
12. Nagino M, Kamiya J, Kanai M, et al. Right trisegment portal vein embolization for biliary tract carcinoma: technique and clinical utility. Surgery. 2000;127(2):155–60.
13. Nagino M, Nimura Y, Kamiya J, et al. Right or left trisegment portal vein embolization before hepatic trisegmentectomy for hilar bile duct carcinoma. Surgery. 1995;117(6):677–81.
14. Farges O, Belghiti J, Kianmanesh R, et al. Portal vein embolization before right hepatectomy: prospective clinical trial. Ann Surg. 2003;237(2):208–17.
15. Hemming AW, Reed AI, Howard RJ, et al. Preoperative portal vein embolization for extended hepatectomy. Ann Surg. 2003;237(5):686–91. discussion 91–3
16. Vauthey JN, Chaoui A, Do KA, et al. Standardized measurement of the future liver remnant prior to extended liver resection: methodology and clinical associations. Surgery. 2000;127(5):512–9.
17. Kishi Y, Abdalla EK, Chun YS, et al. Three hundred and one consecutive extended right hepatectomies: evaluation of outcome based on systematic liver volumetry. Ann Surg. 2009;250(4):540–8.
18. Kubota K, Makuuchi M, Kusaka K, et al. Measurement of liver volume and hepatic functional reserve as a guide to decision-making in resectional surgery for hepatic tumors. Hepatology (Baltimore, Md). 1997;26(5):1176–81.
19. Takagi T, Yokoyama Y, Kokuryo T, Yamaguchi J, Nagino M. Liver regeneration following experimental major hepatectomy with choledochojejunostomy. Br J Surg. 2015;102(11):1410–7.
20. Takagi T, Yokoyama Y, Kokuryo T, Ebata T, Ando M, Nagino M. A clear difference between the outcomes after a major hepatectomy with and without an extrahepatic bile duct resection. World J Surg. 2017;41(2):508–15.
21. Higuchi R, Yamamoto M. Indications for portal vein embolization in perihilar cholangiocarcinoma. J Hepatobiliary Pancreat Sci. 2014;21(8):542–9.

22. Isfordink CJ, Samim M, Braat M, et al. Portal vein ligation versus portal vein embolization for induction of hypertrophy of the future liver remnant: a systematic review and meta-analysis. Surg Oncol. 2017;26(3):257–67.
23. van Lienden KP, van den Esschert JW, de Graaf W, et al. Portal vein embolization before liver resection: a systematic review. Cardiovasc Intervent Radiol. 2013;36(1):25–34.
24. Sugawara G, Ebata T, Yokoyama Y, et al. The effect of preoperative biliary drainage on infectious complications after hepatobiliary resection with cholangiojejunostomy. Surgery. 2013;153(2):200–10.
25. Yokoyama Y, Nagino M, Nishio H, Ebata T, Igami T, Nimura Y. Recent advances in the treatment of hilar cholangiocarcinoma: portal vein embolization. J Hepato-Biliary-Pancreat Surg. 2007;14(5):447–54.
26. Lee KC, Kinoshita H, Hirohashi K, Kubo S, Iwasa R. Extension of surgical indications for hepatocellular carcinoma by portal vein embolization. World J Surg. 1993;17(1):109–15.
27. Mizuno S, Nimura Y, Suzuki H, Yoshida S. Portal vein branch occlusion induces cell proliferation of cholestatic rat liver. J Surg Res. 1996;60(1):249–57.
28. Nagino M, Nimura Y, Kamiya J, et al. Changes in hepatic lobe volume in biliary tract cancer patients after right portal vein embolization. Hepatology (Baltimore, Md). 1995;21(2):434–9.
29. Ebata T, Yokoyama Y, Igami T, Sugawara G, Takahashi Y, Nagino M. Portal vein embolization before extended hepatectomy for biliary cancer: current technique and review of 494 consecutive embolizations. Dig Surg. 2012;29(1):23–9.
30. Wajswol E, Jazmati T, Contractor S, Kumar A. Portal vein embolization utilizing N-butyl cyanoacrylate for contralateral lobe hypertrophy prior to liver resection: a systematic review and meta-analysis. Cardiovasc Intervent Radiol. 2018;41(9):1302–12.
31. Di Stefano DR, de Baere T, Denys A, et al. Preoperative percutaneous portal vein embolization: evaluation of adverse events in 188 patients. Radiology. 2005;234(2):625–30.
32. Kodama Y, Shimizu T, Endo H, Miyamoto N, Miyasaka K. Complications of percutaneous transhepatic portal vein embolization. J Vasc Interv Radiol. 2002;13(12):1233–7.
33. Capussotti L, Muratore A, Ferrero A, Anselmetti GC, Corgnier A, Regge D. Extension of right portal vein embolization to segment IV portal branches. Arch Surg (Chicago, Ill : 1960). 2005;140(11):1100–3.
34. Kim D, Cornman-Homonoff J, Madoff DC. Preparing for liver surgery with "alphabet soup": PVE, ALPPS, TAE-PVE, LVD and RL. Hepatobiliary Surg Nutr. 2020;9(2):136–51.
35. Elias D, De Baere T, Roche A, Mducreux LJ, Lasser P. During liver regeneration following right portal embolization the growth rate of liver metastases is more rapid than that of the liver parenchyma. Br J Surg. 1999;86(6):784–8.
36. Pamecha V, Levene A, Grillo F, Woodward N, Dhillon A, Davidson BR. Effect of portal vein embolisation on the growth rate of colorectal liver metastases. Br J Cancer. 2009;100(4):617–22.
37. Hoekstra LT, van Lienden KP, Doets A, Busch OR, Gouma DJ, van Gulik TM. Tumor progression after preoperative portal vein embolization. Ann Surg. 2012;256(5):812–7. discussion 7–8
38. Klatskin G. Adenocarcinoma of the hepatic duct at its bifurcation within the porta hepatis. An unusual tumor with distinctive clinical and pathological features. Am J Med. 1965;38:241–56.
39. Nagino M, Kanai M, Morioka A, et al. Portal and arterial embolization before extensive liver resection in patients with markedly poor functional reserve. J Vasc Interv Radiol. 2000;11(8):1063–8.
40. Gruttadauria S, Luca A, Mandala L, Miraglia R, Gridelli B. Sequential preoperative ipsilateral portal and arterial embolization in patients with colorectal liver metastases. World J Surg. 2006;30(4):576–8.
41. Nagino M, Yamada T, Kamiya J, Uesaka K, Arai T, Nimura Y. Left hepatic trisegmentectomy with right hepatic vein resection after right hepatic vein embolization. Surgery. 2003;133(5):580–2.
42. Hwang S, Lee SG, Ko GY, et al. Sequential preoperative ipsilateral hepatic vein embolization after portal vein embolization to induce further liver regeneration in patients with hepatobiliary malignancy. Ann Surg. 2009;249(4):608–16.

43. Esposito F, Lim C, Lahat E, et al. Combined hepatic and portal vein embolization as preparation for major hepatectomy: a systematic review. HPB. 2019;21(9):1099–106.
44. Clavien P-A. Hepatic vein embolization for safer liver surgery: insignificant novelty or a breakthrough? Ann Surg. 2020;272(2):206–9.
45. Schnitzbauer AA, Lang SA, Goessmann H, et al. Right portal vein ligation combined with in situ splitting induces rapid left lateral liver lobe hypertrophy enabling 2-staged extended right hepatic resection in small-for-size settings. Ann Surg. 2012;255(3):405–14.
46. Hattori M, Nagino M, Ebata T, Kato K, Okada K, Shimoyama Y. Prospective study of biliary cytology in suspected perihilar cholangiocarcinoma. Br J Surg. 2011;98(5):704–9.
47. Tsuchiya T, Yokoyama Y, Ebata T, et al. Randomized controlled trial on timing and number of sampling for bile aspiration cytology. J Hepatobiliary Pancreat Sci. 2014;21(6):433–8.
48. Nagino M. Value of ALPPS in surgery for Klatskin tumours. BJS. 2019;106(12):1574–5.
49. Nagino M, Kamiya J, Nishio H, Ebata T, Arai T, Nimura Y. Two hundred forty consecutive portal vein embolizations before extended hepatectomy for biliary cancer: surgical outcome and long-term follow-up. Ann Surg. 2006;243(3):364–72.
50. Ebata T, Ito T, Yokoyama Y, et al. Surgical technique of hepatectomy combined with simultaneous resection of hepatic artery and portal vein for perihilar cholangiocarcinoma (with video). J Hepatobiliary Pancreat Sci. 2014;21(8):E57–61.
51. Igami T, Yokoyama Y, Nishio H, et al. A left hepatectomy and caudate lobectomy combined resection of the ventral segment of the right anterior sector for hilar cholangiocarcinoma--the efficacy of PVE (portal vein embolization) in identifying the hepatic subsegment: report of a case. Surg Today. 2009;39(7):628–32.
52. Komada T, Suzuki K, Mizuno T, et al. Efficacy of percutaneous transhepatic portal vein embolization using gelatin sponge particles and metal coils. Acta Radiol Open. 2018;7(4):2058460118769687.
53. Nagino M, Ebata T, Yokoyama Y, et al. Evolution of surgical treatment for perihilar cholangiocarcinoma: a single-center 34-year review of 574 consecutive resections. Ann Surg. 2013;258(1):129–40.

19 Rationale and Techniques for Liver Hypertrophy in Transplant Setting

E. Gringeri, A. Marchini, and U. Cillo

19.1 Introduction

Leveraging hepatic regeneration and evidence from two-stage surgeries, new techniques that integrate these insights have been implemented in the transplant setting.

Liver transplantation (LT) has become increasingly important in the treatment of liver tumors, contributing to the significant growth of the field known as "transplant oncology" [1].

Indication of liver transplantation is nowadays interesting not only for primitive liver cancer (hepatocellular carcinoma (HCC) and intrahepatic cholangiocarcinoma (iCCA)) in cirrhotic patients but also for perihilar cholangiocarcinoma (pCCA), neuroendocrine tumors (NET). and colorectal liver metastases (CRLM) [2]. The transplant oncology era therefore represents a change in the paradigm of the regenerative techniques. The regenerative techniques in fact represented a pushing of the boundaries in borderline resectable patients, while the organ replacement is a new concept.

When the tumor is confined to the liver and unresectable, liver transplantation (LT) enables the most radical excision, eliminates the pro-carcinogenic microenvironment, and restores hepatic metabolic function, which may be impaired due to chronic liver disease or the impact of oncological and surgical treatments. LT can remove occult liver metastases too [3].

Given the extremely limited availability of organs for transplantation, the ability to divide a cadaveric donor liver into two functionally autonomous and transplantable parts (split liver) and the practice of living donor liver transplantation have opened new horizons. The focus on resource optimization and the understanding of

E. Gringeri · A. Marchini · U. Cillo (✉)
Department of Surgery, Oncology and Gastroenterology, Hepatobiliary Surgery and Liver Transplant Unit, Azienda Ospedale Università di Padova, Padova, Veneto, Italy
e-mail: enrico.gringeri@unipd.it; cillo@unipd.it

L. Aldrighetti et al. (eds.), *Liver Regeneration Techniques In Hepatic Surgery*, https://doi.org/10.1007/978-3-032-10997-2_19

hepatic regeneration mechanisms have enabled the development of innovative transplant techniques, such as auxiliary partial orthotopic liver transplantation (APOLT) [4] and resection and partial liver segment 2–3 transplantation with delayed total hepatectomy (RAPID) [5], which allows the use of limited parenchymal portions. These techniques, combined with established methods for hepatic flow control, aim to reduce small-for-size syndrome and have significantly expanded the available therapeutic options.

19.2 From APOLT to RAPID

Auxiliary partial orthotopic liver transplantation (APOLT) is a highly intricate procedure involving an extensive hepatectomy to create sufficient space for placing a partial liver graft in the original liver position.

In 1989 the first APOLT procedure was performed for fulminant hepatic failure in a 33-year-old woman [4]. It was proposed for the treatment of acute liver failure [6], metabolic liver disease [7], and chronic liver disease [8], and later the concept was applied in the transplant oncology field trough RAPID procedure [9].

Indication for APOLT includes metabolic liver disease in children without cirrhosis, as a sort of gene therapy for fulminant hepatic failure. Particularly, in pediatric patients, the concept is to assist the native liver's recovery during a phase of acute, life-threatening insufficiency by providing an additional metabolically functioning parenchyma. This extra parenchyma can serve as a potential bridge to full recovery of native liver function, because it can be removed later, or simply allowed to atrophy without immunosuppression, once the native liver has fully regained its function [10].

Inflammation in the APOLT graft increases intraparenchymal resistance, causing portal flow to divert toward the low-resistance native liver. This can lead to graft atrophy and worsen ischemia. To overcome this problem, portal modulation—reducing the diameter of the portal branch supplying the native liver—can be performed, including through radiological segmental portal embolization.

Sometimes, complete irreversible portal ligation is necessary [11]. Inducing venous congestion in part of the native remnant by ligating the middle hepatic vein close to its outflow in the vena cava might be another option [12].

APOLT, associating liver partition and portal vein ligation for staged hepatectomy (ALPPS), and laparoscopic microwave ablation and portal vein ligation for staged hepatectomy (LAPS) [13] represented the basis for a new technique that integrated the liver regeneration concept with transplantation: the RAPID procedure (Resection And Partial Liver segment II–III transplantation with Delayed total hepatectomy) [5] and later to LD-RAPID [14].

19.3 Resection and Partial Liver Segment 2–3 Transplantation with Delayed Total Hepatectomy: RAPID Procedure

RAPID procedure consists of an auxiliary liver transplantation where a small partial liver graft (namely an LLS graft) is implanted orthotopically after a left hepatectomy of the native liver. Therefore, it conceptually comes from APOLT and two-stage hepatectomy techniques. To encourage rapid regeneration of the transplanted segments, portal flow is diverted toward the future remnant, as in the ALPPS technique. Once the auxiliary future remnant has regenerated quickly, the native liver hepatectomy is completed, similar to a two-stage hepatectomy.

The RAPID procedure has three underlying concepts related with the technique [9]:

1. *Left hepatectomy*: The native liver must be able to tolerate a partial hepatectomy and to sustain liver function while the small partial graft regenerates during the interstage period.
2. *Left lateral graft living donor liver transplantation (LLG LDLT)*: The right portal vein is ligated or transected during the first stage to completely direct the portal blood flow to the graft. The remnant native liver, supplied only by arterial flow, must support the small S2–S3 graft until it has sufficiently regenerated.
3. *Hypersmall graft nursing concept*: Similar to ALPPS for liver tumors, hepatobiliary scintigraphy (showing functional graft function), computed tomography volumetric measurements (showing graft-to-recipient weight ratio (GRWR) >0.8%) and laboratory tests may be used to guide the decision about the timing of the second stage.

19.3.1 RAPID Surgical Technique

The RAPID surgical technique has been previously described in detail [9, 15, 16]. According to the Padova experience, we describe the technique with living donor procurement. Unresectability of the tumor should firstly be confirmed by an international multidisciplinary board. Patient must be a responder to chemotherapy. After ethics committee approval, potential donors are evaluated with estimation of left lateral segment (LLSs) volume.

At the first step, the LLSs procured from the donor are implanted in the recipient in an orthotopic position after a full left hepatectomy (segments 1–4) extended to the left hepatic vein. A tip about the transection plane in the first step is the use of thermal ablation to reduce tumor spillage and the use of a saphenous ring to reduce the risk of kinking for the suprahepatic vein anastomosis [9]. The graft's left hepatic vein is usually anastomosed on the stump of the middle and left hepatic veins. The graft left portal vein is then anastomosed end-to-end with the recipient's left portal vein. Similarly, the left hepatic artery is anastomosed to the stump of the recipient's artery, possibly using operative microscope. Repeated measurements of portal pressures and flow rates are conducted. After ligation of the right portal vein, the pressure in the left portal vein must remain stable below 20 mmHg. Measurements have to be performed with and without clamping of the portal vein to the native liver. If, after clamping the portal vein to the native liver, the pressure rises above 20 mmHg, a splenic artery ligation or a different portal modulation flow has to be put in place. The stump of the left bile duct is connected to a Roux-en-Y loop. The postoperative increase in graft volume is closely monitored. When the volume of the FLR reaches a graft-to-body weight (GRWR) ratio of 1 (usually 2 weeks), it is possible to proceed with the second-stage hepatectomy, which can be performed laparoscopically.

19.3.2 Outcomes of RAPID Procedure

Since RAPID is a recent technique, the results are still not so established. Early results [9] considering 23 non-cirrhotic patients treated with RAPID between 2015 and 2022 in six European centers with unresectable CRLM, unresectable liver metastases of neuroendocrine tumor or liver adenomatosis, receiving a left liver graft (LLG) from a living donor (20 patients), or a split from a cadaveric donor (3 patients) showed a volume increase of 107%, with a kinetic growth rate of 25 mL/day and a median interstage time of 14 days..

Concerning oncologic advantages of liver transplantation, the results of RAPID are good: no donor mortality, low donor morbidity (4.3%), acceptable recipient morbidity (43% ≥ IIIb Clavien–Dindo), and mortality (4.3%) rates [9]. In particular, the results about survival are really encouraging: 90% 1-year overall patient and graft survival and 66.7% 1-year recurrence free survival among patients affected by CRLM, with a median follow up of 696 days.

Selection for RAPID procedure must consider minimization of living donor risk as the most important factor among having a recipient transplant benefit and no waiting list harm, which are the other leading elements with a different weight in cadaveric LT and living donor liver transplantation—right lobe [9].

19.4 Strategies in Technique

19.4.1 Portal Modulation Techniques and Inflow Control

Small-for-size syndrome (SFSS) [17] is an issue of the technique: the graft size with graft inflow and outflow have complex interaction in an effort to meet the metabolic demand of the patient. SFSS is characterized by hepatic insufficiency with hyperbilirubinemia, coagulopathy, ascites, and possibly multiorgan dysfunction. It is extensively being studied in the common liver transplant setting but it is crucial in RAPID technique.

The pathophysiology of this syndrome has many influencing factors [18]:

- *donor and graft factors*: donor age, liver steatosis, small graft (GRWR <0.8; <0.7; <0.6%)
- *transplant surgery factors*: duration of surgery, blood loss during surgery, surgeon experience, medical management, anesthetic management
- *recipient factors*: liver disease severity, lab MELD, portal hypertension, sarcopenia

Prognosis can change according with the degree of SFSS. It can be mild (grade A, pre-SFSS), requiring medical supportive care, which usually recovers, moderate (grade B), with portal hypertension, hyperbilirubinemia with or without ascites, which can be worsened by additional insults after transplantation (such as infections, sepsis, portal steal, thrombosis, acute rejection) or severe (grade C) with liver failure, characterized by hyperbilirubinemia, coagulopathy, with or without encephalopathy with limited or no portal vein or hepatic artery flow with severe graft swelling, leading to graft necrosis with an increased mortality risk and necessity to evaluate retransplantation [18].

The key point is the portal inflow modulation, thus portal pressure/flow should be measured along with hepatic artery flow.

Many graft inflow modulation (GIM) techniques were developed such as spleen inflow modulation techniques (splenic artery ligation, simultaneous splenectomy, splenic devascularization, splenic artery embolization), porto-systemic shunt (spontaneous porto-systemic shunts, hemi-portocaval shunt), and pharmacological approaches (low dose somatostatin, prostaglandin E1, adenosine) [19]. Some of these techniques can be helpful in those patients with auxiliary liver transplantation of small for size grafts in patients with chronic liver disease [8].

Portal inflow modulation by splenic artery ligation/embolization or other porto-systemic shunts is effective in the prevention and treatment of SFSS in the setting of living donors [20]. In the RAPID technique, the portal flow modulation should take into account for a healthy liver with a portal pressure <20 mmHg and flow 100–300 mL/100 g/min, while for a cirrhotic liver with a portal pressure <15 mmHg and flow 100–300 mL/100 g/min [8, 9, 21].

These considerations have significant implications in resective surgery as well, because some surgeons (e.g., Vibert, Cillo) perform portocaval shunts even during extreme resections to reduce portal hyperflow.

19.4.2 Interstage Assessment

As for two-stage hepatectomy, liver function and volume at the interstage can be assessed with hepatobiliary scintigraphy, Indocianin Green (ICG) test, gadoxetic acid-enhanced MRI at preoperative exams, and dynamic MRI [22, 23]. 3D modeling and artificial intelligence models seem to be also effective [24, 25].

The graft-to-recipient weight (GRWR) ratio is expected to be >0.8%, even though some groups described successful use of grafts with a GRWR as low as 0.6% [26, 27].

19.4.3 Pro-regeneration in the Context of "Shift to Left"

Living donor liver transplantation (LDLT) could become a viable resource, although its adoption in the Western world remains limited. To minimize the impact on donors, several groups advocate reducing the extent of donor hepatectomy, shifting from right-lobe to left-lobe or left lateral segment donation ("shift-to-left"). This is particularly relevant for nonestablished indications and could make the procedure more acceptable to both potential donors and recipients. This concept is fundamental for all the above. Left lobe grafts can be transplanted directly, despite a higher risk of small-for-size syndrome, or used in dual-graft LDLT or RAPID procedures, despite technical complexities. In case of dual-graft LDLT, two small grafts obtained from two donors are simultaneously transplanted.

Living donation not only procures a graft for the designed recipient, but at the same time reduces pressure on the deceased donor waiting list, freeing resources for other patients (shift-to-left). The concept of shift-to-left could be applied also to deceased donors: when not required by pediatric recipients, split livers would offer a virtually unlimited additional source of donor organs for this purpose [28].

In high-volume expert centers, right-lobe transplantation, left lateral grafts, RAPID procedures, and dual-graft transplantation should be considered as a range of alternative options. These can be selected based on the patient's specific availability, donor resources, and the characteristics of the recipient [28].

19.5 Conclusions

This comprehensive set of tools, available in the technical arsenal of high-volume expert centers, should be thoughtfully proposed to patients and potential donors. The goal is to achieve the best possible outcomes for recipients with the lowest risk to donors. Additionally, this approach has the potential to judiciously expand transplant indications and enhance curative capacities after transplantation by liver resection in case of disease recurrence.

The key points for RAPID procedure and, in general, in the pro-regeneration techniques in the transplant setting are donor safety, oncologic safety in transection, portal flow modulation/outflow, interstage time (risk of tumor progression, risk of insufficient growth—volume vs. function), second-stage minimization, role of biologic selection, and pathophysiology of coexistent hemilivers. Finally, biology has a key role and the selection should strongly take into account of that, otherwise surgery would be futile.

Split liver technique might serve to expand the donor pool.

Finally, another chapter is the regeneration of the transplanted liver: the feasibility of major liver resections after liver transplantation was exemplarily shown by some [29], who reported almost full compensation of hepatic tissue in one liver transplant recipient shortly after right hepatectomy. The literature about major liver resection in LT is still rare, and more evidence is needed [30].

References

1. Sapisochin G, Hibi T, Toso C, Man K, Berenguer M, Heimbach J, et al. Transplant oncology in primary and metastatic liver tumors: principles, evidence, and opportunities. Ann Surg. 2021;273(3):483–93.
2. Abreu P, Gorgen A, Oldani G, Hibi T, Sapisochin G. Recent advances in liver transplantation for cancer: the future of transplant oncology. JHEP Rep Innov Hepatol. 2019;1(5):377–91.
3. Chávez-Villa M, Ruffolo LI, Al-Judaibi BM, Fujiki M, Hashimoto K, Kallas J, et al. The high incidence of occult carcinoma in total hepatectomy specimens of patients treated for unresectable colorectal liver metastases with liver transplant. Ann Surg. 2023;278(5):e1026–34.
4. Gubernatis G, Pichlmayr R, Kemnitz J, Gratz K. Auxiliary partial orthotopic liver transplantation (APOLT) for fulminant hepatic failure: first successful case report. World J Surg. 1991;15(5):660–5; discussion 665–666.
5. Line PD, Hagness M, Berstad AE, Foss A, Dueland S. A novel concept for partial liver transplantation in nonresectable colorectal liver metastases: the RAPID concept. Ann Surg. 2015;262(1):e5–9.
6. Jaeck D, Boudjema K, Audet M, Chenard-Neu MP, Simeoni U, Meyer C, et al. Auxiliary partial orthotopic liver transplantation (APOLT) in the treatment of acute liver failure. J Gastroenterol. 2002;37(Suppl 13):88–91.
7. Reddy MS, Rajalingam R, Rela M. Revisiting APOLT for metabolic liver disease: a new look at an old idea. Transplantation. 2017;101(2):260–6.
8. Azoulay D, Feray C, Lim C, Salloum C, Conticchio M, Cherqui D, et al. A systematic review of auxiliary liver transplantation of small-for-size grafts in patients with chronic liver disease. JHEP Reports. 2022;4(4):100447.
9. Settmacher U, Ali-Deeb A, Coubeau L, Cillo U, Line PD, Guba M, et al. Auxilliary liver transplantation according to the RAPID procedure in noncirrhotic patients: technical aspects and early outcomes. Ann Surg. 2023;277(2):305–12.
10. Rammohan A, Reddy MS, Narasimhan G, Rajalingam R, Kaliamoorthy I, Shanmugam N, et al. Auxiliary partial orthotopic liver transplantation for selected noncirrhotic metabolic liver disease. Liver Transpl. 2019;25(1):111–8.
11. Yabe S, Nishizawa H, Egawa H, Nakayama H, Okamoto S, Kiuchi T, et al. Portal blood flow and liver regeneration in auxiliary partial orthotopic liver transplantation in a canine model. Eur Surg Res Eur Chir Forsch Rech Chir Eur. 1999;31(1):83–92.
12. Broering DC, Walter J, Bassas AF. Overcoming the portal steal phenomenon in auxiliary partial orthotopic liver transplantation by modulation of the venous outflow of the native liver. Liver Transpl. 2005;11(9):1140–3.
13. Gringeri E, Boetto R, D'Amico FE, Bassi D, Cillo U. Laparoscopic microwave ablation and portal vein ligation for staged hepatectomy (LAPS): a minimally invasive first-step approach. Ann Surg. 2015;261(2):e42–3.
14. Königsrainer A, Templin S, Capobianco I, Königsrainer I, Bitzer M, Zender L, et al. Paradigm shift in the management of irresectable colorectal liver metastases: living donor auxiliary partial orthotopic liver transplantation in combination with two-stage hepatectomy (LD-RAPID). Ann Surg. 2019;270(2):327–32.
15. Lim C, Turco C, Balci D, Savier E, Goumard C, Perdigao F, et al. Auxiliary liver transplantation for cirrhosis: from APOLT to RAPID: a scoping review. Ann Surg. 2022;275(3):551–9.
16. Nadalin S, Settmacher U, Rauchfuß F, Balci D, Königsrainer A, Line PD. RAPID procedure for colorectal cancer liver metastasis. Int J Surg Lond Engl. 2020;82S:93–6.
17. Masuda Y, Yoshizawa K, Ohno Y, Mita A, Shimizu A, Soejima Y. Small-for-size syndrome in liver transplantation: definition, pathophysiology and management. Hepatobiliary Pancreat Dis Int HBPD INT. 2020;19(4):334–41.
18. Parente A, Cho HD, Kim KH, Schlegel A. Association between hepatocellular carcinoma recurrence and graft size in living donor liver transplantation: a systematic review. Int J Mol Sci. 2023;24(7):6224.

19. Cheng P, Li Z, Fu Z, Jian Q, Deng R, Ma Y. Small-for-size syndrome and graft inflow modulation techniques in liver transplantation. Dig Dis Basel Switz. 2023;41(2):250–8.
20. Miller CM, Quintini C, Dhawan A, Durand F, Heimbach JK, Kim-Schluger HL, et al. The international liver transplantation society living donor liver transplant recipient guideline. Transplantation. 2017;101(5):938–44.
21. Balci D, Kirimker EO, Bingol Kologlu M, Ustuner E, Goktug UU, Karadag Erkoc S, et al. A new approach for increasing availability of liver grafts and donor safety in living donor liver transplantation: LD-RAPID procedure in the cirrhotic setting with hepatocellular carcinoma. Liver Transpl. 2021;27(4):590–4.
22. Wang Q, Brismar TB, Gilg S, Jonas E, Nilsson H, Tzortzakakis A, et al. Multimodal perioperative assessment of liver function and volume in patients undergoing hepatectomy for colorectal liver metastasis: a comparison of the indocyanine green retention test, (99m) Tc mebrofenin hepatobiliary scintigraphy and gadoxetic acid enhanced MRI. Br J Radiol. 2022;95(1139):20220370.
23. Ai X, Wang H, Yang Y, Feng Y, Xie X, Zhao X, et al. Four indices on Gd-EOB-DTPA-enhanced MRI can estimate liver functional reserve compared to ICG-R15: a systematic review and meta-analysis. Clin Imaging. 2023;102:1–8.
24. Vicente E, Quijano Y, Duran H, Diaz E, Fabra I, Malave L, et al. Can 3D imaging modeling recognize functional tissue and predict liver failure? A retrospective study based on 3D modelling of the major hepatectomies after hepatic modulation. BMC Surg. 2023;23(1):316.
25. Gerwing M, Schindler P, Katou S, Köhler M, Stamm AC, Schmidt VF, et al. Multi-organ radiomics-based prediction of future remnant liver hypertrophy following portal vein embolization. Ann Surg Oncol. 2023;30(13):7976–85.
26. Wong TCL, Fung JYY, Cui TYS, Sin SL, Ma KW, She BWH, et al. The risk of going small: lowering GRWR and overcoming small-for-size syndrome in adult living donor liver transplantation. Ann Surg. 2021;274(6):e1260–8.
27. Kusakabe J, Yagi S, Sasaki K, Uozumi R, Abe H, Okamura Y, et al. Is 0.6% reasonable as the minimum requirement of the graft-to-recipient weight ratio regardless of lobe selection in adult living-donor liver transplantation? Transplantation. 2021;105(9):2007–17.
28. Cillo U, Furlanetto A, Gringeri E, Bertacco A, Marchini A, Rosso E, et al. Advocating for a “shift-to-left” in transplant oncology: left grafts, RAPID and dual graft. Updates Surg. 2024;77:1889–902.
29. Chari RS, Baker ME, Sue SR, Meyers WC. Regeneration of a transplanted liver after right hepatic lobectomy. Liver Transpl. 1996;2(3):233–4.
30. Pohl JMO, Raschzok N, Eurich D, Pflüger M, Wiering L, Daneshgar A, et al. Outcomes of liver resections after liver transplantation at a high-volume hepatobiliary center. J Clin Med. 2020;9(11):3685.

Part V

Further Insights

Impact of Minimally-Invasive Approaches

20

Hwee-Leong Tan and Brian K. P. Goh

20.1 Introduction

Liver resection has evolved over the past few decades with an improved appreciation of surgical liver anatomy and refinements in technical expertise. One of the key shifts in the field is the growing adoption of minimally-invasive liver resection (MILR) for increasingly complex resections [1–4]. As surgeons mounted their learning curves, MILR has been consistently reported to provide several perioperative benefits compared to open liver resection (OLR) [3, 4]. These include improvements in intraoperative outcomes in terms of blood loss and transfusion requirements, as well as postoperative outcomes such as postoperative morbidity, post-hepatectomy liver failure (PHLF), and length of stay. The enhanced recovery profile of patients after MILR has been shown to be substantial enough to override its higher procedural costs, rendering MILR superior to OLR from a cost-effectiveness standpoint [5, 6].

The application of MILR in the setting of liver resections requiring modulation of the future liver remnant (FLR) such as two-stage hepatectomy (TSH) and associating liver partition and portal vein ligation for staged hepatectomy (ALPPS) has garnered considerable interest [7–10]. The first case of laparoscopic ALPPS was reported in 2012, with a reduction in intra-abdominal adhesions touted as one of the key benefits of the minimally-invasive approach [11]. Minimizing adhesions after stage 1 surgery in both ALPPS and some cases of TSH is particularly attractive as it mitigates a substantial degree of the technical difficulty in subsequent stage 2 surgery [12]. Additionally, extrapolating from the benefits of MILR over OLR for liver resections in general, the reduced morbidity and PHLF that MILR potentially offers

H.-L. Tan · B. K. P. Goh (✉)
Department of Hepatopancreatobiliary and Transplant Surgery, Singapore General Hospital and National Cancer Center Singapore, Singapore, Singapore
e-mail: brian.goh@singhealth.com.sg

L. Aldrighetti et al. (eds.), *Liver Regeneration Techniques In Hepatic Surgery*, https://doi.org/10.1007/978-3-032-10997-2_20

are of particular value in these settings. In ALPPS for instance, PHLF is the leading cause of mortality, and postoperative morbidity after stage 1 ALPPS is a strong predictor for mortality after stage 2 ALPPS [8].

In spite of the potential benefits MILR confers over OLR, substantial concerns over the safety profile of MILR in ALPPS and TSH remain. While MILR in these settings have been reported from centers of expertise [13, 14], liver resections in these settings are usually saddled with substantial tumor burden, the requirement for extensive parenchymal resections, and borderline underlying liver function—factors that are well-recognized contributors to heightened difficulty for MILR as reflected in various difficulty scoring systems [15–20]. Additional technical challenges include the anatomical distortion resulting from induced hypertrophy of the FLR, peri-vascular inflammatory changes (in the use of portal vein embolization), and post-surgical adhesions from a stage 1 surgery [21].

20.2 Evidence for MILR in Staged Hepatectomies

The feasibility of MILR in TSH has been explored in several retrospective cohort studies to date [7]. A bi-institutional, propensity score-matched study of 86 patients who underwent TSH found that those who underwent a laparoscopic approach had lower intraoperative blood loss, postoperative morbidity, and length of hospital stay, as well as earlier administration of postoperative chemotherapy when compared to the open approach [22]. Long-term survival outcomes were similar between both groups. However, patients in the laparoscopic group were more likely to undergo repeat liver resection for disease recurrence, potentially attributable to the reduced adhesions associated with MILR, facilitating repeat resections when necessary [22].

In a similar vein, several comparative studies have sought to evaluate the performance of MILR in the setting of ALPPS in the past decade. Early meta-analyses comparing ALPPS and TSH report a significantly greater increase in FLR volume and frequency of completion of stage 2 associated with ALPPS, with the downside of potentially greater morbidity and mortality [23, 24]. As such, the potential for MILR to reduce surgical morbidity in ALPPS is of particular relevance. A multicenter Italian registry study comparing minimally-invasive ALPPS (MI-ALPPS) with open ALPPS for stage 1 surgery among patients with hepatocellular carcinoma reported several benefits in the MI-ALPPS group including higher rates of hospital discharge after stage 1, lower rates of grade A PHLF after stage 1, lower major morbidity rates after stage 2, and an overall shorter length of hospital stay [25]. On a broader level, earlier systematic reviews of MI-ALPPS found lower rates of major morbidity, mortality, and failure to reach stage 2 when compared to series of open ALPPS in existing literature, although potential selection bias exists in such unadjusted comparisons [26, 27]. A subsequent meta-analysis of nine retrospective cohort studies comparing MI-ALPPS with open ALPSS reported a significantly decreased risk of 90-day mortality and overall length of hospital stay among MI-ALPPS patients, with similar percentage FLR hypertrophy, negative resection margin rates, and PHLF rates [28].

Taken together, the available literature to date suggests that the perioperative benefits of MILR are potentially translatable to TSH and ALPPS. A major caveat to consider, however, is the steep learning curves associated with MILR, as the generalizability of these encouraging results are contingent upon a center's proficiency in MILR [29]. Other than direct procedural complications, inadequate expertise can also manifest as prolonged operative duration when compared to conventional OLR. Prolonged operative time has, in turn, been reported to correlate with an increased risk of postoperative morbidity in MILR, which would likely be poorly tolerated in this patient population [30]. In this respect, robotic liver resection (RLR) may offer an edge over laparoscopic liver resection (LLR) by offering superior dexterity, mitigation of tremor, and fatigue, as well as a high-definition three-dimensional magnified operative visual field [4]. These have translated into a shortened learning curve for RLR, as well as a multitude of perioperative benefits such as decreased blood loss and conversion rates when compared to LLR across various types of liver resection [29, 31–38]. While preliminary reports comparing RLR and OLR for ALPPS have affirmed its feasibility and comparative benefits, further larger scale studies and direct comparisons between LLR and RLR in this setting would be needed to better elucidate their comparative safety and outcomes [39, 40].

20.3 Additional Technical Modifications to Minimize Invasiveness

Beyond operative approach alone, the philosophy of "minimizing invasiveness" has also been extended to other aspects of staged hepatectomies, particularly in ALPPS. To decrease morbidity following stage 1, some surgeons have advocated for a partial parenchymal transaction (partial-ALPPS) as opposed to a full transection in classical ALPPS. This has been demonstrated to achieve comparable FLR hypertrophy with significantly lower morbidity and mortality rates [41, 42]. Alternative means of achieving liver partitioning, such as the use of radiofrequency or microwave assistance, as well as the application of a tourniquet around a parenchymal groove of 1 cm in the future transection line have also been described [43–45]. Further, the use of portal vein embolization in lieu of portal vein ligation in stage 1 has also been utilized to avoid hilar dissection, which poses risks of inadvertent biliary and hepatic arterial injuries [46, 47]. The combination of partial parenchymal transection with portal vein embolization (termed "mini-ALPPS" or "hybrid-ALPPS") has, in turn, been demonstrated to achieved technical success without PHLF, major morbidity, or mortality in small selected patient cohorts [47, 48].

20.4 Conclusion

With continued accrual of experience in staged hepatectomies alongside further refinements and modifications in operative approaches, the potential benefits of MILR and its synergism with other aspects of minimizing invasiveness in staged hepatectomies remains to be affirmed by future studies. Extrapolating from the trajectory of MILR adoption in the field of liver resection thus far, MILR will likely be established as a safe and beneficial stalwart for TSH and ALPPS in the foreseeable future.

References

1. Buell JF, Cherqui D, Geller DA, O'Rourke N, Iannitti D, Dagher I, Koffron AJ, Thomas M, Gayet B, Han HS, Wakabayashi G, Belli G, Kaneko H, Ker CG, Scatton O, Laurent A, Abdalla EK, Chaudhury P, Dutson E, Gamblin C, D'Angelica M, Nagorney D, Testa G, Labow D, Manas D, Poon RT, Nelson H, Martin R, Clary B, Pinson WC, Martinie J, Vauthey JN, Goldstein R, Roayaie S, Barlet D, Espat J, Abecassis M, Rees M, Fong Y, McMasters KM, Broelsch C, Busuttil R, Belghiti J, Strasberg S, Chari RS, World Consensus Conference on Laparoscopic S. The international position on laparoscopic liver surgery: the Louisville Statement, 2008. Ann Surg. 2009;250(5):825–30.
2. Wakabayashi G, Cherqui D, Geller DA, Buell JF, Kaneko H, Han HS, Asbun H, O'Rourke N, Tanabe M, Koffron AJ, Tsung A, Soubrane O, Machado MA, Gayet B, Troisi RI, Pessaux P, Van Dam RM, Scatton O, Abu Hilal M, Belli G, Kwon CH, Edwin B, Choi GH, Aldrighetti LA, Cai X, Cleary S, Chen KH, Schon MR, Sugioka A, Tang CN, Herman P, Pekolj J, Chen XP, Dagher I, Jarnagin W, Yamamoto M, Strong R, Jagannath P, Lo CM, Clavien PA, Kokudo N, Barkun J, Strasberg SM. Recommendations for laparoscopic liver resection: a report from the second international consensus conference held in Morioka. Ann Surg. 2015;261(4):619–29.
3. Abu Hilal M, Aldrighetti L, Dagher I, Edwin B, Troisi RI, Alikhanov R, Aroori S, Belli G, Besselink M, Briceno J, Gayet B, D'Hondt M, Lesurtel M, Menon K, Lodge P, Rotellar F, Santoyo J, Scatton O, Soubrane O, Sutcliffe R, Van Dam R, White S, Halls MC, Cipriani F, Van der Poel M, Ciria R, Barkhatov L, Gomez-Luque Y, Ocana-Garcia S, Cook A, Buell J, Clavien PA, Dervenis C, Fusai G, Geller D, Lang H, Primrose J, Taylor M, Van Gulik T, Wakabayashi G, Asbun H, Cherqui D. The Southampton consensus guidelines for laparoscopic liver surgery: from indication to implementation. Ann Surg. 2018;268(1):11–8.
4. Liu R, Abu Hilal M, Wakabayashi G, Han HS, Palanivelu C, Boggi U, Hackert T, Kim HJ, Wang XY, Hu MG, Choi GH, Panaro F, He J, Efanov M, Yin XY, Croner RS, Fong YM, Zhu JY, Wu Z, Sun CD, Lee JH, Marino MV, Ganpati IS, Zhu P, Wang ZZ, Yang KH, Fan J, Chen XP, Lau WY. International experts consensus guidelines on robotic liver resection in 2023. World J Gastroenterol. 2023;29(32):4815–30.
5. Koh YX, Zhao Y, Tan IE, Tan HL, Chua DW, Loh WL, Tan EK, Teo JY, Au MKH, Goh BKP. Comparative cost-effectiveness of open, laparoscopic, and robotic liver resection: a systematic review and network meta-analysis. Surgery. 2024;176(1):11–23.
6. Koh YX, Zhao Y, Tan IE, Tan HL, Chua DW, Tan EK, Teo JY, Ang KA, Au MKH, Goh BKP. Cost-effectiveness of laparoscopic vs open liver resection: a propensity score-matched single-center analysis of 920 cases. J Am Coll Surg. 2025;241:203–19.
7. Nassar A, Tzedakis S, Dhote A, Strigalev M, Coriat R, Karoui M, Dohan A, Gaillard M, Marchese U, Fuks D. Multiple laparoscopic liver resection for colorectal liver metastases. Cancers (Basel). 2023;15(2):435.
8. Lang H, de Santibanes E, Schlitt HJ, Malago M, van Gulik T, Machado MA, Jovine E, Heinrich S, Ettorre GM, Chan A, Hernandez-Alejandro R, Robles Campos R, Sandstrom P,

Linecker M, Clavien PA. 10th Anniversary of ALPPS-lessons learned and quo Vadis. Ann Surg. 2019;269(1):114–9.
9. Kabir T, Syn N, Goh BKP. Current status of laparoscopic liver resection for the management of colorectal liver metastases. J Gastrointest Oncol. 2020;11(3):526–39.
10. Wang Z, Goh BKP. Editorial comment on: surgical outcomes of two-stage hepatectomy for colorectal liver metastasis: comparison to a benchmark procedure. Hepatobiliary Surg Nutr. 2021;10(4):570–2.
11. Machado MA, Makdissi FF, Surjan RC. Totally laparoscopic ALPPS is feasible and may be worthwhile. Ann Surg. 2012;256(3):e13; author reply e16-19.
12. Cioffi L, Belli G, Izzo F, Fantini C, D'Agostino A, Russo G, Patrone R, Granata V, Belli A. Minimally invasive ALPPS procedure: a review of feasibility and short-term outcomes. Cancers (Basel). 2023;15(6):1700.
13. Wang Z, Loh WL, Goh BKP. Pure laparoscopic associating liver partition and portal vein ligation for staged hepatectomy (ALPPS) for a giant hepatocellular carcinoma (> 15 cm) abutting the liver hilum. J Gastrointest Surg. 2023;27(12):3096–8.
14. Goh BK, Chong D, Teo N-Z. Minimally-invasive 2-stage liver resection with portal vein ligation for bi-lobar colorectal liver metastastes. Surg Gastroenterol Oncol. 2019;24(3):158–61.
15. Ban D, Tanabe M, Ito H, Otsuka Y, Nitta H, Abe Y, Hasegawa Y, Katagiri T, Takagi C, Itano O, Kaneko H, Wakabayashi G. A novel difficulty scoring system for laparoscopic liver resection. J Hepatobiliary Pancreat Sci. 2014;21(10):745–53.
16. Wakabayashi G. What has changed after the Morioka consensus conference 2014 on laparoscopic liver resection? Hepatobiliary Surg Nutr. 2016;5(4):281–9.
17. Hasegawa Y, Wakabayashi G, Nitta H, Takahara T, Katagiri H, Umemura A, Makabe K, Sasaki A. A novel model for prediction of pure laparoscopic liver resection surgical difficulty. Surg Endosc. 2017;31(12):5356–63.
18. Halls MC, Berardi G, Cipriani F, Barkhatov L, Lainas P, Harris S, D'Hondt M, Rotellar F, Dagher I, Aldrighetti L, Troisi RI, Edwin B, Abu Hilal M. Development and validation of a difficulty score to predict intraoperative complications during laparoscopic liver resection. Br J Surg. 2018;105(9):1182–91.
19. Kawaguchi Y, Fuks D, Kokudo N, Gayet B. Difficulty of laparoscopic liver resection: proposal for a new classification. Ann Surg. 2018;267(1):13–7.
20. Linn YL, Wu AG, Han HS, Liu R, Chen KH, Fuks D, Soubrane O, Cherqui D, Geller D, Cheung TT, Edwin B, Aldrighetti L, Abu Hilal M, Troisi RI, Wakabayashi G, Goh BKP, International R, Laparoscopic Liver Resection Study Group I. Systematic review and meta-analysis of difficulty scoring systems for laparoscopic and robotic liver resections. J Hepatobiliary Pancreat Sci. 2023;30(1):36–59.
21. Bozkurt E, Sijberden JP, Abu Hilal M. Safety and feasibility of laparoscopic right or extended right hemi hepatectomy following modulation of the future liver remnant in patients with colorectal liver metastases: a systematic review. J Laparoendosc Adv Surg Tech A. 2023;33(7):654–64.
22. Okumura S, Goumard C, Gayet B, Fuks D, Scatton O. Laparoscopic versus open two-stage hepatectomy for bilobar colorectal liver metastases: a bi-institutional, propensity score-matched study. Surgery. 2019;166(6):959–66.
23. Eshmuminov D, Raptis DA, Linecker M, Wirsching A, Lesurtel M, Clavien PA. Meta-analysis of associating liver partition with portal vein ligation and portal vein occlusion for two-stage hepatectomy. Br J Surg. 2016;103(13):1768–82.
24. Liu Y, Yang Y, Gu S, Tang K. A systematic review and meta-analysis of associating liver partition and portal vein ligation for staged hepatectomy (ALPPS) versus traditional staged hepatectomy. Medicine (Baltimore). 2019;98(15):e15229.
25. Serenari M, Ratti F, Zanello M, Guglielmo N, Mocchegiani F, Di Benedetto F, Nardo B, Mazzaferro V, Cillo U, Massani M, Colledan M, Dalla Valle R, Cescon M, Vivarelli M, Colasanti M, Ettorre GM, Aldrighetti L, Jovine E. Minimally invasive stage 1 to protect against the risk of liver failure: results from the hepatocellular carcinoma series of the associating liver

partition and portal vein ligation for staged hepatectomy Italian registry. J Laparoendosc Adv Surg Tech A. 2020;30(10):1082–9.
26. Melandro F, Giovanardi F, Hassan R, Larghi Laureiro Z, Ferri F, Rossi M, Mennini G, Pawlik TM, Lai Q. Minimally invasive approach in the setting of ALPPS procedure: a systematic review of the literature. J Gastrointest Surg. 2019;23(9):1917–24.
27. Michal K, Sau M, Tamara GMH, Long JR. A better route to ALPPS: minimally invasive vs open ALPPS. Surg Endosc. 2020;34(6):2379–89.
28. Loke S, Ong BDC, Ng J, Kow AWC. Safety and efficacy of minimally invasive associating liver partition and portal vein ligation for staged hepatectomy (ALPPS): a systematic review and meta-analysis. Int J Surg. 2025;111(2):2283–90.
29. Chua D, Syn N, Koh YX, Goh BKP. Learning curves in minimally invasive hepatectomy: systematic review and meta-regression analysis. Br J Surg. 2021;108(4):351–8.
30. Tranchart H, Gaillard M, Chirica M, Ferretti S, Perlemuter G, Naveau S, Dagher I. Multivariate analysis of risk factors for postoperative complications after laparoscopic liver resection. Surg Endosc. 2015;29(9):2538–44.
31. Chiow AKH, Fuks D, Choi GH, Syn N, Sucandy I, Marino MV, Prieto M, Chong CC, Lee JH, Efanov M, Kingham TP, Choi SH, Sutcliffe RP, Troisi RI, Pratschke J, Cheung TT, Wang X, Liu R, D'Hondt M, Chan CY, Tang CN, Han HS, Goh BKP, International R, Laparoscopic Liver Resection Study Group C. International multicentre propensity score-matched analysis comparing robotic versus laparoscopic right posterior sectionectomy. Br J Surg. 2021;108(12):1513–20.
32. Chong CC, Fuks D, Lee KF, Zhao JJ, Choi GH, Sucandy I, Chiow AKH, Marino MV, Gastaca M, Wang X, Lee JH, Efanov M, Kingham TP, D'Hondt M, Troisi RI, Choi SH, Sutcliffe RP, Chan CY, Lai ECH, Park JO, Di Benedetto F, Rotellar F, Sugioka A, Coelho FF, Ferrero A, Long TCD, Lim C, Scatton O, Liu Q, Schmelzle M, Pratschke J, Cheung TT, Liu R, Han HS, Tang CN, Goh BKP, International R, Laparoscopic Liver Resection Study Group I. Propensity score-matched analysis comparing robotic and laparoscopic right and extended right hepatectomy. JAMA Surg. 2022;157(5):436–44.
33. Chong Y, Prieto M, Gastaca M, Choi SH, Sucandy I, Chiow AKH, Marino MV, Wang X, Efanov M, Schotte H, D'Hondt M, Choi GH, Krenzien F, Schmelzle M, Pratschke J, Kingham TP, Giglio M, Troisi RI, Lee JH, Lai EC, Tang CN, Fuks D, D'Silva M, Han HS, Kadam P, Sutcliffe RP, Lee KF, Chong CC, Cheung TT, Liu Q, Liu R, Goh BKP, International R, Laparoscopic Liver Resection Study Group I. An international multicentre propensity score matched analysis comparing between robotic versus laparoscopic left lateral sectionectomy. Surg Endosc. 2023;37(5):3439–48.
34. Krenzien F, Schmelzle M, Pratschke J, Feldbrugge L, Liu R, Liu Q, Zhang W, Zhao JJ, Tan HL, Cipriani F, Hoogteijling TJ, Aghayan DL, Fretland AA, Siow TF, Lim C, Scatton O, Herman P, Coelho FF, Marino MV, Mazzaferro V, Chiow AKH, Sucandy I, Ivanecz A, Choi SH, Lee JH, Gastaca M, Vivarelli M, Giuliante F, Dalla Valle B, Ruzzenente A, Yong CC, Chen Z, Yin M, Fondevila C, Efanov M, Morise Z, Di Benedetto F, Brustia R, Dalla Valle R, Boggi U, Geller D, Belli A, Memeo R, Gruttadauria S, Mejia A, Park JO, Rotellar F, Choi GH, Robles-Campos R, Wang X, Sutcliffe RP, Hasegawa K, Tang CN, Chong CCN, Lee KF, Meurs J, D'Hondt M, Monden K, Lopez-Ben S, Kingham TP, Ferrero A, Ettorre GM, Pascual F, Cherqui D, Zheng J, Liang X, Soubrane O, Wakabayashi G, Troisi RI, Cheung TT, Kato Y, Sugioka A, Dokmak S, D'Silva M, Han HS, Nghia PP, Long TCD, Hilal MA, Chen KH, Fuks D, Aldrighetti L, Edwin B, Goh BKP, International R, Laparoscopic Liver Resection Study Group I. Propensity score-matching analysis comparing robotic versus laparoscopic limited liver resections of the posterosuperior segments: an international multicenter study. Ann Surg. 2024;279(2):297–305.
35. Sucandy I, Rayman S, Lai EC, Tang CN, Chong Y, Efanov M, Fuks D, Choi GH, Chong CC, Chiow AKH, Marino MV, Prieto M, Lee JH, Kingham TP, D'Hondt M, Troisi RI, Choi SH, Sutcliffe RP, Cheung TT, Rotellar F, Park JO, Scatton O, Han HS, Pratschke J, Wang X, Liu R, Goh BKP, International Robotic LLRSGI. Robotic versus laparoscopic left and extended left hepatectomy: an international multicenter study propensity score-matched analysis. Ann Surg Oncol. 2022;29(13):8398–406.

36. Yang HY, Choi GH, Chin KM, Choi SH, Syn NL, Cheung TT, Chiow AKH, Sucandy I, Marino MV, Prieto M, Chong CC, Lee JH, Efanov M, Kingham TP, Sutcliffe RP, Troisi RI, Pratschke J, Wang X, D'Hondt M, Tang CN, Liu R, Park JO, Rotellar F, Scatton O, Sugioka A, Long TCD, Chan CY, Fuks D, Han HS, Goh BKP, the International R, Laparoscopic Liver Resection Study Group I. Robotic and laparoscopic right anterior sectionectomy and central hepatectomy: multicentre propensity score-matched analysis. Br J Surg. 2022;109(4):311–4.
37. Hu J, Guo Y, Wang X, Yeow M, Wu AGR, Fuks D, Soubrane O, Dokmak S, Gruttadauria S, Zimmitti G, Ratti F, Kato Y, Scatton O, Herman P, Aghayan DL, Marino MV, Croner RS, Mazzaferro V, Chiow AKH, Sucandy I, Ivanecz A, Choi SH, Lee JH, Gastaca M, Vivarelli M, Giuliante F, Ruzzenente A, Yong CC, Yin M, Fondevila C, Efanov M, Morise Z, Di Benedetto F, Brustia R, Valle RD, Boggi U, Geller D, Belli A, Memeo R, Mejia A, Park JO, Rotellar F, Choi GH, Robles-Campos R, Hasegawa K, Swijnenburg RJ, Sutcliffe RP, Pratschke J, Lai ECH, Chong CCN, D'Hondt M, Monden K, Lopez-Ben S, Kingham TP, Schmelzle M, Hawksworth J, Peng Y, Ferrero A, Ettorre GM, Cherqui D, Liang X, Wakabayashi G, Troisi RI, Cillo U, Cheung TT, Sugimoto M, Sugioka A, Han HS, Long TCD, Hilal MA, Zhang W, Wei Y, Chen KH, Aldrighetti L, Edwin B, Liu R, Goh BKP, International R, Laparoscopic Liver Resection Study Group I. Propensity score-matched analysis comparing robotic versus laparoscopic minor liver resections of the anterolateral segments: an international multi-center study of 10,517 cases. Ann Surg. 2024:10–1097.
38. Liu Q, Zhang W, Zhao JJ, Syn NL, Cipriani F, Alzoubi M, Aghayan DL, Siow TF, Lim C, Scatton O, Herman P, Coelho FF, Marino MV, Mazzaferro V, Chiow AKH, Sucandy I, Ivanecz A, Choi SH, Lee JH, Prieto M, Vivarelli M, Giuliante F, Dalla Valle B, Ruzzenente A, Yong CC, Chen Z, Yin M, Fondevila C, Efanov M, Morise Z, Di Benedetto F, Brustia R, Dalla Valle R, Boggi U, Geller D, Belli A, Memeo R, Gruttadauria S, Mejia A, Park JO, Rotellar F, Choi GH, Robles-Campos R, Wang X, Sutcliffe RP, Schmelzle M, Pratschke J, Tang CN, Chong CCN, Lee KF, Meurs J, D'Hondt M, Monden K, Lopez-Ben S, Kingham TP, Ferrero A, Ettorre GM, Levi Sandri GB, Saleh M, Cherqui D, Zheng J, Liang X, Mazzotta A, Soubrane O, Wakabayashi G, Troisi RI, Cheung TT, Kato Y, Sugioka A, D'Silva M, Han HS, Nghia PP, Long TCD, Edwin B, Fuks D, Chen KH, Abu Hilal M, Aldrighetti L, Liu R, Goh BKP, International R, Laparoscopic Liver Resection Study Group I. Propensity-score Matched and Coarsened-exact Matched Analysis Comparing Robotic and Laparoscopic Major Hepatectomies: An International Multicenter Study of 4822 Cases. Ann Surg. 2023;278(6):969–75.
39. Guidetti C, Muller PC, Magistri P, Jonas JP, Odorizzi R, Kron P, Guerrini G, Oberkofler CE, Di Sandro S, Clavien PA, Petrowsky H, Di Benedetto F. Full robotic versus open ALPPS: a bi-institutional comparison of perioperative outcomes. Surg Endosc. 2024;38(6):3448–54.
40. Magistri P, Guidetti C, Catellani B, Caracciolo D, Odorizzi R, Frassoni S, Bagnardi V, Guerrini GP, Di Sandro S, Di Benedetto F. Robotic ALPPS for primary and metastatic liver tumours: short-term outcomes versus open approach. Updates Surg. 2024;76(2):435–45.
41. Alvarez FA, Ardiles V, de Santibanes M, Pekolj J, de Santibanes E. Associating liver partition and portal vein ligation for staged hepatectomy offers high oncological feasibility with adequate patient safety: a prospective study at a single center. Ann Surg. 2015;261(4):723–32.
42. Petrowsky H, Gyori G, de Oliveira M, Lesurtel M, Clavien PA. Is partial-ALPPS safer than ALPPS? A single-center experience. Ann Surg. 2015;261(4):e90–2.
43. Robles R, Parrilla P, Lopez-Conesa A, Brusadin R, de la Pena J, Fuster M, Garcia-Lopez JA, Hernandez E. Tourniquet modification of the associating liver partition and portal ligation for staged hepatectomy procedure. Br J Surg. 2014;101(9):1129–34; discussion 1134.
44. Wang Q, Yan J, Feng X, Chen G, Xia F, Li X, Ma K, Bie P. Safety and efficacy of radiofrequency-assisted ALPPS (RALPPS) in patients with cirrhosis-related hepatocellular carcinoma. Int J Hyperth. 2017;33(7):846–52.
45. Cillo U, Gringeri E, Feltracco P, Bassi D, D'Amico FE, Polacco M, Boetto R. Totally laparoscopic microwave ablation and portal vein ligation for staged hepatectomy : a new minimally invasive two-stage hepatectomy. Ann Surg Oncol. 2015;22(8):2787–8.
46. Lai Q, Melandro F, Rossi M. Hybrid partial ALPPS: a feasible approach in case of right Trisegmentectomy and macrovascular invasion. Ann Surg. 2018;267(4):e80–2.

47. de Santibanes E, Alvarez FA, Ardiles V, Pekolj J, de Santibanes M. Inverting the ALPPS paradigm by minimizing first stage impact: the Mini-ALPPS technique. Langenbeck's Arch Surg. 2016;401(4):557–63.
48. Fiorentini G, Ratti F, Cipriani F, Quattromani R, Catena M, Paganelli M, Aldrighetti L. The SMART-ALPPS protocol: strategy to minimize ALPPS risks by targeting invasiveness. Ann Surg Oncol. 2021;28(11):6826–7.

The Dropout Phenomenon in Liver Regeneration

21

Victor Lopez-Lopez, Asunción Lopez Conesa, Roberto Brusadin, Patricia Pastor, Alvaro Navarro, and Ricardo Robles-Campos

21.1 Introduction

Hepatic regeneration techniques are a pivotal procedure in cases where the disease burden prevents a traditional one-stage resection. Nevertheless, sometimes these techniques are not sufficient to achieve an adequate volume (Fig. 21.1). Classical two-stage hepatectomy (TSH) and portal vein embolization (PVE) are traditional strategies to induce future liver remanent (FLR) hypertrophy; however, both methods have limitations in inducing rapid liver growth. Associating liver partition and portal vein ligation for staged hepatectomy (ALPPS) has gained prominence as a salvage technique in complex liver surgeries, particularly following failed conventional TSH or PVE. The emergence of liver venous deprivation (LVD) represents a new alternative for regeneration with promising results, although with a dropout rate that needs further analysis to ensure better criteria selection in the future. This chapter offers a comprehensive analysis of dropout and oncological failure in PVE, TSH, LVD, or even ALPPS, focusing on patient selection, factors influencing interstage progression, and strategies to mitigate dropout.

21.2 Dropout in PVE

PVE is a well-established preoperative procedure aimed at increasing the FLR volume in patients scheduled for major liver resections. The ability of the liver to regenerate after diverting portal flow to the FLR has been known since the twentieth century. While PVE has been shown to be effective in promoting liver hypertrophy,

V. Lopez-Lopez · A. L. Conesa · R. Brusadin · P. Pastor · A. Navarro · R. Robles-Campos (✉)
Department of General, Visceral and Transplantation Surgery, Clinic and University Hospital, Virgen de La Arrixaca, IMIB-Pascual Parrilla, Murcia, Spain
e-mail: Camposrirocam@um.es

L. Aldrighetti et al. (eds.), *Liver Regeneration Techniques In Hepatic Surgery*,
https://doi.org/10.1007/978-3-032-10997-2_21

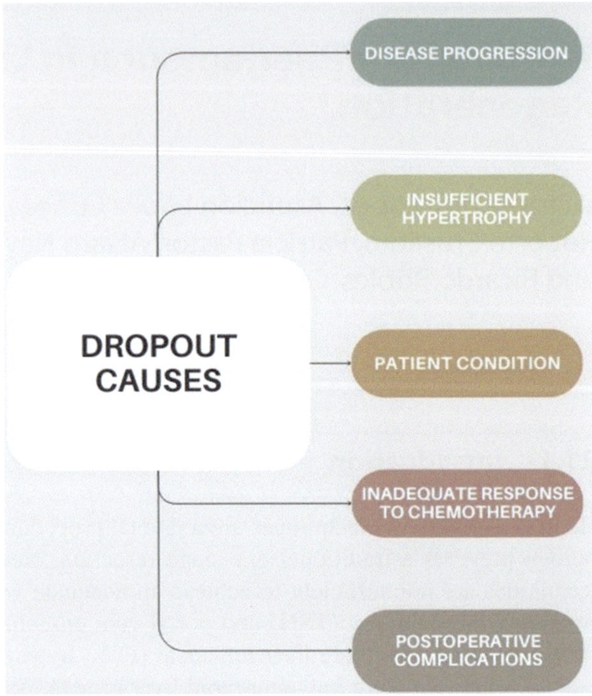

Fig. 21.1 Different causes of dropout in liver regeneration

its dropout rate—defined as the percentage of patients who are unable to proceed to surgery after undergoing PVE—remains a significant concern. According to the literature review, PVE is associated with a percentage increase in FLR (Δ%FLR) of 30–50% with low postoperative morbidity [1, 2]. However, 15–40% of patients are unable to complete surgical resection, mainly due to tumor progression or lack of effective regeneration, resulting in post-hepatectomy liver failure (PHLF). This insufficient liver regeneration seems to be related to the persistence of intraparenchymal portal flow from the FLR to the right deportalized lobe via intrahepatic collaterals, which would dampen the regenerative stimulus induced by PVE.

Several factors may contribute to the dropout phenomenon after PVE. One of the primary concerns is the insufficient hypertrophy of the FLR, which can occur in approximately 15–30% of patient [3]. Abulkhir et al. [4] in a 2008 meta-analysis of 1088 patients operated after PVE showed a Δ%FLR of 9.7–12% with low morbidity (2.2%) and no mortality. Hepatectomy was completed in 85% of patients 29 days after PVE. The main reasons for dropout were liver tumor progression, extrahepatic dissemination, and insufficient hypertrophy of the FLR. Postoperatively, 2.5% of patients experienced transient PHLF and 0.8% experienced fulminant PHLF, leading to patient death. In 2018, another meta-analysis [5] performed on 18 articles including 607 patients who underwent PVE prior to major liver resection. The complication rate was 3.1% and the time from PVE to surgery was 2–10 weeks with a Δ%FLR of 49%. The dropout rate in this study was 24% and again the main reasons for not completing hepatectomy were tumor progression and insufficient FLR hypertrophy. Postoperatively, 4.5% of patients developed PHLF. Also, Broering et al. [6] reported one patient who died of fulminant PHLF 11 days after major liver resection, and Ribero et al. [7] reported six patients with PHLF, one of whom died.

Moreover, the biological behavior of liver tumors plays a crucial role in determining dropout rates. The phenomenon of tumor progression appears in most series, both in the deportalized lobe and the FLR [8, 9]. This appears mainly in patients with bilobar colorectal liver metastases (CRLM), where tumor progression may occur in around 20% of cases during the regeneration period [10, 11]. A systematic review by Esposito et al. [12] highlights that dropout rates are particularly pronounced in patients with advanced liver disease or extensive tumor burden, who are at increased risk of disease progression during the post-PVE waiting period. However, De Graaf et al. [13] conducted a review of clinical and experimental studies and suggested that tumor progression arises equally in both embolized and non-embolized segments. Thus, it appears that it is not portal embolization that is responsible for tumor progression, but rather the long waiting time between PVE and surgery.

In addressing these elevated dropout rates, several strategies have been proposed to enhance the effectiveness of PVE. One current approach is the combination of PVE with other techniques, such as chemotherapy. Some authors [13, 14] resort to the administration of chemotherapy between PVE and surgery, from 1 to 3 cycles. This treatment has been shown to be effective in the Memorial Sloan-Kettering Cancer Center series [15], where tumor progression was greater in PVE without chemotherapy than when chemotherapy was administered during the period of liver regeneration (34% vs. 19%), and this treatment also positively influenced overall survival in the chemotherapy-treated group (50 vs. 24 months). It is vital to emphasize the importance of monitoring tumor response to neoadjuvant therapies, as inadequate response can lead to even higher dropout rates.

Other studies support the combination of PVE with transcatheter arterial chemoembolization (TACE), which may help control tumor growth during the waiting period. This combination has been associated with improved hypertrophy rates and higher resectability, suggesting that multimodal strategies could be helpful in reducing dropout rates [16–18]. The literature also points at the importance of understanding the biological behavior of liver tumors in the context of PVE. Tumor response to neoadjuvant chemotherapy has been identified as a significant factor influencing the likelihood of progression after PVE, emphasizing the need for careful monitoring and management of patients undergoing this procedure [11, 19].

The timing of PVE and the subsequent waiting period before surgery are critical factors influencing failure rates. Research suggests that the regeneration of the FLR typically requires 4–6 weeks, during which time the risk of tumor progression remains a significant concern [19]. In this regard, several studies have suggested an association between longer wait times and increased dropout rates due to tumor growth [1, 20, 21]. Not only the use of imaging but also the use of additional tools, such as functional liver assessment tools, can help identify patients likely to benefit from PVE and those at higher risk of failure, allowing for more tailored preoperative planning [21]. Therefore, the use of advanced imaging techniques to assess FLR growth and functional liver assessment may provide valuable insight into patient selection and timing of surgery [2, 22]. In addition, the presence of underlying liver disease, such as cirrhosis, steatosis, or biliary cancer, significantly affects the likelihood of dropout, as these conditions can interfere with liver regeneration [16, 23].

In conclusion, PVE continues to play an important role in improving the surgical resectability of patients with liver tumors, but dropout rates remain an ongoing challenge. Addressing factors such as inadequate hypertrophy and tumor progression is essential to improve patient outcomes. A refined strategy emphasizing optimal timing of resection, rigorous patient selection, and integration of complementary therapies may help reduce dropout rates. Future research should aim to refine these approaches and investigate innovative techniques to increase the efficacy of PVE.

21.3 Dropout in Two-Stage Hepatectomy

TSH is a method developed to address the unique challenges presented by bilobar CRLM. In cases where cancerous lesions are present across both liver lobes, single-stage resection often fails due to insufficient FLR volume, which is crucial for post-surgical liver function. TSH, first implemented by the Paul Brousse team in 2000, offers a solution by dividing the resection into two steps. This staged approach allows patients with extensive bilobar CRLM to undergo curative resection, aiming to improve survival outcomes that would be otherwise unachievable.

Despite the promise of TSH, dropout remains a significant concern, with reported rates varying between 0% and 36% across studies. Portal vein ligation or embolization are both effective in all cases for obtaining hypertrophy before major liver resection [24]. The study by Imai et al. reported that out of 125 patients initially planned for TSH, 35.2% were unable to proceed to the second stage, with the primary cause being tumor progression during the interstage interval [25]. Specifically, 88.6% of dropouts resulted from disease progression, indicating the aggressive nature of CRLM in these patients. Additional factors contributing to dropout included insufficient hypertrophy of the FLR (6.8%) and deteriorated patient condition or complications after the first stage (2.3%).

To address the high dropout rates in TSH, researchers have developed predictive models that identify key factors contributing to dropout. Independent predictive factors associated with a higher likelihood of dropout. By quantifying these factors, the model enables stratification of patients based on dropout risk, ranging from low-risk patients (10.5% dropout) with none of these factors to high-risk patients with all four factors, who face a 95.5% dropout probability [25].

For high-risk patients, TSH may not be the most suitable approach, as they are more likely to experience disease progression that hinders the second resection stage [26]. The interstage period is particularly sensitive for patients with aggressive CRLM, as the tumor cells can proliferate rapidly. Tumor progression during the FLR hypertrophy phase therefore represents a substantial barrier to completing TSH. Consequently, incomplete TSH not only limits the curative potential but is also associated with markedly poorer survival outcomes, underscoring the necessity of effective patient selection and monitoring strategies to reduce dropout rates.

Interval chemotherapy has emerged as a strategy to manage tumor growth during the hypertrophy phase in TSH. Administered between the first and second stages, interval chemotherapy aims to suppress disease progression, particularly in the FLR, reducing dropout rates and increasing the rate of a successful resection. A systematic review by Raschzok et al. found that interval chemotherapy reduced dropout rates to approximately 18%, compared to dropout rates of 20–40% in patients who did not receive interval chemotherapy [27] (Table 21.1).

While interval chemotherapy shows promise in managing tumor progression, it faces several challenges. Most studies assessing its effectiveness are retrospective, with considerable variation in chemotherapy regimens, patient demographics, and follow-up durations. Additionally, interval chemotherapy introduces potential toxicities and complications, which may hinder FLR hypertrophy and affect patient eligibility for the second stage of TSH. Further research, ideally through randomized controlled trials, is essential to establish standardized protocols that balance tumor control with patient safety, ultimately enabling a more effective use of interval chemotherapy in TSH.

Given the challenges associated with TSH dropout, alternative strategies such as one-stage hepatectomy (OSH) are occasionally considered. OSH eliminates the interstage interval by performing a single, comprehensive resection, which may reduce the chance of tumor progression between stages. However, OSH is generally feasible only for patients with smaller or less extensive disease burden, where an adequate FLR can be maintained after a single operation. Comparative studies indicate that patients who successfully complete TSH or OSH tend to have similar survival rates, suggesting that OSH could be a viable alternative in select cases where the risk of TSH dropout is high [28, 29]. However, due to the limitations of OSH in patients with extensive disease, TSH remains the primary approach for cases where staged resection is necessary to achieve curative outcomes.

Molecular profiling has become an essential component of CRLM management, allowing for refined patient selection and personalized approaches to TSH. Genetic mutations have been associated with poor prognosis and higher recurrence rates, even among patients who complete TSH [30]. The presence of these mutations has been linked to aggressive tumor behavior, which may limit the effectiveness of TSH and increase the likelihood of oncological failure. RAS mutations, for instance, have shown strong correlations with poor oncological outcomes and high recurrence rates. Studies demonstrate that RAS-positive patients often experience limited benefits from TSH, with higher relapse rates compared to RAS-negative patients [31]. Similarly, BRAF mutations are associated with aggressive tumor progression and shorter survival times. This genetic information allows clinicians to tailor treatment options, optimizing TSH for patients with lower oncological risk profiles and reserving alternative treatments for those with high-risk genetic markers [32]. By identifying these molecular profiles, clinicians can better assess which patients are likely to benefit from TSH and who may require alternative treatment strategies.

Table 21.1 Series of Drop-out after two-stage hepatectomy and the related predictive factors

Author, year	Country	No. of patients	Dropout rate (%)	Predictive factors for dropout—univariate	Predictive factors for dropout—multivariate
Tsai, 2010	USA	45	22	Higher tumor number; no preoperative chemo	ND
Narita, 2011	France	76	20	Age ≥70; ≥3 tumors in the FLR; CEA >200 (ng/mL) before PVE	Age ≥70; ≥3 tumors in the FLR
Turrini, 2012	France	42	19	Combined resection of primary tumor; interval chemotherapy	Combined resection of primary tumor
Giulante, 2014	Italy	126	22	Disease progression during chemo	Disease progression during chemo
Faitot, 2015	France	50	24	Male gender; vascular invasion on primary; >5 tumors; segment 1 metastases; need for chemo change; need for >3 curative treatments; microscopic biliary invasion	Nothing
Imai, 2015	France	125	35	CEA >30 (ng/mL); tumor size >40 mm; no. of chemotherapy cycles >12; no. of chemotherapy lines >1; disease progression during first-line chemo	CEA >30 (ng/mL); tumor size >40 mm; no. of chemotherapy cycles >12; disease progression during first-line chemo
Passotl, 2016	USA	109	18	Tumor size >50 mm; no. of chemotherapy cycles >6	No. of chemotherapy cycles >6
Bejjani-Beau, 2017	Worldwide	869	28	No repeat hepatectomy; extrahepatic metastasis; non-R0 resection at first-stage; no preoperative chemo	ND
Quénot, 2018	France	56	38	TRG 4/5; Blazer classification 2; tumor number >6	Blazer classification 2; tumor number >6

Imai et al. [25]

Two-stage hepatectomy represents a critical approach for patients with extensive bilobar CRLM, offering a potential curative option. However, dropout and recurrence remain significant obstacles to achieving long-term survival. By focusing on predictors of dropout and oncological failure, integrating molecular profiling into patient selection, and employing strategies such as interval chemotherapy and ALPPS for high-risk cases, TSH outcomes can be optimized. In addition, interdisciplinary collaboration across oncology, radiology, and surgery is crucial for refining treatment protocols, ensuring that each patient's plan is tailored to their individual disease characteristics and oncological risk factors.

21.4 Dropout in LVD

Several techniques have been proposed to minimize the risk of PHLF, which is the main cause of death after major hepatic surgery. In this sense, Hwang et al. in 2009 described a new interventional radiological technique with the purpose of achieving a greater volumetric increase [33]. This procedure consists of a sequential embolization of the portal vein and a hepatic vein that improves FLR through several mechanisms. The obstruction of hepatic venous outflow following PVE reduces hepatic arterial inflow due to the hepatic arterial buffer response, which can lead to increased damage in the embolized portion of the liver [34]. Consequently, this author demonstrated a greater FLR after sequential embolization than PVE alone. Nevertheless, to complete this technique are necessary two endovascular procedures with a large period between them (1–3 weeks) and this fact could mean a loss of opportunity to undergo hepatectomies due to tumor progression.

Recently, new methods were proposed by Guiu et al. [35] and Le Roy et al. [36] to increase the FRL by performing a simultaneous embolization of the portal vein and the right or right and middle hepatic vein called LVD. These techniques achieve a faster increase of the FLR reducing time in a single technique with acceptable rates of postoperative morbidity. LVD is a relatively new technique that emerged as an alternative to ALPPS with the aim of decrease the morbidity and mortality associated with this surgical technique.

Guiu et al. in 2019 compared FLR-volume (FLR-V) and FLR-function (FLR-F) PVE and LVD and concludes that LVD provides greater FLR-V and FLR-F increase than PVE. At week 3 post-preparation, five patients did not reach the safe FLR-F ($n = 2$ in the LVD and $n = 3$ in the PVE group) but two of these reached the adequate FLR-F threshold at week 5 post-preparation and underwent surgery. The dropout rate in this study was 2% ($n = 1$) due to peritoneal carcinomatosis discovered at surgery [35].

Le Roy et al. reported an LVD dropout of 6 upon 31 patients scheduled for surgery, three of them due to disease progression on imaging and three because of peritoneal carcinomatosis [36]. Bell et al. [37] in a 2022 meta-analysis of eight retrospective studies including 523 patients planned for major hepatectomy following either PVE ($n = 333$) or LVD ($n = 190$) showed a larger increase in hypertrophy of the FLR 66% in the LVD group versus 27% in the PVE group. The percentage of failed to progress to surgery was 13 ($n = 25$) in the LVD group versus 25 ($n = 82$) in the PVE group. The main reason of dropout in patients undergone LVD was disease progression ($n = 22$) on imaging or at the time of surgery while inadequate FLR occurred only in three patients.

Another key concern that emerges from the literature is the time interval between the LVD procedure and surgery. Previous studies have indicated that delayed hepatic hypertrophy following PVE can be a significant factor contributing to increase the dropout rate due to cancer recurrences observed [38, 39]. A key factor in determining if LVD might replace ALPPS in managing FLR is the time required to reach surgery. In addition, it is very important when considering the appropriate clinical contexts in which ALPPS and LVD can be implemented with maximum safety, efficacy, and efficiency [40, 41].

Several researchers have indicated that this interval could be significantly reduced, as increases in FLR volume and function have been noted as early as 7 days after LVD. One major reason for the prolonged delay experienced by patients in some studies may be that the LVD technique is relatively new and is being evaluated against the standards of earlier studies. Specifically, volume measurements are usually taken on days 7 and 21 based on the assumption that the growth effect corresponds to the current radiological standard of care (the longer the wait, the greater the FLR enhancement) [42].

Many still view LVD as an evolving technique that might increase the number of patients eligible for liver resection by reducing the time spent in preparation for surgery. This approach could lead to a quicker and larger FLR while also lowering the risk of complications from tumor progression. The data analyzed and the results obtained to compare ALPPS and LVD are based on indirect evidence in published studies, so more prospective and controlled studies are needed about this topic.

21.5 ALPPS: A Strategy for Reducing Dropout

In some cases, methods such as TSH, PVE, or LVD may fail to induce sufficient liver hypertrophy in the FLR, precluding complete resection. ALPPS has become a critical salvage option, allowing resection in patients who would otherwise face disease progression or poor prognosis. Since its introduction into clinical practice, the ALPPS technique represented a step forward in the liver surgery and it has been described as "one of the most surprising advances in oncological liver surgery so far." Many centers began to use this rapid hypertrophy technique to solve the most important drawback of classic regeneration procedures: the dropout [43]. The first series of ALPPS reported hypertrophy rate never seen before in terms of volume and kinetic growth [44]. These results have led to a significant shortening of interstage time, performing hepatectomy within the first 2 weeks after the first stage, reaching a resectability between 90% and 100%. The main drawback of this novel technique is the high rate of complications and mortality, especially after the first stage, which could also negatively influence the dropout rate.

ALPPS induces rapid hypertrophy through combined portal vein ligation and in situ liver partitioning, which triggers a significant growth response in the FLR by redirecting blood flow and activating regenerative pathways. ALPPS achieves hypertrophy rates of up to 80–90% within 7–14 days, compared to 10–46% seen with TSH or PVE alone [45]. This accelerated hypertrophy is driven by a release of cytokines and growth factors (e.g., IL-6, TNF-α) due to the transection, which promotes both hyperplasia and hypertrophy of hepatocytes. This mechanism makes ALPPS an ideal salvage procedure for patients with insufficient FLR growth following TSH or PVE, as it reduces the waiting time for hypertrophy and lowers the risk of tumor progression during the interval.

In cases of failed TSH, ALPPS provides a second opportunity to achieve resection in patients who otherwise would not meet criteria due to insufficient FLR growth or aggressive tumor progression. ALPPS achieves rapid hypertrophy, allowing for a shorter waiting period and a reduced risk of interstage dropout. In scenarios where TSH fails due to poor FLR growth, ALPPS can facilitate rapid volume increase, enabling resection within days. A case study from the International ALPPS Registry documented a series of patients who, following failed TSH, achieved an average 88% FLR hypertrophy after ALPPS, leading to safe and successful resections [46]. This result underscores the role of ALPPS in overcoming the limitations of TSH, especially in cases where extended waiting periods for hypertrophy increase the likelihood of tumor progression and dropout.

In some salvage cases, inducing hypertrophy in a single liver segment or selectively partitioning the liver has proven beneficial. Monosegment ALPPS, which focuses hypertrophy efforts on one segment, provides a controlled approach to inducing sufficient FLR without exposing the entire liver to extensive transection [47].

The oncological benefits of ALPPS, especially in aggressive tumors or advanced liver disease cases, are closely linked to its ability to enable curative resection in situations of failed TSH or PVE [48]. However, the complexity of these cases often necessitates integration with systemic therapies, such as chemotherapy or immunotherapy, to manage the disease more effectively. Interval chemotherapy between ALPPS stages has been effective in managing residual disease and reducing dropout rates [49]. For patients with aggressive or high-volume tumors, chemotherapy helps control disease progression during the hypertrophy interval, making it a valuable adjunctive treatment. However, clinicians must carefully monitor liver function and potential hepatotoxicity to avoid additional risks during the ALPPS process. Studies indicate that interval chemotherapy, when combined with ALPPS, can improve disease-free survival and reduce recurrence, particularly in patients with CRLM.

Although ALPPS provides a critical option for patients with failed TSH or PVE, it is not without risks, particularly in salvage cases. The rapid hypertrophy induced by ALPPS places significant demands on liver function and can lead to complications, including PHLF, bile leaks, and infections. However, when performed in experienced centers, ALPPS has shown favorable 90-day mortality rates, typically between 0% and 9%, even in complex cases [50].

It is worth remembering that dropout in these patients is related to several factors: the great tumor burden, the characteristics of the liver parenchyma, and finally the general condition of the patients who have usually received previous oncological treatments [51]. Therefore, the main causes of dropout with liver regeneration techniques are the following: disease progression, inappropriate hypertrophy, complications, and mortality.

Despite there is a trend to delay the second stage [52] in most series, hepatectomy is carried out within 2 weeks after the first stage. Some authors had warned about the possible early tumor recurrence with the ALPPS [53]. Although this tumor progression does not influence the dropout rate, considering that it is a recurrence after hepatectomy and not a true disease progression, it could worsen the oncological results. More recent data on long-term outcomes do not confirm these findings. Therefore, the interstage tumor progression does not represent a serious issue of the ALPPS technique. The short interval time between the two stages seems to be one of the great advantages of this complex and controversial technique and seems to solve the issue of tumor progression that is so worrying with classical techniques.

Several meta-analyses show that hypertrophy is significantly higher with ALPPS compared to classic techniques [54]. Regarding other conditions that could negatively influence hypertrophy, it seems that previous chemotherapy is not considered a risk factor. This is especially important considering that most patients who undergo ALPSS are diagnosed with liver metastases from colorectal cancer [55]. ALPPS technique produced a real and effective hypertrophy, and it has also been shown that it works even if applied as a rescue technique. It allows obtaining significant hypertrophy in patients in whom other techniques had previously failed [5, 15].

The Achille's heel of ALPPS is its high complication rates. Since its introduction, the complexity of the technique and the high rate of complications have become evident, even after the first intervention. This high rate of complications inevitably influenced the general condition of the patient and the dropout, given that some patients did not reach the second stage. Changing the paradigm of classic regeneration techniques, the first ALPPS intervention is the longest and most aggressive. To minimize the risks of the first intervention, some less aggressive technical variants have been developed. It could be to achieve similar results in terms of hypertrophy but with fewer complications. Our group was the pioneer in 2011 developing the ALPPS-tourniquet variant, the first variant of ALPPS, published in 2014 [56], and together with other variants such as partial ALPPS, Mini-ALPP or minimally invasive approach reduce the rate of complications. These variants and better patient selection have improved the results of ALPPS. Although there is a tendency toward a higher rate of serious complications with ALPPS, it demonstrates a higher resectability rate, greater hypertrophy, and a significantly shorter time interval compared to PVE, PVL, LVD, and TSH classical techniques, which translates into a clearly lower dropout.

References

1. Masthoff M, Katou S, Köhler M, Schindler P, Heindel W, Wilms C, et al. Portal and hepatic vein embolization prior to major hepatectomy. Z Gastroenterol. 2021;59(1):35–42.
2. Araki K, Shibuya K, Harimoto N, Watanabe A, Tsukagoshi M, Ishii N, et al. A prospective study of sequential hepatic vein embolization after portal vein embolization in patients scheduled for right-sided major hepatectomy: results of feasibility and surgical strategy using functional liver assessment. J Hepatobiliary Pancreat Sci. 2023;30(1):91–101.
3. Luz JHM, Gomes FV, Coimbra E, Costa NV, Bilhim T. Preoperative portal vein embolization in hepatic surgery: a review about the embolic materials and their effects on liver regeneration and outcome. Radiol Res Pract. 2020;2020:9295852.

4. Abulkhir A, Limongelli P, Healey AJ, Damrah O, Tait P, Jackson J, et al. Preoperative portal vein embolization for major liver resection: a meta-analysis. Ann Surg. 2008;247(1):49–57.
5. Wajswol E, Jazmati T, Contractor S, Kumar A. Portal vein embolization utilizing N-butyl cyanoacrylate for contralateral lobe hypertrophy prior to liver resection: a systematic review and meta-analysis. Cardiovasc Intervent Radiol. 2018;41(9):1302–12.
6. Broering DC, Hillert C, Krupski G, Fischer L, Mueller L, Achilles EG, et al. Portal vein embolization vs. portal vein ligation for induction of hypertrophy of the future liver remnant. J Gastrointest Surg. 2002;6(6):905–13; discussion 13.
7. Ribero D, Abdalla EK, Madoff DC, Donadon M, Loyer EM, Vauthey JN. Portal vein embolization before major hepatectomy and its effects on regeneration, resectability and outcome. Br J Surg. 2007;94(11):1386–94.
8. Elias D, De Baere T, Roche A, Mducreux, Leclere J, Lasser P. During liver regeneration following right portal embolization the growth rate of liver metastases is more rapid than that of the liver parenchyma. Br J Surg. 1999;86(6):784–8.
9. Kokudo N, Tada K, Seki M, Ohta H, Azekura K, Ueno M, et al. Proliferative activity of intrahepatic colorectal metastases after preoperative hemihepatic portal vein embolization. Hepatology. 2001;34(2):267–72.
10. Kobayashi K, Yamaguchi T, Denys A, Perron L, Halkic N, Demartines N, et al. Liver venous deprivation compared to portal vein embolization to induce hypertrophy of the future liver remnant before major hepatectomy: a single center experience. Surgery. 2020;167(6):917–23.
11. Simoneau E, Hassanain M, Shaheen M, Aljiffry M, Molla N, Chaudhury P, et al. Portal vein embolization and its effect on tumour progression for colorectal cancer liver metastases. Br J Surg. 2015;102(10):1240–9.
12. Esposito F, Lim C, Lahat E, Shwaartz C, Eshkenazy R, Salloum C, et al. Combined hepatic and portal vein embolization as preparation for major hepatectomy: a systematic review. HPB. 2019;21(9):1099–106.
13. de Graaf W, van den Esschert JW, van Lienden KP, van Gulik TM. Induction of tumor growth after preoperative portal vein embolization: is it a real problem? Ann Surg Oncol. 2009;16(2):423–30.
14. Goéré D, Farges O, Leporrier J, Sauvanet A, Vilgrain V, Belghiti J. Chemotherapy does not impair hypertrophy of the left liver after right portal vein obstruction. J Gastrointest Surg. 2006;10(3):365–70.
15. Fischer C, Melstrom LG, Arnaoutakis D, Jarnagin W, Brown K, D'Angelica M, et al. Chemotherapy after portal vein embolization to protect against tumor growth during liver hypertrophy before hepatectomy. JAMA Surg. 2013;148(12):1103–8.
16. Tustumi F, Ernani L, Coelho FF, Bernardo WM, Junior SS, Kruger JAP, et al. Preoperative strategies to improve resectability for hepatocellular carcinoma: a systematic review and meta-analysis. HPB. 2018;20(12):1109–18.
17. Zhang CW, Dou CW, Zhang XL, Liu XQ, Huang DS, Hu ZM, et al. Simultaneous transcatheter arterial chemoembolization and portal vein embolization for patients with large hepatocellular carcinoma before major hepatectomy. World J Gastroenterol: WJG. 2020;26(30):4489–500.
18. Choi JH, Hwang S, Lee YJ, Kim KH, Ko GY, Gwon DI, et al. Prognostic effect of preoperative sequential transcatheter arterial chemoembolization and portal vein embolization for right hepatectomy in patients with solitary hepatocellular carcinoma. Korean J Hepatobiliary Pancreat Surg. 2015;19(2):59–65.
19. Lin Q, Chen D, Li K, Fan X, Cai Q, Lin W, et al. Case report: massive hepatocellular carcinoma complete surgical resection after portal vein embolization and multimodality therapy. Front Radiol. 2022;2:858963.
20. Sparrelid E, Hasselgren K, Røsok BI, Larsen PN, Schultz NA, Carling U, et al. How should liver hypertrophy be stimulated? A comparison of upfront associating liver partition and portal vein ligation for staged hepatectomy (ALPPS) and portal vein embolization (PVE) with rescue possibility. Hepatobiliary Surg Nutr. 2021;10(1):1–8.
21. Bell R, Begum S, Prasad R, Taura K, Dasari BVM. Volume and flow modulation strategies to mitigate post-hepatectomy liver failure. Front Oncol. 2022;12:1021018.

22. Onishi Y, Isoda H, Ohno T, Shimizu H, Shimada K, Taura K, et al. Future liver remnant hypertrophy rate in portal vein embolization before left trisectionectomy: a retrospective cohort study. Abdom Radiol(New York). 2022;47(2):878–84.
23. Imamura H, Adachi T, Matsushima H, Ishimaru H, Fukumoto M, Yoshino K, et al. Analysis of the clinical course in a population of patients with biliary tract cancer diagnosed as unresectable after portal vein embolization: a case series. Kurume Med J. 2024;70(1.2):77–81.
24. Robles R, Marín C, Lopez-Conesa A, Capel A, Perez-Flores D, Parrilla P. Comparative study of right portal vein ligation versus embolisation for induction of hypertrophy in two-stage hepatectomy for multiple bilateral colorectal liver metastases. Eur J Surg Oncol. 2012;38(7):586–93.
25. Imai K, Allard MA, Baba H, Adam R. Optimal patient selection for successful two-stage hepatectomy of bilateral colorectal liver metastases. Ann Gastroenterol Surg. 2021;5(5):634–8.
26. Lam VW, Laurence JM, Johnston E, Hollands MJ, Pleass HC, Richardson AJ. A systematic review of two-stage hepatectomy in patients with initially unresectable colorectal liver metastases. HPB (Oxford). 2013;15(7):483–91.
27. Raschzok N, Moosburner S, Blank M, Krenzien F, Lurje G, Schöning W, et al. Is interval chemotherapy safe and does it improve the outcome of patients with colorectal liver metastases undergoing multimodal two-stage hepatectomy? – a systematic literature review. BMC Cancer. 2024;24(1):1260.
28. Viganò L, Torzilli G, Cimino M, Imai K, Vibert E, Donadon M, et al. Drop-out between the two liver resections of two-stage hepatectomy. Patient selection or loss of chance? Eur J Surg Oncol. 2016;42(9):1385–93.
29. Torzilli G, Viganò L, Cimino M, Imai K, Vibert E, Donadon M, et al. Is enhanced one-stage hepatectomy a safe and feasible alternative to the two-stage hepatectomy in the setting of multiple bilobar colorectal liver metastases? A comparative analysis between two pioneering centers. Dig Surg. 2018;35(4):323–32.
30. Nassar A, Tzedakis S, Marchese U, Naveendran G, Sindayigaya R, Gaillard M, et al. Factors of oncological failure in two stage hepatectomy for colorectal liver metastases. Eur J Surg Oncol. 2024;50(1):107267.
31. Margonis GA, Vauthey JN. Precision surgery for colorectal liver metastases: current knowledge and future perspectives. Ann Gastroenterol Surg. 2022;6(5):606–15.
32. Tosi F, Magni E, Amatu A, Mauri G, Bencardino K, Truini M, et al. Effect of KRAS and BRAF mutations on survival of metastatic colorectal cancer after liver resection: a systematic review and meta-analysis. Clin Colorectal Cancer. 2017;16(3):e153–e63.
33. Hwang S, Lee SG, Ko GY, Kim BS, Sung KB, Kim MH, et al. Sequential preoperative ipsilateral hepatic vein embolization after portal vein embolization to induce further liver regeneration in patients with hepatobiliary malignancy. Ann Surg. 2009;249(4):608–16.
34. Guiu B, Chevallier P, Denys A, Delhom E, Pierredon-Foulongne MA, Rouanet P, et al. Simultaneous trans-hepatic portal and hepatic vein embolization before major hepatectomy: the liver venous deprivation technique. Eur Radiol. 2016;26(12):4259–67.
35. Guiu B, Quenet F, Panaro F, Piron L, Cassinotto C, Herrerro A, et al. Liver venous deprivation versus portal vein embolization before major hepatectomy: future liver remnant volumetric and functional changes. Hepatobiliary Surg Nutr. 2020;9(5):564–76.
36. Le Roy B, Gallon A, Cauchy F, Pereira B, Gagnière J, Lambert C, et al. Combined biembolization induces higher hypertrophy than portal vein embolization before major liver resection. HPB (Oxford). 2020;22(2):298–305.
37. Bell RJ, Hakeem AR, Pandanaboyana S, Davidson BR, Prasad RK, Dasari BVM. Portal vein embolization versus dual vein embolization for management of the future liver remnant in patients undergoing major hepatectomy: meta-analysis. BJS Open. 2022;6(6):zrac131.
38. Cassese G, Troisi RI, Khayat S, Benoudifa B, Quenet F, Guiu B, et al. Liver venous deprivation versus portal vein embolization before major hepatectomy for colorectal liver metastases: a retrospective comparison of short- and medium-term outcomes. J Gastrointest Surg. 2023;27(2):296–305.

39. Kim D, Cornman-Homonoff J, Madoff DC. Preparing for liver surgery with "Alphabet Soup": PVE, ALPPS, TAE-PVE, LVD and RL. Hepatobiliary Surg Nutr. 2020;9(2):136–51.
40. Deshayes E, Piron L, Bouvier A, Lapuyade B, Lermite E, Vervueren L, et al. Study protocol of the HYPER-LIV01 trial: a multicenter phase II, prospective and randomized study comparing simultaneous portal and hepatic vein embolization to portal vein embolization for hypertrophy of the future liver remnant before major hepatectomy for colorectal liver metastases. BMC Cancer. 2020;20(1):574.
41. Heil J, Korenblik R, Heid F, Bechstein WO, Bemelmans M, Binkert C, et al. Preoperative portal vein or portal and hepatic vein embolization: DRAGON collaborative group analysis. Br J Surg. 2021;108(7):834–42.
42. Gavriilidis P, Marangoni G, Ahmad J, Azoulay D. Simultaneous portal and hepatic vein embolization is better than portal embolization or ALPPS for hypertrophy of future liver remnant before major hepatectomy: a systematic review and network meta-analysis. Hepatobiliary Pancreat Dis Int. 2023;22(3):221–7.
43. Wicherts DA, Miller R, de Haas RJ, Bitsakou G, Vibert E, Veilhan LA, et al. Long-term results of two-stage hepatectomy for irresectable colorectal cancer liver metastases. Ann Surg. 2008;248(6):994–1005.
44. Schadde E, Ardiles V, Slankamenac K, Tschuor C, Sergeant G, Amacker N, et al. ALPPS offers a better chance of complete resection in patients with primarily unresectable liver tumors compared with conventional-staged hepatectomies: results of a multicenter analysis. World J Surg. 2014;38(6):1510–9.
45. Au KP, Chan ACY. Current status of associating liver partition with portal vein ligation for staged hepatectomy: comparison with two-stage hepatectomy and strategies for better outcomes. World J Gastroenterol. 2019;25(43):6373–85.
46. Enne M, Schadde E, Björnsson B, Hernandez Alejandro R, Steinbruck K, Viana E, et al. ALPPS as a salvage procedure after insufficient future liver remnant hypertrophy following portal vein occlusion. HPB (Oxford). 2017;19(12):1126–9.
47. Schadde E, Malagó M, Hernandez-Alejandro R, Li J, Abdalla E, Ardiles V, et al. Monosegment ALPPS hepatectomy: extending resectability by rapid hypertrophy. Surgery. 2015;157(4):676–89.
48. Robles-Campos R, Brusadin R, López-Conesa A, López-López V, Navarro-Barrios Á, López-Espín JJ, et al. Long-term outcome after conventional two-stage hepatectomy versus tourniquet-ALPPS in colorectal liver metastases: a propensity score matching analysis. World J Surg. 2019;43(9):2281–9.
49. Alvarez FA, Ardiles V, Chara C, de Santibañes M, Sánchez Clariá R, Pekolj J, et al. Adjuvant chemotherapy is associated with better oncological outcomes after ALPPS for colorectal liver metastases. Updates Surg. 2024;76(3):855–68.
50. Linecker M, Björnsson B, Stavrou GA, Oldhafer KJ, Lurje G, Neumann U, et al. Risk adjustment in ALPPS is associated with a dramatic decrease in early mortality and morbidity. Ann Surg. 2017;266(5):779–86.
51. Lopez-Lopez V, Linecker M, Caballero-Llanes A, Reese T, Oldhafer KJ, Hernandez-Alejandro R, et al. Liver histology predicts liver regeneration and outcome in ALPPS: novel findings from a multicenter study. Ann Surg. 2024;279(2):306–13.
52. Hernandez-Alejandro R, Bertens KA, Pineda-Solis K, Croome KP. Can we improve the morbidity and mortality associated with the associating liver partition with portal vein ligation for staged hepatectomy (ALPPS) procedure in the management of colorectal liver metastases? Surgery. 2015;157(2):194–201.
53. Oldhafer KJ, Donati M, Jenner RM, Stang A, Stavrou GA. ALPPS for patients with colorectal liver metastases: effective liver hypertrophy, but early tumor recurrence. World J Surg. 2014;38(6):1504–9.
54. Eshmuminov D, Raptis DA, Linecker M, Wirsching A, Lesurtel M, Clavien PA. Meta-analysis of associating liver partition with portal vein ligation and portal vein occlusion for two-stage hepatectomy. Br J Surg. 2016;103(13):1768–82.

55. Lopez-Lopez V, Linecker M, Cruz J, Brusadin R, Lopez-Conesa A, Machado MA, et al. Liver growth prediction in ALPPS – a multicenter analysis from the international ALPPS registry. Liver Int. 2022;42(12):2815–29.
56. Robles R, Parrilla P, López-Conesa A, Brusadin R, de la Peña J, Fuster M, et al. Tourniquet modification of the associating liver partition and portal ligation for staged hepatectomy procedure. Br J Surg. 2014;101(9):1129–34; discussion 34.

Management of Postoperative Liver Failure

22

Gianluca Rompianesi and Roberto Troisi

22.1 Introduction

Post-hepatectomy liver failure (PHLF) is among the most feared and serious complications following liver resection. Defined by the International Study Group of Liver Surgery (ISGLS) as a postoperative decline in the liver's synthetic, excretory, and detoxifying functions, it typically presents after postoperative Day 5 with rising serum bilirubin and INR. While grade A cases are often self-limiting, grades B and C carry significant morbidity and mortality, with grade C associated with death rates exceeding 50% [1].

Advances in preoperative planning and surgical technique have lowered the incidence of PHLF in high-volume centers. However, once liver failure occurs, its management remains challenging, with no curative treatment available aside from liver transplantation. As such, the possible therapeutic approaches continue to evolve, incorporating established supportive care and novel regenerative strategies [2].

This chapter addresses the therapeutic management of established post-hepatectomy liver failure, with a focus on evidence-based strategies aimed at supporting hepatic recovery, stabilizing systemic function, and identifying appropriate candidates for advanced interventions, including liver transplantation.

22.2 Non-Liver-Directed Supportive Measures

Early management of PHLF prioritizes stabilization of the hemodynamic and metabolic functions, alongside extrahepatic organs support. The clinical events that require active management include impaired ammonia clearance, hypoglycemia

G. Rompianesi · R. Troisi (✉)
HPB, Minimally Invasive, Robotic and Transplant Surgery Unit, Federico II University Hospital of Naples, Naples, Italy

L. Aldrighetti et al. (eds.), *Liver Regeneration Techniques In Hepatic Surgery*, https://doi.org/10.1007/978-3-032-10997-2_22

from reduced gluconeogenesis, and lactic acidosis. Additional complications may include acute respiratory distress syndrome (ARDS), adrenal insufficiency, sepsis, catabolism, cerebral edema, and acute kidney injury (AKI).

Patients with moderate to severe PHLF (ISGLS grade B or C) often require care in a high-dependency or intensive care setting, where continuous monitoring and prompt initiation of organ support therapies—such as vasopressors, renal replacement therapy, or mechanical ventilation—can be implemented. This critical care model reflects the multidisciplinary approach increasingly advocated in liver failure management [3–5].

22.2.1 Hemodynamic Stabilization

Hemodynamic disturbances in PHLF arise from systemic vasodilation, altered vascular tone, and compromised hepatic perfusion. The therapeutic goal is to maintain adequate oxygen delivery to vital organs while avoiding volume overload, which may exacerbate liver congestion and impair recovery. A mean arterial pressure (MAP) of 65 mmHg is generally targeted [6]. Volume resuscitation should be guided by dynamic indices or bedside ultrasound, avoiding excessive fluid administration. Balanced crystalloids are preferred over normal saline to prevent hyperchloremic acidosis and to limit exacerbation of metabolic acidosis, frequently observed due to impaired lactate metabolism [7].

Norepinephrine is usually the vasopressor of choice, as it restores perfusion pressure while preserving splanchnic circulation [8]. If a higher support is needed, vasopressin could be added to further ameliorate the vascular tone. In cases of persistent hypotension despite fluid resuscitation and vasopressor support, relative adrenal insufficiency should be suspected, and a trial of low-dose corticosteroids—such as hydrocortisone 200 mg/day—may be warranted, particularly in the setting of septic shock [9].

Albumin infusions can enhance effective intravascular volume and support oncotic pressure, especially in the context of hypoalbuminemia or refractory ascites [10].

22.2.2 Nutritional Support

Nutritional therapies play a fundamental role in the management of PHLF, supporting hepatic regeneration and limiting catabolic stress. In the setting of acute liver dysfunction, energy consumption is elevated, and early muscle breakdown can compromise immune function and recovery [11].

Whenever possible, enteral nutrition should be initiated within 24–48 h to preserve gut barrier integrity and reduce the risk of infection. Parenteral support is reserved for patients with gastrointestinal intolerance. Caloric requirements typically range from 25 to 30 kcal/kg/day, with protein intake of 1.2–1.5 g/kg/day to maintain nitrogen balance and prevent sarcopenia. Protein restriction, once commonly recommended in hepatic encephalopathy to reduce ammonia production, is now generally unwarranted, as it may impair nitrogen balance and delay recovery. BCAA-enriched formulations are preferred in encephalopathic patients because they bypass hepatic metabolism and serve as an alternative energy source for skeletal muscle and the brain, thereby reducing ammonia levels and supporting neurocognitive function [12].

Glucose levels should be closely monitored, as glycemic instability is common in PHLF. Hypoglycemia, resulting from impaired hepatic gluconeogenesis, requires prompt correction and may necessitate continuous dextrose infusion, an intervention often indicative of advanced liver dysfunction and associated with worse prognosis. Conversely, hyperglycemia, frequently driven by stress-induced insulin resistance and glucose infusions, should also be avoided, as it may exacerbate systemic inflammation, increase the risk of infection, and impair wound healing. A target blood glucose range of 150–180 mg/dL is generally recommended to minimize both metabolic stress and the risks associated with overtreatment [3].

22.2.3 Infection Control

Infection is a frequent and serious complication in PHLF, often accelerating clinical deterioration. Hepatic dysfunction impairs innate immunity by reducing pathogen clearance, altering complement synthesis, and disrupting Kupffer cell activity [13]. This vulnerability is amplified by invasive procedures, biliary drainage, and prolonged ICU exposure.

Bacterial infections—particularly biliary, pulmonary, and bloodstream—are common and may be polymicrobial. Infected collections and cholangitis further compromise hepatic function and increase the risk of multiorgan failure. Empiric broad-spectrum antibiotics should be initiated promptly when infection is suspected and adjusted according to culture results [14]. Daily reassessment, including imaging when indicated, is essential to identify evolving sources.

Routine removal of unnecessary catheters and drains is critical to reduce device-related infections. Fungal infections, especially *Candida* spp., should be considered in patients with prolonged antibiotic use or parenteral nutrition. Empirical antifungal therapy may be warranted in selected high-risk cases [15].

22.2.4 Coagulopathy Management

Coagulopathy is a common feature of PHLF, reflecting impaired hepatic synthesis of clotting factors and, often, concurrent thrombocytopenia. Despite elevated INR values, the risk of spontaneous bleeding is generally lower than expected, due to a rebalanced but fragile hemostatic system in liver dysfunction. Management should therefore be guided by clinical context rather than isolated laboratory abnormalities. Indeed, routine correction of coagulopathy is not indicated in the absence of active bleeding or planned invasive procedures. In such settings, administration of fresh frozen plasma, cryoprecipitate, or vitamin K may be appropriate [12, 16].

Thromboelastography (TEG) or rotational thromboelastometry (ROTEM) can provide a more accurate functional assessment of coagulation status and guide targeted transfusion strategies, helping to avoid unnecessary use of blood products [17].

Given the dual risk of bleeding and thrombosis in this population, a balanced approach to coagulation management is essential, ideally in collaboration with hematology or critical care teams.

22.2.5 Renal and Pulmonary Support

Renal and pulmonary dysfunction frequently coexist with PHLF and may precipitate or aggravate multiorgan failure. AKI occurs in a significant proportion of patients and is associated with poor prognosis. Contributing factors include hypoperfusion, systemic inflammation, and nephrotoxic exposures [2]. Early identification and avoidance of precipitating factors are essential. Volume status should be carefully optimized, and nephrotoxic agents minimized. Renal replacement therapy (RRT) is indicated for refractory fluid overload, hyperkalemia, or severe acidosis, and may also assist in managing hyperammonemia [18].

Pulmonary complications range from volume-related pulmonary edema to acute respiratory distress syndrome (ARDS), often secondary to infection or systemic inflammation. Lung-protective ventilation strategies and judicious fluid management are key. In severe cases, mechanical ventilation may be required to stabilize gas exchange and reduce the work of breathing [19].

Integrated renal and respiratory support, in close coordination with critical care teams, is often necessary in advanced PHLF, both to stabilize systemic physiology and to allow time for hepatic recovery or consideration of liver transplantation.

22.3 Liver-Directed Therapies

22.3.1 Pharmacological Support

To date, no pharmacologic agent has been shown to reverse or definitively improve the prognosis of post-hepatectomy liver failure (PHLF). However, several drugs have been used empirically or in investigational settings with the aim of limiting hepatocellular injury, modulating systemic inflammation, and supporting regenerative pathways. While their efficacy remains unproven, selected therapies may have a role in specific clinical scenarios.

N-acetylcysteine (NAC)

NAC is well established in the management of acetaminophen-induced acute liver failure due to its antioxidant properties and ability to restore hepatic glutathione stores. In the context of PHLF, its proposed benefits include improved hepatic microcirculation, reduced oxidative stress, and protection against ischemia–reperfusion injury [20]. Although high-quality evidence is lacking, several centers use NAC empirically, particularly in cases suggestive of hypoxic or ischemic liver damage [21]. Its favorable safety profile and low cost support its inclusion in the early management of selected patients.

Prostaglandin E1 (PGE1)
PGE1 has vasodilatory and anti-inflammatory effects, with experimental studies suggesting a potential hepatoprotective role through enhanced sinusoidal perfusion and cytoprotective action on hepatocytes. Some clinical studies, mainly in Asian populations, have reported improved liver function parameters, but robust randomized trials are lacking [22]. Moreover, its short half-life and potential for hypotension limit its widespread adoption. At present, PGE1 remains investigational and is not routinely used in most Western centers.

Hepatotropic Growth Factors
Growth factors such as hepatocyte growth factor (HGF), epidermal growth factor (EGF), and vascular endothelial growth factor (VEGF) are critical mediators of liver regeneration. Preclinical models have shown promising results in promoting hepatocyte proliferation and enhancing functional recovery [2]. However, clinical translation has been slow, and these agents are not yet available for routine use. Their potential application lies primarily in experimental settings or as adjuncts in regenerative medicine platforms.

Ammonia-Lowering Agents
Although not directly hepatoprotective, agents targeting ammonia metabolism may be used in patients with hepatic encephalopathy secondary to PHLF. Nonabsorbable disaccharides (e.g., lactulose), oral antibiotics (e.g., rifaximin), and L-ornithine L-aspartate (LOLA) help reduce systemic ammonia levels by promoting its elimination through alternative pathways [23]. While these therapies can improve mental status, their impact on overall outcome in PHLF remains unclear and should not delay more definitive interventions.

In summary, pharmacologic therapy in PHLF remains supportive in nature. Its use should be individualized, guided by the presumed etiology of liver dysfunction, the presence of encephalopathy or hypoperfusion, and the overall therapeutic goals whether recovery, stabilization, or bridging to transplantation.

22.3.2 Extracorporeal Liver Support Systems

Extracorporeal liver support (ELS) systems have been designed to provide temporary detoxification in patients with acute or acute-on-chronic liver failure, and may be considered in selected cases of PHLF. These therapies aim to reduce the burden of circulating toxins—particularly albumin-bound substances—modulate systemic inflammation, and stabilize organ function in critically ill patients. In this context,

ELS may serve as a bridge to hepatic regeneration or, when appropriate, to liver transplantation. Several systems have been proposed, with two main platforms currently employed in clinical practice.

Molecular Adsorbent Recirculating System (MARS)
MARS is the most widely used albumin-based dialysis platform. It combines hemodialysis with albumin-containing dialysate to remove protein-bound toxins such as bilirubin, bile acids, and cytokines. MARS has been shown to transiently improve biochemical parameters and encephalopathy in acute liver failure, but its impact on survival remains unproven. In PHLF, its use is largely empirical and reserved for selected patients with severe hyperbilirubinemia or refractory hepatic encephalopathy, particularly when liver transplantation is under consideration [24].

Prometheus System
Prometheus is another extracorporeal device that incorporates high-flux hemodialysis and fractionated plasma separation with adsorption. It offers a broader spectrum of detoxification, but similar to MARS, survival benefits have not been convincingly demonstrated. Its use is less widespread due to technical complexity and limited availability [25].

Despite the lack of definitive outcome data, ELS may be considered in highly selected patients as a supportive measure when standard therapy fails or as a bridge to transplant. Patient selection, timing, and institutional experience are key determinants of efficacy.

22.3.3 Biliary and Vascular Interventions

In selected cases, persistent or worsening PHLF may be driven by mechanical or vascular complications that are potentially reversible. Timely identification and correction of such conditions can significantly improve hepatic function and, in some cases, prevent further deterioration or the need for liver transplantation.

Biliary complications—including anastomotic strictures, retained stones, ischemic cholangiopathy, or bile leaks—are not uncommon following major hepatic resections, particularly those involving biliary-enteric reconstruction or vascular isolation of a segment. Biliary obstruction impairs bile excretion, favors cholangitis, and perpetuates hepatocellular injury. When suspected, early imaging with MRCP or contrast-enhanced CT should be obtained. Intervention may involve endoscopic retrograde cholangiopancreatography (ERCP) with sphincterotomy, bile ducts stenting, stone extraction, or percutaneous transhepatic biliary drainage (PTBD) in cases where endoscopic access is not feasible. Prompt decompression of the biliary system is essential to reduce cholestasis, resolve infection, and promote hepatic recovery [12].

Vascular complications, although less frequent, may have dramatic consequences. Hepatic artery thrombosis can lead to ischemic necrosis, especially in the setting of marginal perfusion or complex biliary reconstruction. Portal vein stenosis or thrombosis may impair inflow to the liver remnant, while hepatic vein outflow obstruction (e.g., following right hepatectomy or ALPPS procedures) can exacerbate sinusoidal congestion and impede regeneration. These conditions should be suspected in patients with unexplained hepatic decompensation, ascites, or rapidly rising transaminases. Doppler ultrasound is often the first-line investigation, but CT angiography or MR venography provide superior anatomical definition. When feasible, percutaneous interventions such as thrombolysis, angioplasty, or stent placement may restore vascular patency and prevent irreversible damage [16, 26].

Decision-making should be rapid and multidisciplinary, involving hepatobiliary surgeons, interventional radiologists, and hepatologists. In patients with anatomically correctable causes of hepatic failure, targeted interventions may represent the most effective form of therapy—potentially reversing the trajectory of organ dysfunction and obviating the need for transplantation.

22.3.4 Liver Transplantation

Liver transplantation (LT) represents the only definitive treatment for irreversible PHLF. However, its role in this setting is complex and constrained by multiple clinical, technical, and oncological considerations. Unlike acute liver failure of medical origin, PHLF typically develops in postoperative patients who have not been evaluated for LT preoperatively and may have undergone major resections for malignant disease, factors that can limit eligibility for listing [27].

Indeed, candidacy for LT is further challenged by the oncologic context, particularly in patients with non-early-stage hepatocellular carcinoma or colorectal liver metastases, where the risk of recurrence may preclude transplant [28]. Moreover, the rapid evolution of PHLF often limits the window for comprehensive evaluation and organ allocation. Recent surgical history also adds technical complexity due to adhesions, altered anatomy, and ongoing inflammation, increasing perioperative risk.

Despite these limitations, LT has been successfully performed in highly selected patients, especially those with benign disease, favorable tumor biology, or low recurrence risk. A recent pooled analysis reported that approximately 17.5% of PHLF-related liver transplants were performed using living donors, highlighting the feasibility and growing role of this approach. Living donor liver transplantation (LDLT) offers the unique advantage of timely graft availability without impacting the deceased-donor pool, a particularly relevant aspect in rapidly deteriorating cases. However, its use must carefully balance donor safety, technical complexity, and the overall prognosis of the recipient.

Early identification of candidates is crucial, particularly in patients with grade C PHLF and signs of progressive hepatic insufficiency despite maximal supportive care. Indicators such as persistent hyperbilirubinemia, worsening coagulopathy, rising lactate, encephalopathy, and unresponsive synthetic failure may prompt referral for transplant evaluation. Bridging therapies, including extracorporeal liver support, may help stabilize patients while assessment and allocation proceed.

In selected cases dominated by complications of portal hypertension—such as refractory ascites, renal dysfunction, or hepatic congestion—transjugular intrahepatic portosystemic shunt (TIPS) may be considered as a temporizing measure [29]. Although not routinely indicated in PHLF, portosystemic shunting—including TIPS—has been described in the context of small-for-size syndrome and severe portal hypertension, particularly when transplantation is delayed or not feasible. While most data derive from surgical shunt techniques, TIPS may represent a minimally invasive alternative in selected cases, though evidence remains limited [30]. Its use should be carefully balanced against the risk of precipitating or worsening hepatic encephalopathy.

Innovative surgical strategies inspired by the principles of auxiliary liver transplantation have also been explored in the setting of PHLF. A possible approach is LD-RAPID (Living Donor—Resection and Partial Liver Transplantation with Delayed Total Hepatectomy), in which a partial graft—typically segments 2–4—is implanted from a living donor while the diseased native liver is left in place. This technique allows temporary support with the potential for progressive graft dominance or native liver recovery. Another strategy, RAVAS (Rescue ALPPS and Vascularized Auxiliary Segmental Transplantation), involves the implantation of a segmental graft—often segments 2–3—in cases of failed ALPPS or insufficient liver remnant, with or without delayed resection of the native liver. While both procedures are technically demanding and remain largely anecdotal, they reflect a growing interest in hybrid, regenerative-compatible transplant paradigms tailored to complex postoperative liver failure scenarios [31].

Institutional protocols and access to transplantation may vary considerably, making early multidisciplinary communication essential. In conclusion, while liver transplantation remains feasible only in a limited subset of patients with PHLF, it can be life-saving when appropriately indicated. Early recognition, timely referral, and precise candidate selection are critical to optimizing its benefit—particularly when advanced strategies such as living donation or auxiliary techniques are available.

22.4 Emerging and Investigational Therapies

While current treatment strategies for PHLF are predominantly supportive, a growing body of research is focused on developing innovative approaches that may 1 day complement or replace existing therapies. These investigational strategies aim to enhance hepatocyte regeneration, modulate the immune response, and provide metabolic support, with the ultimate goal of improving transplant-free survival in patients with limited hepatic reserve.

22.4.1 Cellular and Stem Cell Therapies

Cell-based therapies are among the most actively investigated approaches to liver failure. Hepatocyte transplantation has shown potential in preclinical models and early clinical studies, particularly for metabolic disorders and acute liver injury.

More recently, mesenchymal stem cells (MSCs) and induced pluripotent stem cells (iPSCs) have attracted attention for their regenerative and immunomodulatory properties [32]. These cells may contribute to hepatic repair by secreting trophic factors, modulating inflammation, and promoting endogenous regeneration. However, challenges related to cell sourcing, engraftment, scalability, and long-term safety remain unresolved.

22.4.2 Bioartificial Liver Devices

Bioartificial liver (BAL) systems combine extracorporeal detoxification with a biological component—usually encapsulated hepatocytes or hepatic cell lines—to replicate some of the metabolic functions of the liver. Devices such as HepatAssist and ELAD have undergone clinical testing with mixed results. While improvements in encephalopathy and biochemical parameters have been reported, a consistent survival benefit has not been demonstrated [33, 34]. Nevertheless, continued refinement of these platforms may eventually yield bridge-to-recovery or bridge-to-transplant options for patients with PHLF unresponsive to conventional support.

22.4.3 Normothermic Perfusion and Ex Situ Liver Support

Normothermic machine perfusion (NMP) is an advanced organ preservation modality that maintains the liver in a metabolically active state ex situ by circulating oxygenated, nutrient-enriched perfusate at physiological temperature. Originally developed to optimize graft assessment and minimize ischemia–reperfusion injury in transplantation, NMP has since evolved into a versatile platform with broader potential applications.

Emerging experimental strategies have begun to explore the use of perfused human or xenogeneic livers as temporary biological support systems capable of providing ex vivo detoxification, synthetic activity, and metabolic stabilization. In this setting, NMP-based systems may serve as an interim bridge—either to transplant allocation or to spontaneous recovery—particularly in patients with acute hepatic decompensation, including those with post-hepatectomy liver failure [35].

Although still at a preclinical or investigational stage, ex situ liver perfusion offers a promising intermediary between conventional bioartificial liver devices and functional liver replacement. Furthermore, it may facilitate advanced interventions such as graft reconditioning, pharmacologic manipulation, or integration into auxiliary and segmental transplantation protocols. As technology and translational experience advance, the therapeutic scope of machine perfusion may expand to include not only organ preservation but also extracorporeal hepatic support in critical care settings.

In summary, emerging therapies for PHLF remain experimental but reflect a growing commitment to regenerative medicine and precision liver support. As these strategies evolve, they may expand the therapeutic arsenal available to hepatobiliary surgeons and critical care teams, offering new hope for patients with limited options.

22.5 Conclusion

Post-hepatectomy liver failure remains a formidable challenge in hepatobiliary surgery, often arising despite optimal operative technique and perioperative management. Once established, its treatment requires timely recognition and a coordinated, multidisciplinary approach centered on supportive care. Hemodynamic stabilization, nutritional support, infection control, and organ support form the foundation of management, while selected patients may benefit from liver-specific interventions such as biliary or vascular decompression, extracorporeal support, or liver transplantation.

Although no curative therapy exists outside of transplantation, the field is evolving. Novel regenerative strategies, cell-based therapies, and advanced perfusion technologies are under active investigation and may, in the future, broaden the therapeutic landscape. Until then, early intervention, individualized care, and referral to experienced centers remain the cornerstones of improving outcomes in this high-risk setting.

Bibliography

1. Rahbari NN, Garden OJ, Padbury R, Brooke-Smith M, Crawford M, Adam R, et al. Posthepatectomy liver failure: a definition and grading by the International Study Group of Liver Surgery (ISGLS). Surgery. 2011;149(5):713–24.
2. Sparrelid E, Olthof PB, Dasari BVM, Erdmann JI, Santol J, Starlinger P, et al. Current evidence on posthepatectomy liver failure: comprehensive review. BJS Open. 2022;6(6):zrac142.
3. Maiwall R, Kulkarni AV, Arab JP, Piano S. Acute liver failure. Lancet. 2024;404(10454):789–802.
4. Van Den Broek MAJ, Olde Damink SWM, Dejong CHC, Lang H, Malagó M, Jalan R, et al. Liver failure after partial hepatic resection: definition, pathophysiology, risk factors and treatment. Liver Int. 2008;28(6):767–80.
5. Colle I, Verhelst X, Vanlander A, Geerts A, Vlierberghe HV, Berrevoet F, et al. Pathophysiology and management of post resection liver failure. Acta Chir Belg. 2013;113(3):155–61.
6. Van Eldere A, Pirani T. Liver intensive care for the general intensivist. Anaesthesia. 2023;78(7):884–901.
7. Arab JP, Pizarro M, Solis N, Sun H, Thevananther S, Arrese M. Mild hypothermia does not affect liver regeneration after partial hepatectomy in mice. Liver Int. 2009;29(3):344–8.
8. Gupta T, Saini A, Gaur V, Goel A. Comparative study of terlipressin and noradrenaline as vasopressors in patients with acute-on-chronic liver failure and septic shock: a randomized controlled trial. J Clin Exp Hepatol. 2025;15(3):102494.
9. Evans L, Rhodes A, Alhazzani W, Antonelli M, Coopersmith CM, French C, et al. Surviving sepsis campaign: international guidelines for management of sepsis and septic shock 2021. Intensive Care Med. 2021;47(11):1181–247.
10. Imamura H. One thousand fifty-six hepatectomies without mortality in 8 years. Arch Surg. 2003;138(11):1198.

11. Bischoff SC, Bernal W, Dasarathy S, Merli M, Plank LD, Schütz T, et al. ESPEN practical guideline: clinical nutrition in liver disease. Clin Nutr. 2020;39(12):3533–62.
12. Qadan M, Garden JO, Corvera CU, Visser BC. Management of postoperative hepatic failure. J Am Coll Surg. 2016;222(2):195–208.
13. Zigmond E, Samia-Grinberg S, Pasmanik-Chor M, Brazowski E, Shibolet O, Halpern Z, et al. Infiltrating monocyte-derived macrophages and resident Kupffer cells display different ontogeny and functions in acute liver injury. J Immunol. 2014;193(1):344–53.
14. Dong Y, Sun D, Wang Y, Du Q, Zhang Y, Han R, et al. Evaluation of the current guidelines for antibacterial therapy strategies in patients with cirrhosis or liver failure. BMC Infect Dis. 2022;22(1):23.
15. Venkatakrishnan G, Amma BSPT, Menon RN, Rajakrishnan H, Surendran S. Infections in acute liver failure – assessment, prevention, and management. Best Pract Res Clin Gastroenterol. 2024;73:101958.
16. Søreide JA, Deshpande R. Post hepatectomy liver failure (PHLF) – recent advances in prevention and clinical management. Eur J Surg Oncol. 2021;47(2):216–24.
17. Mancuso A, Fung K, Cox D, Mela M, Patch D, Burroughs AK. Assessment of blood coagulation in severe liver disease using thromboelastography. Blood Coagul Fibrinolysis. 2003;14(2):211–6.
18. Slack AJ, Auzinger G, Willars C, Dew T, Musto R, Corsilli D, et al. Ammonia clearance with haemofiltration in adults with liver disease. Liver Int. 2014;34(1):42–8.
19. Herrero R, Sánchez G, Asensio I, López E, Ferruelo A, Vaquero J, et al. Liver–lung interactions in acute respiratory distress syndrome. Intensive Care Med Exp. 2020;8(S1):48.
20. Jegatheeswaran S, Siriwardena AK. Experimental and clinical evidence for modification of hepatic ischaemia–reperfusion injury by N-acetylcysteine during major liver surgery. HPB. 2011;13(2):71–8.
21. Kemp R, Mole J, Gomez D. Current evidence for the use of *N*-acetylcysteine following liver resection. ANZ J Surg. 2018;88(6):E486–90.
22. Une Y, Shimamura T, Uchino J. Effect of prostaglandin E1 on hepatic function after hepatectomy in patients with chronic liver disease. Clin Ther. 1995;17(6):1118–25.
23. Balzano T. Active clinical trials in hepatic encephalopathy: something old, something new and something borrowed. Neurochem Res. 2023;48(8):2309–19.
24. Kanjo A, Ocskay K, Gede N, Kiss S, Szakács Z, Párniczky A, et al. Efficacy and safety of liver support devices in acute and hyperacute liver failure: a systematic review and network meta-analysis. Sci Rep. 2021;11(1):4189.
25. Kotulski M, Patkowski W, Grodzicki M, Zieniewicz K. Results of treatment of patients with acute liver failure by albumin dialysis using the Prometheus system. Transplantation. 2020;104(S3):S493–3.
26. Jaffe V, Lygidakis NJ, Blumgart LH. Acute portal vein thrombosis after right hepatic lobectomy: successful treatment by thrombectomy. J Br Surg. 1982;69(4):211–1.
27. Azoulay D, Desterke C, Bhangui P, Serrablo A, De Martin E, Cauchy F, et al. Rescue liver transplantation for posthepatectomy liver failure: a systematic review and survey of an international experience. Transplantation. 2024;108:947–57.
28. Sparrelid E, Thorsen T, Sauter C, Jorns C, Stål P, Nordin A, et al. Liver transplantation in patients with post-hepatectomy liver failure – a Northern European multicenter cohort study. HPB. 2022;24(7):1138–44.
29. Ripoll C, Rauchfuss F, Aschenbach R, Settmacher U, Zipprich A. Transjugular intrahepatic portosystemic shunt for the patients on the liver transplant list. Liver Transpl. 2025;31(1):105–16.
30. Kinaci E, Kayaalp C. Portosystemic shunts for “too small-for-size syndrome” after liver transplantation: a systematic review. World J Surg. 2016;40(8):1932–40.
31. Angelico R, Siragusa L, Serenari M, Scalera I, Kauffman E, Lai Q, et al. Rescue liver transplantation after post-hepatectomy acute liver failure: a systematic review and pooled analysis. Transplant Rev. 2023;37(3):100773.
32. Liu Z, Ren J, Qiu C, Wang Y, Zhang T. Application of mesenchymal stem cells in liver fibrosis and regeneration. Liver Res. 2024;8(4):246–58.

33. He YT, Qi YN, Zhang BQ, Li JB, Bao J. Bioartificial liver support systems for acute liver failure: a systematic review and meta-analysis of the clinical and preclinical literature. World J Gastroenterol. 2019;25(27):3634–48.
34. Kumar A, Tripathi A, Jain S. Extracorporeal bioartificial liver for treating acute liver diseases. J Extra Corpor Technol. 2011;43(4):195–206.
35. Czigany Z, Shirini K, Putri AJ, Longchamp AE, Bhusal S, Kamberi S, et al. Bridging therapies—ex vivo liver xenoperfusion and the role of machine perfusion: an update. Xenotransplantation. 2025;32(1):e70011.

Future of Regenerative Hepatology 23

Javier Martínez-García, Álvaro Blanes-Rodríguez, Sandra Melitón-Barbancho, Marta Sáinz-Viartola, and Pedro M. Baptista

23.1 Introduction to Regenerative Hepatology

The liver, as the primary organ responsible for metabolic homeostasis and detoxification, possesses a unique self-repair capacity. However, the prevalence of acute or chronic end-stage liver diseases (ESLD) continues to increase worldwide, largely due to factors such as alcohol abuse, viral hepatitis, and metabolic dysfunction-associated steatotic liver disease (MASLD). These liver disorders can eventually lead to loss of liver function and architecture resulting in advanced stages of liver disease, such as cirrhosis and hepatocellular carcinoma (HCC), where the liver's regenerative capacity is overwhelmed and it is unable to recover vital functionality [1]. Currently, liver transplantation is the only definitive treatment for most ESLD, but it is limited by the scarcity of donor organs, its high cost, and associated

J. Martínez-García
Health Research Institute of Aragón (IIS Aragón), Zaragoza, Spain

Multiscale in Mechanical and Biological Engineering (M2BE), Universidad de Zaragoza, Zaragoza, Spain
e-mail: jmartinez@iisaragon.es

Á. Blanes-Rodríguez · S. Melitón-Barbancho · M. Sáinz-Viartola
Health Research Institute of Aragón (IIS Aragón), Zaragoza, Spain

P. M. Baptista (✉)
Health Research Institute of Aragón (IIS Aragón), Zaragoza, Spain

Center for Biomedical Research Network Liver and Digestive Diseases (CIBERehd), Zaragoza, Spain

Biomedical Engineering Department, Universidad Carlos III de Madrid, Madrid, Spain

Fundación ARAID, Zaragoza, Spain
e-mail: pmbaptista@iisaragon.es

L. Aldrighetti et al. (eds.), *Liver Regeneration Techniques In Hepatic Surgery*,
https://doi.org/10.1007/978-3-032-10997-2_23

morbidity. This lack of alternatives for liver repair underscores the need to explore new approaches to regenerative hepatology further (Fig. 23.1) [2].

Over the past decades, breakthroughs in stem cell research and the development of advanced biotechnologies and biomaterials have contributed to the interest in exploring different approaches to induce and enhance liver regeneration. At the forefront of these are cell-based therapies, gene therapy and editing tools, and liver bioengineering. First, cell-based therapy aims to restore lost functionality due to damaged liver tissue by engrafting functionally mature parenchymal and/or

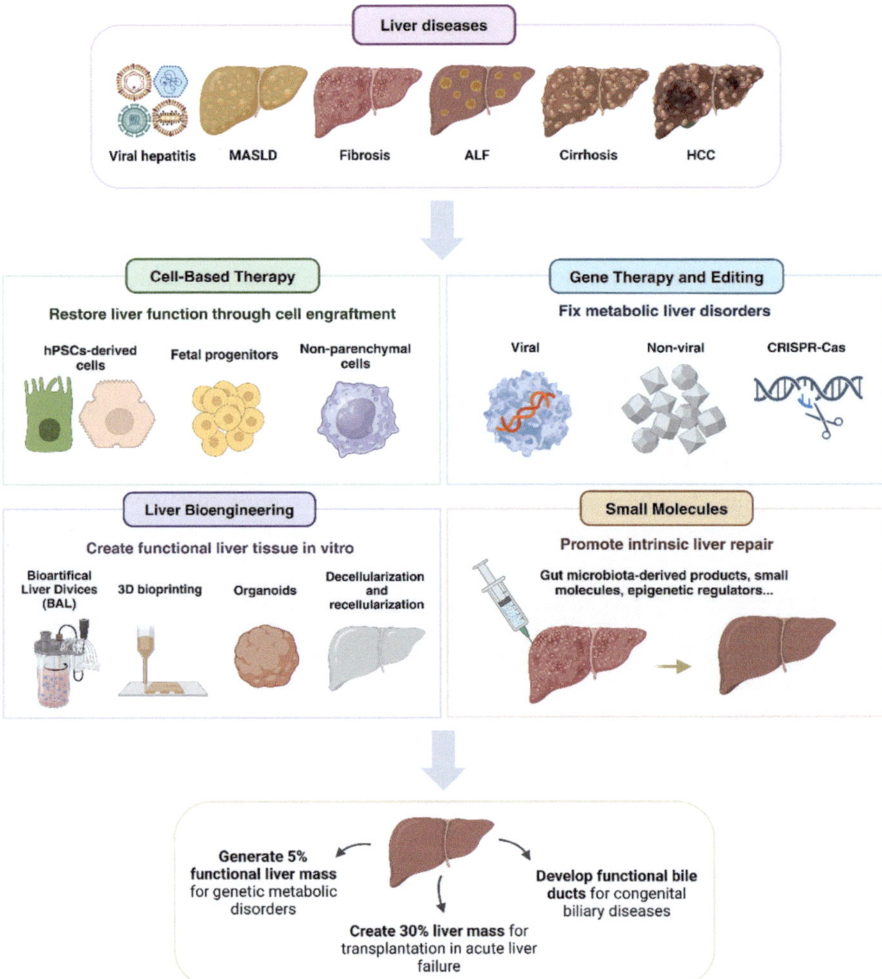

Fig. 23.1 Overview of regenerative hepatology strategies to restore hepatic function in liver diseases. (Figure created with BioRender.com). ALF acute liver failure, HCC hepatocellular carcinoma, MASLD metabolic dysfunction-associated steatotic liver disease, PSCs pluripotent stem cells

non-parenchymal liver cells [3, 4]. Currently, it has demonstrated significant potential as a bridge to transplantation or as a pathway to an endogenous cure in cases of acute liver failure (ALF). However, its applicability as a long-term solution faces several challenges, such as the maturity and functionality of the liver cells used [5], as well as the cells being able to engraft properly into the tissue by mitigating inflammation, fibrosis, and modification of the extracellular matrix of the organ [4, 6]. Second, gene therapy represents another promising strategy for congenital hepatic and biliary metabolic disorders as it allows to correct liver function impairment, thereby reducing liver damage and promoting tissue regeneration [7]. Similarly, gene editing tools such as CRISPR-Cas enable in situ correction of mutations responsible for liver damage, effectively halting disease progression [8]. Nevertheless, this strategy faces some limitations, such as toxicity induced by high doses of viral vectors, immune rejection, and the requirement for immunosuppressants [9]. Finally, liver bioengineering aims to create functional liver tissue in vitro. Advances in technologies such as organoids, three-dimensional (3D) bioprinting, or decellularization and recellularization of liver scaffolds favor the development of bioengineered organs that mimic the liver microenvironment and liver function [10]. However, liver bioengineering faces significant challenges, including achieving efficient organ vascularization and ensuring the engraftment and functionality of liver cells. Overcoming these hurdles is critical to establishing viable alternatives to liver donation in liver transplantation and addressing the high mortality and morbidity rates associated with prolonged time on the organ transplant waiting list [11, 12].

In addition to these cornerstone approaches, small molecules remain a widely explored strategy in regenerative hepatology, offering ways to stimulate intrinsic liver repair mechanisms. Products derived from the gut microbiota, such as short-chain fatty acids, vitamins, and secondary bile acids, have demonstrated hepatoprotective effects [13]. Similarly, small molecules such as mitogen-activated protein kinase 4 (MKK4) inhibitors, FGF21 analogs, selective thyroid hormone receptor-β, and glucagon-like peptide 1 (GLP1) agonists have shown a potential to reduce liver fibrosis and mitigate hepatic steatosis and inflammation, respectively [14–17]. Finally, epigenetic regulators, such as histone deacetylase inhibitors, have shown an effect on liver regeneration and fibrosis with great potential for treating HCC [18].

Together, these strategies reflect the broad nature of regenerative hepatology approaches and underscore the necessity for ongoing research to refine and integrate these therapies. This would enable the creation of 5% functional liver mass for the treatment of genetic metabolic disorders, the development of functional bile ducts to address congenital biliary diseases, and, finally, the creation of at least 30% liver mass for transplantation in patients with ALF or acute-on-chronic liver failure (ACLF), leading to the incorporation of these therapies into clinical practice.

23.2 Cell-Based Therapies

Liver diseases, including ALF, ACLF, and ESLD, impose substantial global health and economic burdens. Orthotopic liver transplantation (OLT) remains the only definitive treatment; however, the limited availability of donor organs restricts its widespread application [19]. In response, innovative cell-based therapies have emerged as promising alternatives to reduce reliance on invasive surgical procedures and address the donor shortage. These therapies aim to restore liver function by replacing damaged hepatocytes or remodeling the hepatic microenvironment to facilitate host liver regeneration. Recent advancements in hepatocyte encapsulation, hepatocyte transplantation (HTx), mesenchymal stem cell (MSC) therapy, liver organoids, and pluripotent stem cells (PSCs) are paving the way for transformative strategies in liver disease management [20].

23.2.1 Hepatocyte Transplantation

An optimistic alternative to liver transplantation, particularly for metabolic disorders and acute liver injury, is HTx. Functioning as cellular gene therapy, transplanted hepatocytes can restore metabolic functions with as little as 1–2.5% of total liver mass. Clinical successes include temporary metabolic stability in patients with Crigler–Najjar syndrome [19]. Despite these advancements, challenges such as low engraftment rates, immune rejection, and limited availability of high-quality hepatocytes hinder broader clinical application. Enhancements in cryopreservation and the use of anti-apoptotic agents have improved cell viability, enabling the development of more consistent "off-the-shelf" solutions [21]. Additionally, liver preconditioning techniques, such as sinusoidal disruption to induce endothelial cell apoptosis, promote donor cell integration. Another notable advancement is the encapsulation of hepatocytes in alginate beads, which mitigates immune rejection and enhances cell viability by allowing extrahepatic transplantation [20]. In a study by Dhawan et al., eight pediatric patients with ALF received intraperitoneal infusions of alginate-encapsulated hepatocytes. Four patients achieved full recovery without the need for transplantation, and three were successfully bridged to OLT. The encapsulated hepatocytes remained viable and functionally intact upon retrieval, demonstrating the safety and feasibility of this approach as both a standalone solution and a bridge to transplantation [22].

23.2.2 Mesenchymal Stem Cell Therapy

MSCs have gained attention in the last decades for their regenerative and immunomodulatory properties. Derived from sources such as bone marrow, umbilical cord, and adipose tissue, MSCs can modulate the hepatic microenvironment by reducing inflammation, suppressing fibrosis, and promoting hepatocyte proliferation through the secretion of growth factors such as interleukin-10, transforming growth factor-beta, and prostaglandin E2 [23]. Clinical trials have demonstrated significant improvements in liver function markers, including MELD scores and serum albumin levels, following MSC infusion. A pivotal study with a 75-month follow-up on 219 cirrhotic patients revealed enhanced survival rates, improved liver function, and no increase in tumor incidence or major adverse events [24]. MSCs are particularly effective in treating ACLF, where they help control inflammation and fibrosis, thereby reducing mortality. In a randomized trial involving 110 ACLF patients, MSC infusion led to significant improvements in liver function and infection control and reduced mortality at 24 weeks post-treatment [25]. Furthermore, preclinical studies suggest that co-transplantation of MSCs with hepatocytes enhances liver repair by providing both cellular replacement and environmental remodeling, offering a dual mechanism of action that targets comprehensive liver regeneration [26].

23.2.3 Future Directions in Cell Therapy

23.2.3.1 Human Pluripotent Stem Cells

PSCs-based technology, including cell sources such as embryonic stem cells (ESCs) and induced pluripotent stem cells (iPSCs), has emerged in recent decades, holding great promise for generating hepatocyte-like cells (HLCs) and cholangiocyte-like cells (CLCs). These cells can be derived in vitro and transplanted to replace damaged liver tissues [20]. While HLCs exhibit partial functionality, further advancements are necessary to achieve full maturation comparable to primary hepatocytes. Carpentier's team demonstrated that iPSC-derived cells facilitated 15% liver regeneration in urokinase-type plasminogen activator immunodeficient mice [27]. Similarly, studies from the University of Cambridge successfully repaired bile duct injuries in human liver models using cholangiocyte organoids derived from hPSCs [28]. Continued improvements in differentiation protocols and bioengineering techniques are expected to enhance the clinical viability of hPSC-derived cells, paving the way for their integration into therapeutic regimens.

23.2.3.2 Fetal Progenitors

Fetal liver progenitor (FLP) cells are another promising source due to their high proliferative capacity and ability to differentiate into hepatocytes and cholangiocytes. Preclinical studies have shown successful engraftment and liver repopulation in animal models, with significant liver mass restoration and reduced fibrosis [20]. For instance, transplantation of human FLPs effectively reduced liver fibrosis in animal models [29]. However, ethical concerns and limited availability pose significant challenges for their clinical use. Advances in in vitro expansion techniques for FLP cells may offer scalable alternatives, potentially overcoming these limitations and enabling broader application in liver regeneration therapies [30].

23.2.3.3 Liver Organoids

Liver organoids, 3D structures derived from stem or adult cells, provide a more physiologically relevant model than traditional two-dimensional cell cultures. These organoids mimic liver architecture and function, making them suitable for transplantation and regenerative purposes [31]. Bioengineering advancements, such as encapsulating organoids in hydrogels or extracellular matrix (ECM) components, have enhanced their viability and integration into host tissues. Forbes et al. successfully rescued bile duct structure and function in a mouse model of biliary disease using organoids constructed from purified human biliary epithelial cells (hBECs) [32]. This was also previously performed by Sampaziotis et al. by repairing segments of biliary trees of human livers preserved ex vivo under normothermic machine perfusion [28]. Additionally, organoids are valuable platforms for drug testing and disease modeling, with potential applications in personalized medicine [33]. Due to their potential, researchers have explored their use in bridging patients to transplantation and providing long-term liver support, highlighting their versatility and therapeutic potential [34].

23.2.3.4 Non-parenchymal Cells

Non-parenchymal cells, including liver sinusoidal endothelial cells (LSECs) and macrophages, are crucial for liver regeneration and homeostasis. LSECs contribute to the vascular niche and promote hepatocyte engraftment through paracrine signaling, while macrophages facilitate debris clearance, modulate inflammation, and support tissue repair [20]. Franchesca Moroni et al. evaluated the safety and feasibility of autologous monocyte-derived macrophage infusion in patients with compensated liver cirrhosis, suggesting potential antifibrotic and regenerative effects [35]. Therapeutic strategies focusing on non-parenchymal cells aim to optimize the hepatic microenvironment, thereby enhancing the efficacy of hepatocyte and stem cell transplantation. For example, co-transplanting macrophages with MSCs or organoids has synergistic effects in preclinical models, improving liver regeneration and reducing fibrosis [35, 36].

23.3 Gene Therapy and Gene Editing Tools

Advances in genetic engineering in the field of genetic engineering have led to the rise of new technologies, such as gene therapy that prove to be a promising strategy for treating genetic diseases. Gene therapy is often classified as based on viral or nonviral vectors. In the following sections, the major advances in liver-targeted gene therapy will be described according to the vector type.

23.3.1 Viral Liver-Targeted Gene Therapy

Gene therapy based on viral vectors has advantages such as increased efficiency in transduction and long-term expression of the transgene of interest. In the 1990s, the first successful clinical trials in patients with familial hypercholesterolemia were conducted using a retroviral vector. However, this success was limited since this therapy raised safety concerns [37]. To increase the efficacy and safety of liver-targeted therapies, research with adeno-associated viral (AAV) vectors was initiated. Liver-targeted gene therapy based on AAV vectors has achieved positive preclinical outcomes for treating monogenic liver disorders such as hemophilia B, Wilson's disease, and cholestatic diseases, among others [38–40]. There are currently AAV vector-based therapies approved for clinical use, such as Roctavian and Giroctocogene for hemophilia A [41, 42], or Hemgenix and BEQVEZ for hemophilia B therapy, which have successfully increased the expression and activity of the clotting factor involved, thereby reducing bleeding in patients [43, 44].

However, AAV viral vectors continue to face several obstacles, such as toxicity associated with the use of high doses of the viral vectors, as has occurred in a clinical trial of gene therapy for myotubular myopathy with some unexpected deaths due to liver failure [45]. Therefore, the future of research in the use of this type of viral vector involves reducing immunogenicity, dosage optimization, genotoxicity prevention, and improving the vectors.

One of the strategies being explored in recent years to reduce the immunogenicity of AAV vectors is to incorporate immunoinhibitory sequences of internal immune sensors, such as a reduced number of CpG motifs, into the vector genome [46]. Another strategy is the combined treatment with nanoparticles encapsulating immunosuppressants such as rapamycin to prevent the induction of anti-capsid cell and humoral-mediated responses. In addition, this strategy has proven to be efficient for the administration of repeated doses of the vector in mice and nonhuman primates [47]. Finally, another strategy is the elimination of neutralizing antibodies using IgG-degrading endopeptidases [48].

Moreover, strategies such as the codon optimization that could increase the efficiency of transgene expression, resulting in higher production of the therapeutic protein, are being addressed to achieve the optimization and reduction of the doses of the viral vector [40]. Another strategy to increase the potency of the vectors is the incorporation of promoters that allow for stronger expression and reduce the viral dose needed to achieve the desired therapeutic effect and the possible risk of toxicity from the use of high doses. Alternatively, inducible promoters could be introduced that allow controlled and safe expression of the transgene of interest by mimicking physiological regulation, which would avoid undesired effects of overexpression induced by constitutive promoters, as well as silencing of expression and exacerbated immune responses [49].

23.3.2 Nonviral Liver-Targeted Gene Therapy

The need for gene therapies based on nonviral vectors has arisen to reduce the toxicity associated with high doses of viral vectors. These nonviral vectors have advantages such as a much better safety profile, the ease of large-scale production, and the theoretically unlimited genome size to be administered. The most widely used nonviral vector-based strategy is the use of small interfering RNAs (siRNAs) that enable gene silencing. Currently, six siRNA drugs have been approved for clinical use: (1) Givosiran to ameliorate acute hepatic porphyria attacks, (2) Lumasiran and

Nedosiran for the treatment of primary hyperoxaluria 1, (3) Inclisiran for hyperlipidemia and hypercholesterolemia, and lastly, (4) Vutrisiran and Patisiran for the treatment of hereditary transthyretin-mediated amyloidosis [50–54]. The success of these products has led to further research into this type of technology. However, siRNA-based therapy requires periodic readministration of treatment to maintain therapeutic effect [55].

The most commonly addressed alternative for gene therapy based on nonviral vectors currently involves lipid nanoparticles that encapsulate messenger RNA (mRNA) that, using the cell's machinery, leads to the expression of the therapeutic protein of interest. As a significant advantage over viral vectors, mRNA-based therapy reduces the potential risks associated with genotoxicity and immunogenicity [56]. In the field of liver-targeted gene therapy, it was first used in treating methylmalonic acidemia in 2017, achieving increased liver function and reduced toxicity in mice [57]. Since then, many preclinical studies have shown very promising results of mRNA-based gene therapy in monogenic liver disorders [58, 59]. However, the main limitation of this strategy is that expression is not sustained over time and requires weekly administration to maintain the therapeutic effect.

23.3.3 Gene Editing

Gene editing has emerged in recent decades as a revolutionary alternative for the treatment of monogenic disorders. Indeed, the arrival of CRISPR/Cas9-based technologies has transformed regenerative medicine by demonstrating its great potential in preclinical studies targeting liver diseases such as hemophilia and phenylketonuria over the last decade [60]. However, the presence of this innovative approach in liver-targeted clinical trials has been limited to three studies based on the use of zinc finger nucleases [8]. As difficulties arise when therapeutic efficacy requires the integration of therapeutic genetic material into the genome by homology-dependent recombination, the clinical success of these classical gene-editing tools is hampered by the low efficiency of recombination and the transient effect of expression [61].

In recent years, Gillmore et al. have demonstrated groundbreaking results for treating transthyretin amyloidosis with CRISPR technology [62]. However, despite the potential of this gene editing tool, it is necessary to reduce the potential genotoxicity associated with undesired cuts in off-target regions. Alternatively, new tools based on CRISPR technology, such as Base editing and Prime editing, have been developed to improve the safety and efficiency of cutting or rewriting the genetic information to correct the monogenic disorder.

Base editing has shown therapeutic efficacy for treating liver diseases in mice and nonhuman primates [63, 64]. The first clinical trial in human patients using base editing technology has been registered this year (NCT05398029). This study aims to determine the safety profile and therapeutic potential for the treatment of familial hypercholesterolemia by disrupting PCSK9 and then lowering blood levels of LDL cholesterol and PCSK9. Although this approach is very promising, it must avoid off-target base editing. Therefore, by overcoming the limitations associated with

DNA cutting and off-target editing, improving repair pathways and the enzymes involved in the process, as well as achieving safe and efficient in vivo through enhancements in the delivery vehicles used in patients, CRISPR-derived gene editing tools could represent a genetic revolution, potentially leading to multiple gene therapy products for the clinical treatment of hereditary diseases.

23.4 Liver Bioengineering

23.4.1 Bioartificial Liver Devices

Artificial liver support systems (ALSS) offer critical treatment options for patients with liver failure by mimicking the detoxification functions of the liver. The main extracorporeal albumin dialysis (ECAD) systems in use include the Molecular Adsorbent Recirculating System (MARS) and the Advanced Organ Support (ADVOS) system, both of which can help in managing symptoms such as hepatic encephalopathy and jaundice [65]. MARS has been widely studied and shown to aid in multiple liver failure conditions [66]. ADVOS, introduced in 2013, enhances detoxification by regenerating albumin through temperature and pH adjustments, showing comparable effectiveness and safety to MARS in in vitro studies [67]. Plasma exchange is another system that improves outcomes in acute liver failure by reducing systemic inflammation and removing harmful molecules. Recent trials show benefits for transplant-free survival and improved organ function, with large Phase 3 trials currently underway [68]. However, these systems face limitations in providing long-term support, high operational costs, and limited evidence of improved survival rates, especially compared to liver transplantation. Ongoing research focuses on combining ECAD systems with stem-cell technology and bioartificial components to enhance ALSS's regenerative capacity and accessibility [65].

In recent years, ex situ organ preservation machines have gained interest in potentially repairing damaged organs and assessing organ function. Examples are the hypothermic ex situ oxygenated perfusion machine (HOPE) and the normothermic perfusion machine (NMP) [69, 70]. This NMP technology has succeeded in preserving a liver discarded for transplantation into a patient and restoring the patient's quality of life for at least 1 year [70]. Additionally, this technology allows the incorporation of pharmacological treatments such as defatting agents, gene therapy products, and cell therapies to improve the biological parameters of the discarded liver [71, 72], making it suitable for transplantation.

23.4.2 Whole Liver Bioengineering

The field of liver bioengineering has made significant advancements, particularly in the development of decellularized extracellular matrix (dECM) scaffolds, which can be later recellularized with parenchymal and non-parenchymal cells to ultimately create bioengineered livers for research, therapeutic, or transplantation purposes. These scaffolds, which maintain the liver's intricate architecture and biochemical cues, offer promising frameworks for cell repopulation [73]. However, ensuring cell removal methods do not damage critical ECM proteins remains a significant challenge, as excessive treatment can degrade cell attachment sites and biochemical signals. Beyond these technical issues, long-term scaffold stability and immune acceptance are also significant concerns. Even though decellularization reduces immunogenicity by removing cellular material, immune responses can still occur [74]. Other applications for dECM could include the fabrication of hydrogels [75] and the production of decellularized tissue discs or cubes for in vitro studies, allowing a microenvironment and cell–cell and cell–matrix interaction more similar to that found in vivo [76–78].

The primary challenge lies in effectively repopulating these dECM scaffolds with diverse liver cell types, including parenchymal cells such as hepatocytes, hepatocyte-like cells derived from hPSCs, or fetal progenitors, or non-parenchymal cells such as endothelial cells, LSECs, immune cells, among others, in an approach that replicates liver microarchitecture. Current techniques employ perfusion-based seeding and advanced growth media, but a physiologically precise spatial organization of cells remains elusive [79]. Baptista et al. demonstrated that targeting different cell types to specific liver regions improves compartmentalization, which is essential for liver functionality [11]. Future research is focused on refining cell placement and distribution techniques to enhance cell viability and functionality within the scaffold. However, one of the major challenges in recellularizing a liver is establishing a vascular tree with endothelial cells, as the liver's extensive capillary network is critical for the supply of nutrients and oxygen that determines metabolic zonation. The leap from revascularizing small to large animal livers has been exceptionally complex. A key example is the work by Pla-Palacín et al., which developed a method to recellularize porcine livers with endothelial and mesenchymal stem cells [80]. The most significant advancement in bioengineered liver perfusion to this day has been made by Higashi et al., who achieved 28 days of successful vascular perfusion in decellularized pig livers seeded with porcine aorta endothelial cells and primary hepatocytes, marking a milestone in human-sized bioengineered liver development for therapeutic applications [81].

On the other hand, repopulating a liver scaffold with parenchymal cells remains a significant challenge, primarily due to the substantial number of hepatocyte-like cells required to adequately populate large animal models. Such cells must also exhibit functional activity and maintain viability within the scaffold over an extended period. Studies using primary hepatocytes reported short-term functionality [74]. Recent efforts in the organoid field have addressed this issue. Schneeberger et al. reported the large-scale expansion of intrahepatic cholangiocyte organoids (ICOs) in spinner flasks, which showed promise for scalable cell generation [77]. Noteworthy, fetal progenitors and hPSCs may involve loss of functionality and maturity, ethical dilemmas regarding their procurement, as well as the associated risk of tumorgenesis [82]. Future work in recellularization focuses on using growth factors and specialized ECM coatings to promote stable, mature vascular networks that can integrate with a fully differentiated parenchyma [74].

23.4.3 Bile Duct Bioengineering

Bile duct bioengineering aims to create functional bile duct tissues for modeling and drug testing of cholangiopathies and eventually to be used as alternatives to liver transplantation [83]. The primary challenge in bile duct bioengineering lies in recreating the intricate structure and function of bile duct tissues formed by cholangiocytes, as well as the scaffold choice to be repopulated [84]. Cholangiocyte-based organoids, including ICOs, represent a significant advancement in liver tissue engineering. However, long-term engraftment and functionality remain challenging, which has been addressed by different works. Roos et al. developed branching cholangiocyte organoids raised in Matrigel that could be used to study bile duct development [85]. Wang et al. showed the differentiation and functional characterization of ICOs into cholangiocyte-like cells in hollow fiber membranes generating 3D duct structures [86]. Nonetheless, in vitro studies still exhibit variability in their morphological characteristics and functional assays. While bioengineered bile ducts have already been transplanted to mouse [87], future work is oriented toward large animal models.

References

1. Zuñiga-Aguilar E, Ramírez-Fernández O. Fibrosis and hepatic regeneration mechanism. Transl Gastroenterol Hepatol. 2022;7:9–9. https://doi.org/10.21037/tgh.2020.02.21.
2. Papatheodoridi M, Mazza G, Pinzani M. Regenerative hepatology: in the quest for a modern Prometheus? Dig Liver Dis. 2020;52(10):1106–14. https://doi.org/10.1016/j.dld.2020.08.001.
3. Vogel KR, Kennedy AA, Whitehouse LA, Gibson KM. Therapeutic hepatocyte transplant for inherited metabolic disorders: functional considerations, recent outcomes and future prospects. J Inherit Metab Dis. 2014;37(2):165–76. https://doi.org/10.1007/s10545-013-9656-5.
4. Meng F, Wang K, Aoyama T, et al. Interleukin-17 signaling in inflammatory, Kupffer cells, and hepatic stellate cells exacerbates liver fibrosis in mice. Gastroenterology. 2012;143(3):765–76.e3. https://doi.org/10.1053/j.gastro.2012.05.049.
5. Nguyen MP, Jain V, Iansante V, Mitry RR, Filippi C, Dhawan A. Clinical application of hepatocyte transplantation: current status, applicability, limitations, and future outlook. Expert Rev Gastroenterol Hepatol. 2020;14(3):185–96. https://doi.org/10.1080/17474124.2020.1733975.
6. Tacke F. Targeting hepatic macrophages to treat liver diseases. J Hepatol. 2017;66(6):1300–12. https://doi.org/10.1016/j.jhep.2017.02.026.
7. Martínez-García J, Molina A, González-Aseguinolaza G, Weber ND, Smerdou C. Gene therapy for acquired and genetic cholestasis. Biomedicines. 2022;10(6):1238. https://doi.org/10.3390/biomedicines10061238.
8. Zabaleta N, Torella L, Weber ND, Gonzalez-Aseguinolaza G. mRNA and gene editing: late breaking therapies in liver diseases. Hepatology. Published online April 2022. https://doi.org/10.1002/hep.32441.
9. Baruteau J, Waddington SN, Alexander IE, Gissen P. Gene therapy for monogenic liver diseases: clinical successes, current challenges and future prospects. J Inherit Metab Dis. 2017;40(4):497–517. https://doi.org/10.1007/s10545-017-0053-3.

10. Baptista PM, Moran E, Vyas D, Shupe T, Soker S. Liver regeneration and bioengineering. In: Regenerative medicine applications in organ transplantation. Elsevier; 2014. p. 391–400. https://doi.org/10.1016/B978-0-12-398523-1.00027-6.
11. Baptista PM, Siddiqui MM, Lozier G, Rodriguez SR, Atala A, Soker S. The use of whole organ decellularization for the generation of a vascularized liver organoid. Hepatology. 2011;53(2):604–17. https://doi.org/10.1002/hep.24067.
12. Moran EC, Dhal A, Vyas D, Lanas A, Soker S, Baptista PM. Whole-organ bioengineering: current tales of modern alchemy. Transl Res. 2014;163(4):259–67. https://doi.org/10.1016/j.trsl.2014.01.004.
13. Huang W, Ma K, Zhang J, et al. Nuclear receptor-dependent bile acid signaling is required for normal liver regeneration. Science (1979). 2006;312(5771):233–6. https://doi.org/10.1126/science.1121435.
14. Zwirner S, Abu Rmilah AA, Klotz S, et al. First-in-class MKK4 inhibitors enhance liver regeneration and prevent liver failure. Cell. 2024;187(7):1666–684.e26. https://doi.org/10.1016/j.cell.2024.02.023.
15. Alkhouri N, Herring R, Kabler H, et al. Safety and efficacy of combination therapy with semaglutide, cilofexor and firsocostat in patients with non-alcoholic steatohepatitis: a randomised, open-label phase II trial. J Hepatol. 2022;77(3):607–18. https://doi.org/10.1016/j.jhep.2022.04.003.
16. Harrison SA, Bashir MR, Guy CD, et al. Resmetirom (MGL-3196) for the treatment of non-alcoholic steatohepatitis: a multicentre, randomised, double-blind, placebo-controlled, phase 2 trial. Lancet. 2019;394(10213):2012–24. https://doi.org/10.1016/S0140-6736(19)32517-6.
17. Loomba R, Sanyal AJ, Kowdley KV, et al. Randomized, controlled trial of the FGF21 analogue pegozafermin in NASH. N Engl J Med. 2023;389(11):998–1008. https://doi.org/10.1056/NEJMoa2304286.
18. Fernández-Barrena MG, Arechederra M, Colyn L, Berasain C, Avila MA. Epigenetics in hepatocellular carcinoma development and therapy: the tip of the iceberg. JHEP Rep. 2020;2(6):100167. https://doi.org/10.1016/j.jhepr.2020.100167.
19. Dwyer BJ, Macmillan MT, Brennan PN, Forbes SJ. Cell therapy for advanced liver diseases: repair or rebuild. J Hepatol. 2021;74(1):185–99. https://doi.org/10.1016/j.jhep.2020.09.014.
20. Hu XH, Chen L, Wu H, et al. Cell therapy in end-stage liver disease: replace and remodel. Stem Cell Res Ther. 2023;14(1):141. https://doi.org/10.1186/s13287-023-03370-z.
21. Mahieu-Caputo D, Allain JE, Branger J, et al. Repopulation of athymic mouse liver by cryopreserved early human fetal hepatoblasts. Hum Gene Ther. 2004;15(12):1219–28. https://doi.org/10.1089/hum.2004.15.1219.
22. Dhawan A, Chaijitraruch N, Fitzpatrick E, et al. Alginate microencapsulated human hepatocytes for the treatment of acute liver failure in children. J Hepatol. 2020;72(5):877–84. https://doi.org/10.1016/j.jhep.2019.12.002.
23. Khan S, Mahgoub S, Fallatah N, Lalor PF, Newsome PN. Liver disease and cell therapy: advances made and remaining challenges. Stem Cells. 2023;41(8):739–61. https://doi.org/10.1093/stmcls/sxad029.
24. Shi M, Li YY, Xu RN, et al. Mesenchymal stem cell therapy in decompensated liver cirrhosis: a long-term follow-up analysis of the randomized controlled clinical trial. Hepatol Int. 2021;15(6):1431–41. https://doi.org/10.1007/s12072-021-10199-2.
25. Liang LB, Feng CJ, Hong QW, et al. Allogeneic bone marrow-derived mesenchymal stromal cells for hepatitis B virus-related acute-on-chronic liver failure: a randomized controlled trial. Hepatology. 2017;66(1):209–19. https://doi.org/10.1002/hep.29189.
26. Ho CM, Chen YH, Chien CS, et al. Hepatocyte and mesenchymal stem cell co-transplantation in rats with acute liver failure. Korean J Transplant. 2020;34(2):100–8. https://doi.org/10.4285/kjt.2020.34.2.100.
27. Carpentier A, Tesfaye A, Chu V, et al. Engrafted human stem cell–derived hepatocytes establish an infectious HCV murine model. J Clin Invest. 2014;124(11):4953–64. https://doi.org/10.1172/JCI75456.

28. Sampaziotis F, Muraro D, Tysoe OC, et al. Cholangiocyte organoids can repair bile ducts after transplantation in the human liver. Science (1979). 2021;371(6531):839–46. https://doi.org/10.1126/science.aaz6964.
29. Zheng JF. Transplantation of fetal liver epithelial progenitor cells ameliorates experimental liver fibrosis in mice. World J Gastroenterol. 2006;12(45):7292. https://doi.org/10.3748/wjg.v12.i45.7292.
30. Sharma M, Kulkarni A, Sasikala M, et al. Long-term outcome of autologous hematopoietic stem cell infusion in cirrhosis: waning effect over time. J Clin Transl Hepatol. 2020;8(4):1–6. https://doi.org/10.14218/JCTH.2020.00052.
31. Zhao J, Zhi Y, Ren H, Wang J, Zhao Y. Emerging biotechnologies for engineering liver organoids. Bioact Mater. 2025;45:1–18. https://doi.org/10.1016/j.bioactmat.2024.11.002.
32. Hallett JM, Ferreira-Gonzalez S, Man TY, et al. Human biliary epithelial cells from discarded donor livers rescue bile duct structure and function in a mouse model of biliary disease. Cell Stem Cell. 2022;29(3):355–71.e10. https://doi.org/10.1016/j.stem.2022.02.006.
33. Song X, Hou K, Zhou H, Yang J, Cao T, Zhang J. Liver organoids and their application in liver cancer research. Regen Ther. 2024;25:128–37. https://doi.org/10.1016/j.reth.2023.12.011.
34. Harrison SP, Siller R, Tanaka Y, et al. Scalable production of tissue-like vascularized liver organoids from human PSCs. Exp Mol Med. 2023;55(9):2005–24. https://doi.org/10.1038/s12276-023-01074-1.
35. Moroni F, Dwyer BJ, Graham C, et al. Safety profile of autologous macrophage therapy for liver cirrhosis. Nat Med. 2019;25(10):1560–5. https://doi.org/10.1038/s41591-019-0599-8.
36. Liu J. In vitro co-culture models for studying organoids-macrophages interaction: the golden technology of cancer immunotherapy. Am J Cancer Res. 2024;14(7):3222–40. https://doi.org/10.62347/BQFH7352.
37. Marshall E. CLINICAL TRIALS: gene therapy death prompts review of adenovirus vector. Science (1979). 1999;286(5448):2244–5. https://doi.org/10.1126/science.286.5448.2244.
38. Nathwani AC, Tuddenham EGD, Rangarajan S, et al. Adenovirus-associated virus vector–mediated gene transfer in hemophilia B. N Engl J Med. 2011;365(25):2357–65. https://doi.org/10.1056/NEJMoa1108046.
39. Murillo O, Luqui DM, Gazquez C, et al. Long-term metabolic correction of Wilson's disease in a murine model by gene therapy. J Hepatol. 2016;64(2):419–26. https://doi.org/10.1016/j.jhep.2015.09.014.
40. Weber ND, Odriozola L, Martínez-García J, et al. Gene therapy for progressive familial intrahepatic cholestasis type 3 in a clinically relevant mouse model. Nat Commun. 2019;10(1):5694. https://doi.org/10.1038/s41467-019-13614-3.
41. Mahlangu J, Kaczmarek R, von Drygalski A, et al. Two-year outcomes of valoctocogene roxaparvovec therapy for hemophilia A. N Engl J Med. 2023;388(8):694–705. https://doi.org/10.1056/NEJMoa2211075.
42. Leavitt AD, Konkle BA, Stine KC, et al. Giroctocogene fitelparvovec gene therapy for severe hemophilia A: 104-week analysis of the phase 1/2 Alta study. Blood. 2024;143(9):796–806. https://doi.org/10.1182/blood.2022018971.
43. Pipe SW, Leebeek FWG, Recht M, et al. Gene therapy with etranacogene dezaparvovec for hemophilia B. N Engl J Med. 2023;388(8):706–18. https://doi.org/10.1056/NEJMoa2211644.
44. Cuker A, Kavakli K, Frenzel L, et al. Gene therapy with fidanacogene elaparvovec in adults with hemophilia B. N Engl J Med. 2024;391(12):1108–18. https://doi.org/10.1056/NEJMoa2302982.
45. Wilson JM, Flotte TR. Moving forward after two deaths in a gene therapy trial of myotubular myopathy. Hum Gene Ther. 2020;31(13–14):695–6. https://doi.org/10.1089/hum.2020.182.
46. Chan YK, Wang SK, Chu CJ, et al. Engineering adeno-associated viral vectors to evade innate immune and inflammatory responses. Sci Transl Med. 2021;13(580):eabd3438. https://doi.org/10.1126/scitranslmed.abd3438.
47. Meliani A, Boisgerault F, Hardet R, et al. Antigen-selective modulation of AAV immunogenicity with tolerogenic rapamycin nanoparticles enables successful vector re-administration. Nat Commun. 2018;9(1):4098. https://doi.org/10.1038/s41467-018-06621-3.

48. Ros-Gañán I, Hommel M, Trigueros-Motos L, et al. Optimising the IgG-degrading enzyme treatment regimen for enhanced adeno-associated virus transduction in the presence of neutralising antibodies. Clin Transl Immunol. 2022;11(2):e1375. https://doi.org/10.1002/cti2.1375.
49. Martínez-García J, Molina M, Odriozola L, et al. A minimal bile salt excretory pump promoter allows bile acid-driven physiological regulation of transgene expression from a gene therapy vector. Cell Biosci. 2022;12(1):79. https://doi.org/10.1186/s13578-022-00803-9.
50. Sardh E, Harper P, Balwani M, et al. Phase 1 trial of an RNA interference therapy for acute intermittent porphyria. N Engl J Med. 2019;380(6):549–58. https://doi.org/10.1056/NEJMoa1807838.
51. McGregor TL, Hunt KA, Yee E, et al. Characterising a healthy adult with a rare HAO1 knockout to support a therapeutic strategy for primary hyperoxaluria. Elife. 2020;9:e54363. https://doi.org/10.7554/eLife.54363.
52. Machin N, Ragni MV. An investigational RNAi therapeutic targeting antithrombin for the treatment of hemophilia A and B. J Blood Med. 2018;9:135–40. https://doi.org/10.2147/JBM.S159297.
53. Adams D, Tournev IL, Taylor MS, et al. Efficacy and safety of vutrisiran for patients with hereditary transthyretin-mediated amyloidosis with polyneuropathy: a randomized clinical trial. Amyloid. 2023;30(1):18–26. https://doi.org/10.1080/13506129.2022.2091985.
54. Baum MA, Langman C, Cochat P, et al. PHYOX2: a pivotal randomized study of nedosiran in primary hyperoxaluria type 1 or 2. Kidney Int. 2023;103(1):207–17. https://doi.org/10.1016/j.kint.2022.07.025.
55. Moscoso CG, Steer CJ. The evolution of gene therapy in the treatment of metabolic liver diseases. Genes (Basel). 2020;11(8):915. https://doi.org/10.3390/genes11080915.
56. Sahin U, Karikó K, Türeci Ö. mRNA-based therapeutics – developing a new class of drugs. Nat Rev Drug Discov. 2014;13(10):759–80. https://doi.org/10.1038/nrd4278.
57. An D, Schneller JL, Frassetto A, et al. Systemic messenger RNA therapy as a treatment for methylmalonic acidemia. Cell Rep. 2017;21(12):3548–58. https://doi.org/10.1016/j.celrep.2017.11.081.
58. Jiang L, Berraondo P, Jericó D, et al. Systemic messenger RNA as an etiological treatment for acute intermittent porphyria. Nat Med. 2018;24(12):1899–909. https://doi.org/10.1038/s41591-018-0199-z.
59. Jiang L, Park JS, Yin L, et al. Dual mRNA therapy restores metabolic function in long-term studies in mice with propionic acidemia. Nat Commun. 2020;11(1):5339. https://doi.org/10.1038/s41467-020-19156-3.
60. Sharma G, Sharma AR, Bhattacharya M, Lee SS, Chakraborty C. CRISPR-Cas9: a preclinical and clinical perspective for the treatment of human diseases. Mol Ther. 2021;29(2):571–86. https://doi.org/10.1016/j.ymthe.2020.09.028.
61. Harmatz P, Prada CE, Burton BK, et al. First-in-human in vivo genome editing via AAV-zinc-finger nucleases for mucopolysaccharidosis I/II and hemophilia B. Mol Ther. 2022;30(12):3587–600. https://doi.org/10.1016/j.ymthe.2022.10.010.
62. Gillmore JD, Gane E, Taubel J, et al. CRISPR-Cas9 in vivo gene editing for transthyretin amyloidosis. N Engl J Med. 2021;385(6):493–502. https://doi.org/10.1056/NEJMoa2107454.
63. Villiger L, Grisch-Chan HM, Lindsay H, et al. Treatment of a metabolic liver disease by in vivo genome base editing in adult mice. Nat Med. 2018;24(10):1519–25. https://doi.org/10.1038/s41591-018-0209-1.
64. Musunuru K, Chadwick AC, Mizoguchi T, et al. In vivo CRISPR base editing of PCSK9 durably lowers cholesterol in primates. Nature. 2021;593(7859):429–34. https://doi.org/10.1038/s41586-021-03534-y.
65. Saliba F, Bañares R, Larsen FS, et al. Artificial liver support in patients with liver failure: a modified DELPHI consensus of international experts. Intensive Care Med. Published online September 6, 2022. https://doi.org/10.1007/s00134-022-06802-1.
66. Camus C, Locher C, Saliba F, et al. Outcome of patients treated with molecular adsorbent recirculating system albumin dialysis: a national multicenter study. JGH Open. 2020;4(4):757–63. https://doi.org/10.1002/jgh3.12359.

67. Fuhrmann V, Weber T, Roedl K, et al. Advanced organ support (ADVOS) in the critically ill: first clinical experience in patients with multiple organ failure. Ann Intensive Care. 2020;10(1):96. https://doi.org/10.1186/s13613-020-00714-3.
68. Tan EXX, Wang MX, Pang J, Lee GH. Plasma exchange in patients with acute and acute-on-chronic liver failure: a systematic review. World J Gastroenterol. 2020;26(2):219–45. https://doi.org/10.3748/wjg.v26.i2.219.
69. Muller X, Schlegel A, Kron P, et al. Novel real-time prediction of liver graft function during hypothermic oxygenated machine perfusion before liver transplantation. Ann Surg. 2019;270(5):783–90. https://doi.org/10.1097/SLA.0000000000003513.
70. Clavien PA, Dutkowski P, Mueller M, et al. Transplantation of a human liver following 3 days of ex situ normothermic preservation. Nat Biotechnol. Published online May 31, 2022. https://doi.org/10.1038/s41587-022-01354-7.
71. Sousa Da Silva RX, Borrego LB, Lenggenhager D, et al. Defatting of human livers during long-term ex situ normothermic perfusion. Novel strategy to rescue discarded organs for transplantation. Ann Surg. Published online July 27, 2023. https://doi.org/10.1097/SLA.0000000000006047.
72. Cabanes-Creus M, Liao SHY, Gale Navarro R, et al. Harnessing whole human liver ex situ normothermic perfusion for preclinical AAV vector evaluation. Nat Commun. 2024;15(1):1876. https://doi.org/10.1038/s41467-024-46194-y.
73. Brovold M, Almeida JI, Pla-Palacín I, et al. Naturally-derived biomaterials for tissue engineering applications. In: Novel biomaterials for regenerative medicine; 2018. p. 421–49. https://doi.org/10.1007/978-981-13-0947-2_23.
74. Afzal Z, Huguet EL. Bioengineering liver tissue by repopulation of decellularised scaffolds. World J Hepatol. 2023;15(2):151–79. https://doi.org/10.4254/wjh.v15.i2.151.
75. Zhu L, Yuhan J, Yu H, Zhang B, Huang K, Zhu L. Decellularized extracellular matrix for remodeling bioengineering organoid's microenvironment. Small. 2023;19(25):2207752. https://doi.org/10.1002/smll.202207752.
76. DuBray BJ, Conzen KD, Upadhya GA, et al. Novel in vitro model for studying hepatic ischemia-reperfusion injury using liver cubes. Surgery. 2012;152(2):247–53. https://doi.org/10.1016/j.surg.2012.02.012.
77. Schneeberger K, Sánchez-Romero N, Ye S, et al. Large-scale production of LGR5-positive bipotential human liver stem cells. Hepatology. 2020;72(1):257–70. https://doi.org/10.1002/hep.31037.
78. Vyas D, Baptista PM, Brovold M, et al. Self-assembled liver organoids recapitulate hepatobiliary organogenesis in vitro. Hepatology. Published online 2018. https://doi.org/10.1002/hep.29483.
79. Mir T, Alzhrani A, Nakamura M, et al. Whole liver derived acellular extracellular matrix for bioengineering of liver constructs: an updated review. Bioengineering. 2023;10(10):1126. https://doi.org/10.3390/bioengineering10101126.
80. Pla-Palacín I, Sainz-Arnal P, Morini S, Almeida M, Baptista PM. Liver bioengineering using decellularized whole-liver scaffolds. In: Decellularized scaffolds and organogenesis: methods and protocols; 2017. p. 293–305. https://doi.org/10.1007/7651_2017_98.
81. Higashi H, Yagi H, Kuroda K, et al. Transplantation of bioengineered liver capable of extended function in a preclinical liver failure model. Am J Transplant. 2022;22(3):731–44. https://doi.org/10.1111/ajt.16928.
82. Telles-Silva KA, Pacheco L, Chianca F, et al. iPSC-derived cells for whole liver bioengineering. Front Bioeng Biotechnol. 2024;12:1338762. https://doi.org/10.3389/fbioe.2024.1338762.
83. Wang Z, Faria J, Penning LC, Masereeuw R, Spee B. Tissue-engineered bile ducts for disease modeling and therapy. Tissue Eng Part C Methods. 2021;27(2):59–76. https://doi.org/10.1089/ten.tec.2020.0283.
84. Buisson EM, Jeong J, Kim HJ, Choi D. Regenerative medicine of the bile duct: beyond the myth. Int J Stem Cells. 2019;12(2):183–94. https://doi.org/10.15283/ijsc18055.

85. Roos FJM, van Tienderen GS, Wu H, et al. Human branching cholangiocyte organoids recapitulate functional bile duct formation. Cell Stem Cell. 2022;29(5):776–94.e13. https://doi.org/10.1016/j.stem.2022.04.011.
86. Wang Z, Faria J, van der Laan LJW, Penning LC, Masereeuw R, Spee B. Human cholangiocytes form a polarized and functional bile duct on hollow fiber membranes. Front Bioeng Biotechnol. 2022;10:868857. https://doi.org/10.3389/fbioe.2022.868857.
87. Sampaziotis F, Justin AW, Tysoe OC, et al. Reconstruction of the mouse extrahepatic biliary tree using primary human extrahepatic cholangiocyte organoids. Nat Med. 2017;23(8):954–63. https://doi.org/10.1038/nm.4360.

MIX
Papier aus verantwortungsvollen Quellen
Paper from responsible sources
FSC® C105338

If you have any concerns about our products,
you can contact us on
ProductSafety@springernature.com

In case Publisher is established outside the EU,
the EU authorized representative is:
Springer Nature Customer Service Center GmbH
Europaplatz 3, 69115 Heidelberg, Germany

Printed by Libri Plureos GmbH
in Hamburg, Germany